Marine Natural Products and Obesity

Marine Natural Products and Obesity

Special Issue Editors

Ralph Urbatzka
Vítor Vasconcelos

MDPI • Basel • Beijing • Wuhan • Barcelona • Belgrade

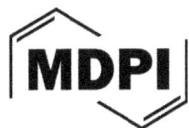

MDPI

Special Issue Editors

Ralph Urbatzka
CIIMAR—Interdisciplinary Centre of
Marine and Environmental Research
Portugal

Vítor Vasconcelos
CIIMAR—Interdisciplinary Centre of
Marine and Environmental Research
Portugal

Editorial Office
MDPI
St. Alban-Anlage 66
4052 Basel, Switzerland

This is a reprint of articles from the Special Issue published online in the open access journal *Marine Drugs* (ISSN 1660-3397) from 2018 to 2019 (available at: https://www.mdpi.com/journal/marinedrugs/special_issues/marine_obesity)

For citation purposes, cite each article independently as indicated on the article page online and as indicated below:

LastName, A.A.; LastName, B.B.; LastName, C.C. Article Title. *Journal Name* **Year**, *Article Number*, Page Range.

ISBN 978-3-03921-191-3 (Pbk)
ISBN 978-3-03921-192-0 (PDF)

Cover image courtesy of Ralph Urbatzka and Vítor Vasconcelos.

Contents

About the Special Issue Editors

Ralph Urbatzka, Assistant Researcher, graduated in Biology in 2002 (University of Cologne, Germany) and received his PhD in 2007 in Molecular Biology from the Humboldt-University Berlin, Germany. He moved in 2008 to the CIIMAR, Interdisciplinary Centre of Marine and Environmental Research in Porto, Portugal and works since 2013 in the BBE Blue Biotechnology and Ecotoxicology Group. His current research interests focus on marine biotechnology, and more specifically on the bioactivity screening of marine organism for the discovery of novel compounds with activities towards human diseases (cancer, obesity, diabetes, hepatic steatosis) and the deciphering of their molecular mechanism.

Vítor Vasconcelos, Full Professor—Faculty of Sciences of Porto University and director of CIIMAR—Interdisciplinary Center of Marine and Environmental Research. Director of the Group of Blue Biotechnology and Ecotoxicology (LEGE lab). Director of the PhD Program on Marine Biotechnology and Aquaculture at the University of Porto and University of Minho, Portugal. Main research focus on cyanobacteria secondary metabolites and their uses: toxins and molecules with biotechnological applications. Responsible for the LEGE culture collection comprising more than 1000 strains of cyanobacteria and microalgae. Published 340 papers in Toxicology and Biotechnology.

Preface to "Marine Natural Products and Obesity"

Obesity and related co-morbidities are increasing worldwide and pose a serious health problem. Changes in lifestyle and diet would be the best remedies to fight obesity; however, many people will still rely on medical aid. Marine organisms have been prolific in the production of bioactive compounds for many diseases, e.g., cancer, and promise to be an excellent source for natural-derived molecules and novel nutraceuticals.

This Special Issue of Marine Drugs highlights advances of research regarding marine natural products and obesity. Contributions in the form of research publications range from the isolation of novel compounds from marine resources, the elucidation of molecular mechanism of marine, bioactive compounds up to clinical trials in humans. As novel resources, cyanobacteria demonstrated relevant bioactivities towards various metabolic diseases, and chlorophyll derivatives from marine cyanobacteria were shown to possess lipid-reducing activities. New aromatic bisabolane-related compounds were isolated from a marine sponge and reduced the neutral lipid content in the zebrafish model. Advances on molecular mechanism for marine natural products with beneficial effects on obesity are presented for diphlorethohydroxycarmalol isolated from brown algae, for omega-3 poly unsaturated fatty acids (PUFAs), chitosan oligosaccharides, fucoidans from brown seaweeds and from collagen peptides derived from skate skin. Beneficial effects of Spirulina and collagen peptides from skate skin were demonstrated in clinical trials in humans. Additionally, a proteomics methodology for target dereplication was improved and applied to decipher the molecular targets of 132-hydroxypheophytine a, previously isolated from a marine cyanobacteria with lipid reducing activity. Finally, a review covers the anti-obesity and anti-diabetes effects from a brown alga (*Ishige okamurae*).

Ralph Urbatzka, Vítor Vasconcelos
Special Issue Editors

marine drugs

MDPI

Article

Commercial Fucoidans from *Fucus vesiculosus* Can Be Grouped into Antiadipogenic and Adipogenic Agents

Ruth Medeiros Oliveira [1,2], Rafael Barros Gomes Câmara [2,3], Jessyka Fernanda Santiago Monte [1], Rony Lucas Silva Viana [1], Karoline Rachel Teodosio Melo [1], Moacir Fernandes Queiroz [1], Luciana Guimarães Alves Filgueira [1], Lila Missae Oyama [4] and Hugo Alexandre Oliveira Rocha [1,*]

[1] Departamento de Bioquímica, Universidade Federal do Rio Grande do Norte, Natal, Rio Grande do Norte 59.078-970, Brazil; ruth.oliveira@ifrn.edu.br (R.M.O.); jessykamonte@gmail.com (J.F.S.M.); rony_lucas@hotmail.com (R.L.S.V.); melo.krt@gmail.com (K.R.T.M.); moacirfqn@gmail.com (M.F.Q.); lucianagalves@hotmail.com (L.G.A.F.)
[2] Instituto Federal de Educação, Ciência e Tecnologia do Rio Grande do Norte, Caicó, Rio Grande do Norte 59.300-000, Brazil; rafael_bgc@yahoo.com.br
[3] Escola Multicampi de Ciências Médicas, Universidade Federal do Rio Grande do Norte, Caicó, Rio Grande do Norte 59.300-000, Brazil
[4] Departamento de Fisiologia, Universidade Federal de São Paulo—Escola Paulista de Medicina, São Paulo 04023-060, Brazil; lmoyama@gmail.com
* Correspondence: hugo@cb.ufrn.br; Tel.: +55-84-3215-3416

Received: 29 March 2018; Accepted: 25 May 2018; Published: 4 June 2018

Abstract: *Fucus vesiculosus* is a brown seaweed used in the treatment of obesity. This seaweed synthesizes various bioactive molecules, one of them being a sulfated polysaccharide known as fucoidan (FF). This polymer can easily be found commercially, and has antiadipogenic and lipolytic activity. Using differential precipitation with acetone, we obtained four fucoidan-rich fractions (F0.5/F0.9/F1.1/F2.0) from FF. These fractions contain different proportions of fucose:glucuronic acid:galactose:xylose:sulfate, and also showed different electrophoretic mobility and antioxidant activity. Using 3T3-L1 adipocytes, we found that all samples had lipolytic action, especially F2.0, which tripled the amount of glycerol in the cellular medium. Moreover, we observed that FF, F1.0, and F2.0 have antiadipogenic activity, as they inhibited the oil red staining by cells at 40%, 40%, and 50%, respectively. In addition, they decreased the expression of key proteins of adipogenic differentiation (C/EBPα, C/EBPβ, and PPARγ). However, F0.5 and F0.9 stimulated the oil red staining at 80% and increased the expression of these proteins. Therefore, these fucoidan fractions have an adipogenic effect. Overall, the data show that F2.0 has great potential to be used as an agent against obesity as it displays better antioxidant, lipolytic and antiadipogenic activities than the other fucoidan fractions that we tested.

Keywords: 3T3-L1 cells; fucan; lipolytic; obesity; brown seaweed

1. Introduction

Fucus vesiculosus is a brown seaweed commonly found in coastal wetlands, in temperate or cold waters of the Atlantic and Pacific oceans. It was shown that *F. vesiculosus* intake helps women with abnormal menstrual cycles, and health problems associated with their periods [1]. Other author also reported that consumption of this seaweed promotes a decrease in body weight [2,3]. This seaweed has various active elements in its composition, of which fucoidan is one of the best known.

The presence of fucoidan in *F. vesiculosus* was demonstrated in 1913, and was initially called fucoidin [4]. Years later, it was suggested that the term be changed to fucoidan [5].

The structure of fucoidan (FF) from *F. vesiculosus* was last reviewed by Patankar et al. [6]. It was suggested that it possesses a central core formed by α-L-fucose (1,3)-linked, sulfated at C4. In addition, several branching points (every two or three fucose residues) were present in α-(1,2) or α-(1,4)-linked, on the main chain.

Currently, it is easy to acquire fucoidan from *F. vesiculosus*, as a multinational company sells it commercially. In part, this may explain the large amount of research and the number of activities ascribed to this sulfated polysaccharide, including antilipemic [7,8], and antiadipogenic activities [9,10].

Adipogenesis is a process of cell differentiation in which mesenchymal stem cells differentiate into adipocytes, with this process initially involving a stage where cells "compromise" with the adipocyte line [11]. In the next step, differentiation occurs, and the pre-adipocytes develop into mature adipocytes. The process of differentiation is complex and involves the participation of hundreds of proteins, although two proteins particularly play a crucial role in this event: C/EBPα, a protein of the CCAAT-enhancer binding protein class, and PPARγ, a peroxisome proliferator activated receptor [12].

Although pre-adipocyte primary cultures are an important tool for understanding the mechanisms of adipocyte differentiation, these cells have low mitogenic capacity and lose their ability to differentiate over time under culture conditions [13]. Therefore, the development of studies on adipogenesis is carried out mainly by the use of cellular models, such as the murine 3T3-L1 and 3T3-F442A (pre-adipocyte) lines. These cells, when stimulated to differentiate into adipocytes, follow the same metabolic pathways of differentiation of mesenchymal cells [14].

By using a differentiation cocktail based on insulin, dexamethasone, isobutylmethylxanthine, and fetal bovine serum, it is possible to obtain mature adipocytes from a 3T3-L1 culture. The actions of these compounds result in the initial events of differentiation, represented by the expression of CCAAT-enhancer binding proteins [13–15]. Afterwards, the cells return to their cell cycles, undergo clonal expansion in a regulated manner, and enter a terminal differentiation process by activation of PPARγ and C/EBPα [16]. Besides, the differentiation of these cells takes place in precisely controlled sequential stages: cell cycle arrest, clonal expansion, and differentiation (first phase and second phase of activation of transcriptional factors), by activating hundreds of previously silenced genes [15].

Studies with pre-adipocyte 3T3-L1 cells showed that fucoidan from *F. vesiculosus* inhibits adipogenesis. Real-time polymerase chain reaction (PCR) data showed that fucoidan reduced mRNA expression of C/EBPα and PPARγ by 22.6% and 17.6%, respectively [9].

FF from *F. vesiculosus* can be fractionated, with certain fractions showing very similar activities to each other [10]. Moreover, Nishino et al. [17] reported that some fucoidan fractions showed much greater activity than others did. However, antiadipogenic activity across different fucoidan populations has not yet been evaluated. With this in mind, we obtained four different fucoidan-rich fractions of commercial fucoidan from *F. vesiculosus* and, assessed them for their adipogenic activity.

2. Results

2.1. Obtaining Different Fractions of Fucoidan (FF)

Using differential precipitation with acetone, we obtained four fractions from FF. These were called F0.5, F0.9, F1.1, and F2.0 corresponding to 4.5%, 35.2%, 22.0% and 38.3% of the material, respectively (Table 1). Chemical analysis and sulfated polysaccharide yield are summarized in Table 1. Data show that mannose and glucose were not found in the samples, whereas fucose, glucuronic acid, galactose and xylose were found in all samples. The data also showed fucose was the major component present in all fractions, whereas the relative amounts of other monosaccharides vary according to the fraction. Thus, the relative amounts of these sugars vary according to the fraction.

When the sulfate content of the samples was quantified, it was observed that there is no significant difference between F1.1 and F2.0. Although F1.1 and F2.0 both have the same sulfate content, they were precipitated with different volumes of acetone. This is probably because the sulfated polysaccharide conformation interferes during the precipitation process.

To confirm this hypothesis, the fucoidan-rich fractions were subjected to agarose gel electrophoresis in 1,3 diamineacetate (PDA) buffer. Figure 1 shows an agarose gel stained with toluidine blue. It is possible to see that all the fractions have a predominant band. For F0.9, F1.1, and F2.0, the bands display different electrophoretic mobilities.

Table 1. Chemical composition of fucoidan (FF) and its fractions. Fuc: fucose; Gluc acid: glucuronic acid; Gal: galactose; Xyl: xylose; Man: mannose; Gluc: glucose; n.d—not detected. Different letters ([a,b,c,d]) indicate a significant difference ($p < 0.05$) between the samples. Each value is the mean ± standard deviation (SD) of three determinations and from three independent assays.

Sulfated Polysaccharides	Yield (%)	Sulfate (%)	Molar Ratio					
			Fuc	Gluc Acid	Gal	Xyl	Man	Gluc
FF	-	23.70% ± 0.04 [a]	1.0	0.7	0.4	0.2	n.d	n.d
F0.5	4.5	12.70% ± 0.08 [b]	1.0	0.2	0.3	0.5	n.d	n.d
F0.9	35.2	17.40% ± 0.02 [c]	1.0	0.8	0.2	0.6	n.d	n.d
F1.1	22.0	20.30% ± 0.05 [d]	1.0	0.2	0.4	0.2	n.d	n.d
F2.0	38.3	20.40% ± 0.04 [d]	1.0	0.1	0.3	0.1	n.d	n.d

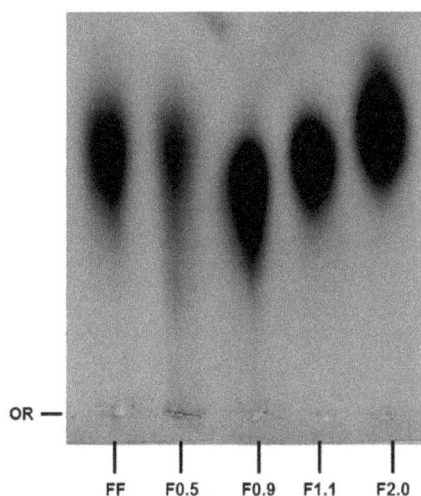

Figure 1. Staining pattern of the polysaccharides after agarose gel electrophoresis, stained with toluidine blue. About 5 µL (50 µg) of each sample was applied in agarose gel prepared in diaminopropane acetate buffer and subjected to electrophoresis, as described in methods. OR—origin. This figure is representative of three separate tests made independently.

2.2. Antioxidant Activities

The antioxidant activity of samples was evaluated in vitro by the total antioxidant capacity test (TAC). All samples showed antioxidant activity, though the values were significantly different from each other, particularly for F2.0 fucoidan, which was approximately 400 ± 12.0 equivalents of ascorbic acid. This is nearly double the values obtained for FF and F0.9, which were 189 ± 10.0 and 172 ± 11.0 ascorbic acid equivalents, respectively. The value identified for F1.1 was found to be significantly lower than the two mentioned above (150 ± 8.0 equivalents). The value obtained for F0.5 was around 38 ± 2.0 equivalents, the lowest recorded in this study. There was positive Pearson correlation coefficient between the sulfated content of fractions and TAC ($P = 0.566$).

2.3. 3T3-L1 Cell Viability

As the 3T3-L1 line (pre-adipocytes) is the main cell model used for the study of adipogenesis, it was first necessary to assess the effects of the samples on the viability of these cells. The results are shown in Figure 2.

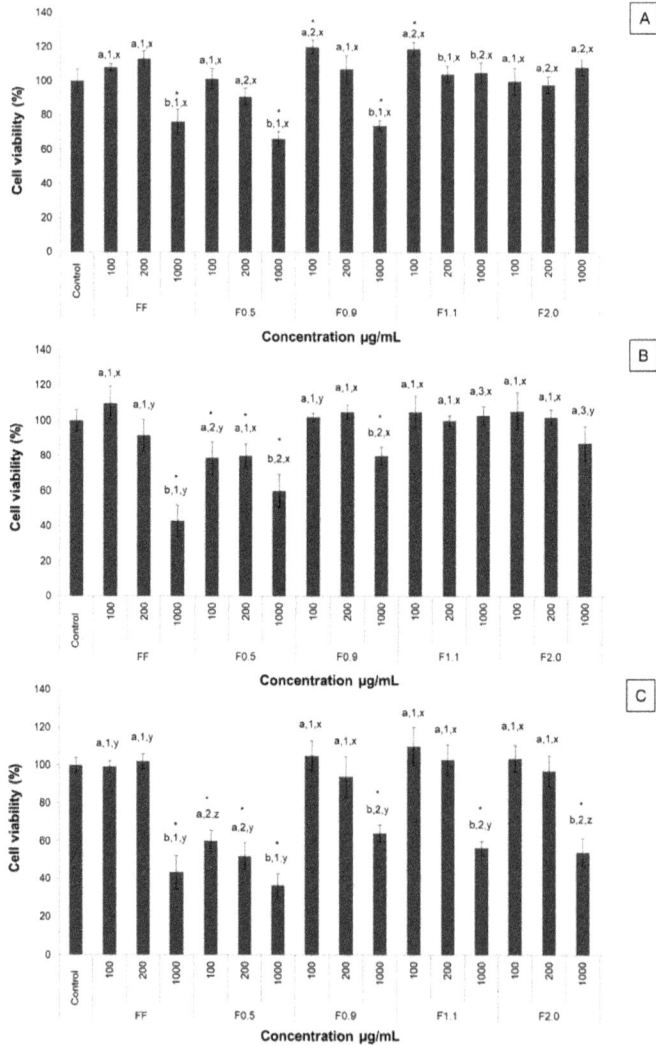

Figure 2. The effects of FF, F0.5, F0.9, F1.1, and F2.0 on 3T3-L1 cell viability. (**A**) 24 h; (**B**) 48 h; (**C**) 72 h. Each value is the mean ± SD of three determinations and from three independent assays. Different letters ([a,b]) indicate a significant difference ($p < 0.05$) between different concentrations of the same sample; Different numbers ([1,2,3]) indicate a significant difference ($p < 0.05$) between the same concentration of each sample; Different letters ([x,y,z]) indicate a significant difference ($p < 0.05$) between the same concentration in different times (24, 48 and 72 h). Asterisks (*) indicate a significant difference ($p < 0.05$) between the concentrations of any sample and the control.

Over a period of 24 h (Figure 2A), it was observed that there was a reduction in cell viability (~30%) when the cells were cultured in the presence of FF, F0.5, and F0.9 at the highest concentration tested (1000 µg/mL). A similar effect was observed after 48 h. On the other hand, cytotoxicity (decrease in MTT (3-(4,5-dimethylthiazol-2-yl)2,5-diphenil tetrazolium bromide) reduction by 20%) was also identified using F0.5 at lower concentrations (100 and 200 µg/mL) (Figure 2B). The cytotoxic effects observed with the use of F0.5 was more pronounced after 72 h (Figure 2C), since there was a decrease in the MTT reduction by 40%, 48%, and 64%, using F0.5 in concentrations of 100, 200, and 1000 µg/mL, respectively. The same was also observed with the use of FF, F1.1, and F2.0 (all at 1000 µg/mL), when there was a decrease in MTT reduction of ~55%. Thus, a concentration of 200 µg/mL was selected for use in the following tests relating to the antiadipogenic effects of fucoidans.

2.4. Evaluation of the Antiadipogenic Effects of Samples

Figure 3 shows that samples had different effects on adipocyte differentiation. As shown in the images below, FF, F1.1, and F2.0 were able to reduce the amounts of neutral lipids within cells, a fact evidenced by the reduced labeling of the cells.

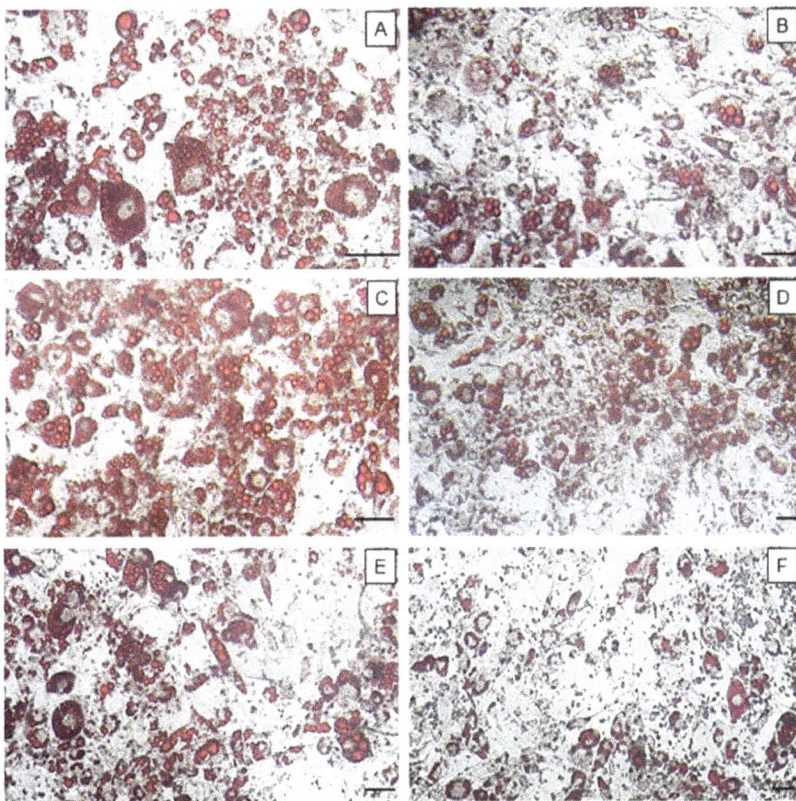

Figure 3. Adipocytes stained with the dye, oil red O. 10× magnification. (**A**) Control; (**B**) FF; (**C**) F0.5; (**D**) F0.9; (**E**) F1.1; (**F**) F2.0. Bar = 60 µm. This figure is representative of three separate tests made independently.

To confirm what was observed by optical microscopy, the oil red O was eluted from the inside of the cells and quantified (Figure 4). As the oil red O dye has an affinity for neutral lipids (triglycerides), the more fat (triglycerides) that is accumulated in the adipocyte the greater the amount of dye within the cell and vice versa. Thus, it was observed that FF induced an approximately 40% reduction of triglyceride in the cells. F2.0 reduced the amount of triglyceride within the adipocytes by approximately 50% and this effect was more pronounced than that observed for FF. An unprecedented result was observed with F0.5, which induced the accumulation of oil red by approximately 80% more than the control group.

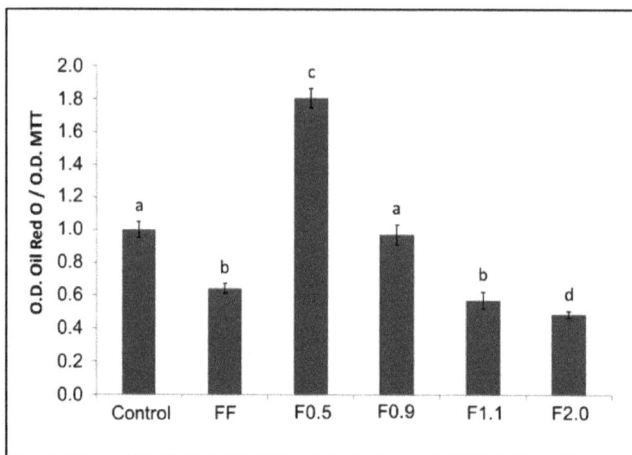

Figure 4. Oil red O content. Each value is the mean ± SD of three determinations and from three independent assays. Different letters ([a,b,c,d]) indicate a significant difference ($p < 0.05$) between the concentration tested (200 µg/mL) of all samples. O.D. (Optical density).

To understand the biochemical mechanisms by which these fucoidans act, the expression of key proteins of adipogenesis: C/EBPα, C/EBPβ, and PPARγ of the 3T3-l1 cells was evaluated. Figure 5 shows an immunoblot (Figure 5A) of these proteins. The results obtained from the densitometry of this blot are shown in Figure 5B.

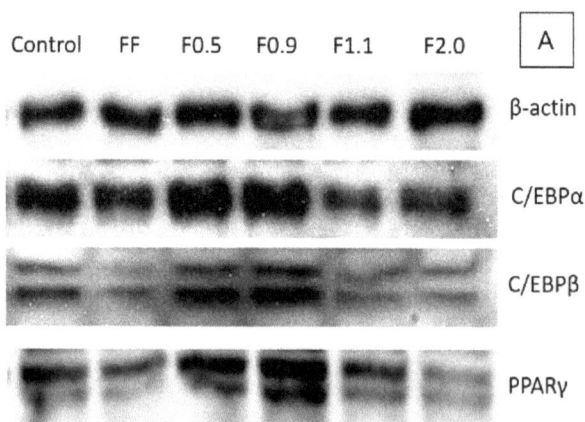

Figure 5. *Cont.*

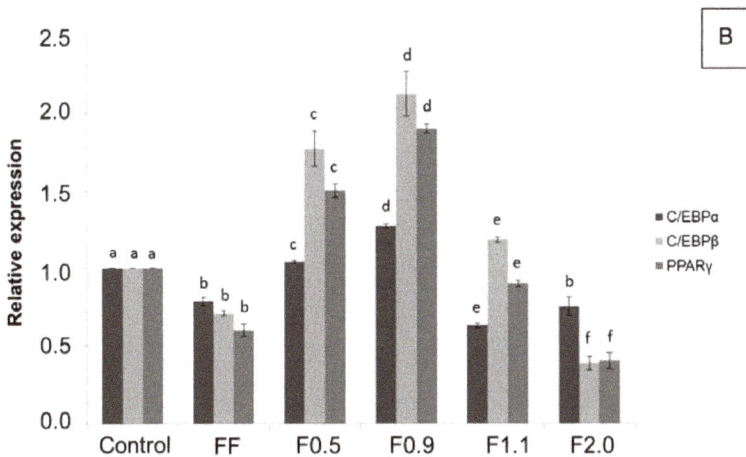

Figure 5. (A) The effects of FF, F0.5, F0.9, F1.1, and F2.0 on the expression of adipocyte markers. Equal amounts of protein (50 µg) were used for Western blot analysis, for the detection of β-actin, C/EBPα, C/EBPβ, and PPARγ. These gels are representative of three separate tests made independently; **(B)** Represents the expression relative to the control value. Different letters ([a,b,c,d,e,f]) indicate a significant difference ($p < 0.05$) between the expression of the same marker for different samples. The control corresponds to cells that were not exposed to fucoidans. Each value is the mean ± SD of three determinations and from three independent assays.

The expressions of these three proteins were altered when the cells were incubated with fucoidans (Figure 5B). F0.5 and F0.9 mainly stimulated the expression of C/EBPβ and PPAR gamma. However, F2.0 reduced the expression of all three proteins evaluated herein, particularly for C/EBPβ and PPARγ, by approximately 55% when compared to the control. In regards to F1.1, we take special note of the particularly strong reduction of C/EBPα expression. These data are in agreement with the oil red test and confirm that F0.5 and F0.9 are adipogenic agents, while F2.0 and F1.1 are antiadipogenic agents.

2.5. Evaluation of the Effects of Samples on Lipolysis

In order to evaluate the potential of the samples to induce lipid hydrolysis in adipocytes, specifically in triglycerides, free glycerol in the culture medium from untreated cells (control), and from cells treated with the fucoidans (200 µg/mL) was quantified. The results are shown in Figure 6.

As illustrated in Figure 6, all samples induced lipolysis. F0.5 was able to induce the mobilization of triglycerides after only 15 days of differentiation, while F0.9 showed a discreet effect by the ninth day of differentiation and after 15 days of culture. Twice as much glycerol in the medium of cells treated with F0.9 than for the control group was found. F1.1 needed only nine days of differentiation to achieve such an effect, i.e., double the lipolysis in comparison with the control group, with this potential being maintained throughout the differentiation process. In turn, F2.0 showed the strongest lipolytic effect, as it was able to increase the breakdown of triglycerides by three times after only nine days of differentiation. Despite the slight decrease in its potential to induce lipolysis during the differentiation process, we also observed 2.5 times more glycerol in the medium of the cells treated with F2.0 than in the control group at the end of the test.

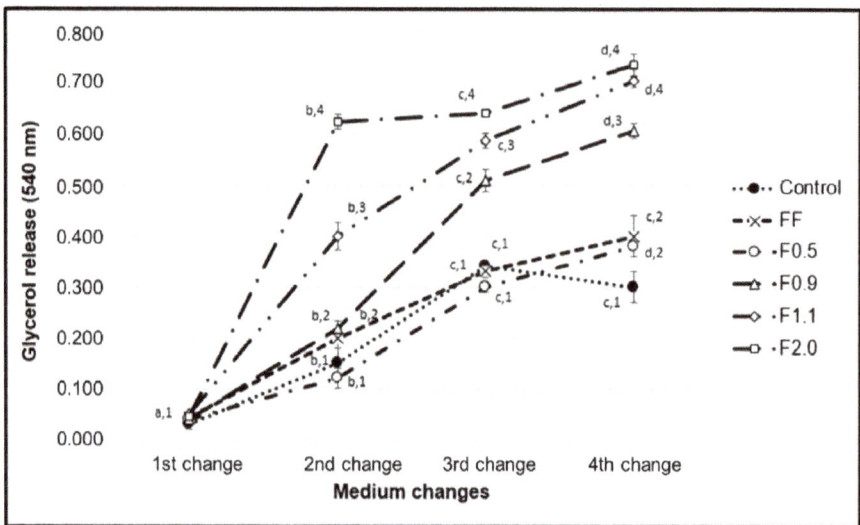

Figure 6. The content of glycerol released into the medium. Each value is the mean ± SD of three determinations and from three independent assays. Different letters ([a,b,c,d]) indicate a significant difference ($p < 0.05$) between the changes of the medium for same sample; Different numbers ([1,2,3,4]) indicate a significant difference ($p < 0.05$) between the same change of the medium in the different samples.

3. Discussion

Using differential precipitation with acetone, we acquired four different fractions of commercial fucoidan (FF) from *Fucus vesiculosus*. Other fucoidans were also separated into different fractions by the use of acetone, such as fucoidan from *Spatoglossum schröederi* [18], *Dictyopteris delicatula* [19], and *Dictyota menstrualis* [20]. Acetone separates the different polysaccharides because it competes with them for water molecules. Therefore, the smaller the interaction of the polysaccharide with water, the smaller the amount of acetone that should be added to the solution to precipitate it. Generally, the interactions between sulfated polysaccharides and water partly depend on the amount of charges on the polysaccharide, with the least negatively charged being the first to be precipitated.

Figure 1 shows that fucoidans fractions have different electrophoretic mobilities. In this electrophoresis system, the buffer used (PDA) includes 1,3-diaminopropane in its constitution, which is positively charged at pH 9.0. These positively charged buffers are able to link with the negatively charged groups of the polysaccharides that are exposed, such as sulfates, thus neutralizing them. However, the formation of this complex depends not only on the negatively charged groups of the sulfated polysaccharide, but also on the spatial conformation that the molecule takes in the system, and the effects that it has on how the sulfated polysaccharide exhibits its charged groups. Therefore, the amines do not form complexes with all sulfate groups, but only those that are exposed. In this way, the polysaccharide's mobility depends on the sulfate groups that have not formed complexes. A classic example is the behavior of chondroitin and heparin, two sulfated polysaccharides that are structurally similar, although heparin is more strongly sulfated. However, in the electrophoresis system with PDA, heparin has a much lower electrophoretic mobility than chondroitin [21]. In a previous study it was shown that commercial fucoidan was composed of fucose, glucose, galactose, mannose, xylose, glucuronic acid and sulfate [17]. Of these monosaccharides we find neither glucose nor mannose in FF. This is probably because the composition of commercial fucoidans should vary. So, we also did not find these two monosaccharides in the fractions. In addition, the relative proportion of glucuronic acid, xylose and galactose was different in each sample. Overall, these data lead us to propose that we have obtained four different fucoidan-rich fractions from *F. vesiculosus*.

Qi et al. [22] suggested that the antioxidant activity of fucoidan is related to the degree of sulfation: the more sulfated the polysaccharide, the more active it is. However, the data from the TAC test did not agree with those suggested by these authors. In addition, there was a weak Pearson correlation coefficient between the sulfated content of fractions and TAC. Furthermore, the data submitted by various authors that evaluated the antioxidant capacity of fucoidans obtained from other brown seaweed [19,23–25] indicate that the structure of fucoidans, as well as the exposure of the oxidizable groups along the molecule, are more important factors for the antioxidant capacity of these polymers than the number of sulfate groups.

The antiadipogenic activity of the fucoidan (FF) from *F. vesiculosus* had previously been reported [9]. However, the fucoidan fraction constituents of FF have not yet been evaluated in isolation for their antiadipogenic potential. In this work, we observed that these fractions had different effects on adipocyte differentiation.

Since oil red O has an affinity for neutral lipids (triglycerides), the greater the amount of fat (triglycerides) accumulated within adipocytes, the more dye will be observed within that cell, and vice versa. FF promoted a reduction of triglycerides in cells of around 40%. This value was highly similar to that observed by other authors, for example by Kim et al. [26]. In 2009, they reported that a commercial fucoidan was able to reduce the incorporation of oil red O by adipocytes in 39.7%, at a concentration of 200 µg/mL [9]. An unprecedented result was observed for F0.5 and F0.9, which induced the accumulation of triglycerides to approximately 80% more, compared to the control group. On the other hand, F2.0 fucoidan reduced the amount of triglycerides within adipocytes by approximately 50%, with this effect being more pronounced than that observed using FF.

To better understand the biochemical mechanism by which these fucoidans act, we verified the expression of key regulatory proteins of adipogenesis: C/EBPα, C/EBPβ, and PPARγ, as it has been reported that commercial fucoidan affects these enzymes [9,26]. In agreement with the results of the oil red O test, F0.5 and F0.9 caused an acute increase, mainly in the expression of C/EBPβ and PPARγ, in comparison to the control, confirming that these two compounds are adipogenic agents. However, F1.1 and F2.0 caused a reduction in the expression of these proteins, which in turn led to a reduction in the amount of triglycerides inside the adipocytes, as observed in the oil red O test.

The effects caused by fucoidans on gene expression and adipogenesis regulatory proteins have been previously reported in the literature, corroborating our results. FF was reported to reduce preadipocyte differentiation in adipocytes by reducing the expression of certain genes, including *PPARγ* [26], and *C/EBPα*, by 22.6% and 17.6%, respectively [9].

F1.1 and F2.0 were able to induce the release of triglycerides from the interior of the adipocytes (Figure 6). The molecular pathways by which these fucoidans act was not suggested, but fucoidan is known to stimulate the activity of hormone-sensitive lipase (LSH) [8]. LSH regulates lipolytic activity within adipocytes, and the phosphorylation of this enzyme leads to its activation with consequent hydrolysis of the triglycerides stored inside these cells, which subsequently release their glycerol and fatty acids [27]. Therefore, we believe that the LSH activation pathway may be the target of fucoidan activity demonstrated in our work. We intend to investigate this hypothesis in future work.

Anti-obesity drugs, besides causing a series of undesired effects, may possibly contribute to the onset of cardiovascular diseases [28]. Thus, the search for new agents that are effective against obesity and present lower health risks remains a priority [29]. We believe that *Fucus vesiculosus* fucoidan and its fractions could potentially be used to develop future treatments for obesity. We hope that our work will contribute to this end.

9

4. Materials and Methods

4.1. Materials

Commercial fucoidan extracted from *Fucus vesiculosus*, monoclonal mouse anti-β-actin antibody, 3-Isobutyl-1-methylxanthine, dexamethasone, insulin, and free glycerol reagent were obtained from Sigma-Aldrich® (St. Louis, MO, USA). Sodium bicarbonate, culture media components [minimum essential Dulbecco's modified Eagle medium (DMEM)], non-essential amino acids, fetal bovine serum, sodium pyruvate, and phosphate buffered saline [PBS] were purchased from Invitrogen Corporation (Burlington, ON, USA). Monoclonal rabbit anti-CEBPα, anti-CEBPβ, anti-PPAR-γ and anti-rabbit and anti-mouse horseradish peroxidase-conjugated secondary antibodies were obtained from Cell Signaling Technology (Beverly, MA, USA). Other solvents and chemicals used in this study were of analytical grade.

4.2. Cell Culture

3T3-L1 preadipocyte cells were purchased from the cell bank of Rio de Janeiro, RJ, Brazil (CR089-BCRJ/UFRJ), and maintained with 10% fetal bovine serum (FBS)/DMEM containing 4.5 g/L glucose, 100 U/mL penicillin, 0.1 mg/mL streptomycin, and 0.25 mg/mL amphotericin B at 37 °C in 5% CO_2 incubator.

4.3. Obtaining Different Populations of FF from F. vesiculosus

Four grams of FF were solubilized into 0.25 M sodium chloride. To this solution was added increasing volumes of acetone to precipitate the different fucoidans. To obtain fucoidan F0.5, for example, 0.5 volumes of ice-cold acetone was added to this solution slowly and under gentle agitation, and then held at 4 °C for 12 h. The precipitate formed was collected by centrifugation at 8000× *g* for 15 min at 4 °C. Acetone was added to the supernatant until a precipitated material appeared. Like this, we used the acetone volumes of 0.9, 1.1 and 2.0, calculated from the initial solution, and the operations repeated as above.

4.4. Determination of Sulfate Content and Monosaccharide Composition of Fucoidans

In order to determine the amount of sulfate, the fucoidan samples were hydrolyzed (4 N HCl for 6 h at 100 °C), and then the sulfate amount was given by turbidimetry at 500 nm by the gelatin/barium method as described early [23]. Sodium sulfate was used as standard.

To determine the best hydrolysis condition, the polysaccharides were hydrolyzed with 0.5, 1, 2, and 4 M, respectively, for various lengths of time (0.5; 1; 2; and 4 h), at 100 °C and the amount of reducing sugars of each condition was determined as described early [23]. Hydrolysis with 2 M HCl for 2 h producing the best reducing sugar yields.

After acid hydrolysis (2 M HCl for 2 h, 100 °C), sugar composition was determined by a LaChrom Elite® HPLC system from VWR-Hitachi (Hitachi Co., Tokyo, Japan) with a refractive index detector (RI detector model L-2490, Hitachi Co., Tokyo, Japan). A LichroCART® 250-4 column (250 mm × 40 mm, Merck, Darmstadt, Germany) packed with Lichrospher® 100 NH_2 (5 µm, Merck, Darmstadt, Germany) was coupled to the system. The sample mass used was 0.2 mg and analysis time was 25 min. The following sugars were analyzed as references: arabinose, fructose, fucose, galactose, glucose, glucosamine, glucuronic acid, mannose, and xylose.

4.5. Agarose Gel Electrophoresis

Agarose gel electrophoresis of the fucoidans was performed in 0.6% agarose gel (7.5 cm × 10 cm × 0.2 cm thick) prepared in 0.05 M 1.3-diaminopropane acetate buffer pH 9.0, as previously described [20]. Aliquots of the samples (50 µg) were applied to the gel and subjected to electrophoresis. The gel was fixed with 0.1% cetyltrimethylammonium bromide solution for 2 h, dried, and stained for 15 min with 0.1% toluidine blue in 1% acetic acid in 50% ethanol. The gel was then destained with the same solution without the dye.

4.6. Determination of Total Antioxidant Capacity (TAC)

This assay is based on the reduction of Mo^{6+} to Mo^{5+} by samples and subsequent formation of a green phosphate-molybdate complex at acid pH [19,23]. Tubes containing extracts and reagent solution (0.6 M sulfuric acid, 28 mM sodium phosphate and 4 mM ammonium molybdate) were incubated at 95 °C for 90 min. After the mixture had cooled to room temperature, the absorbance of each solution was measured at 695 nm against a blank. The TAC was accounted in ascorbic acid milligrams/sample grams, described as equivalent of ascorbic acid.

4.7. MTT Assay

The 3T3-L1 cell capacity to reduce MTT after fucoidan exposure was evaluated in vitro according to the method described earlier [19]. This method is based on the reduction of MTT to formazan crystals by living cells. Briefly, 5×10^3 3T3-L1 cells/well were plated in a 96-well plate. For which well 100 μL DMEM medium with 10% FBS was the final volume used. The cells grew up (95% air, 5% CO_2, 37 °C) until 80% confluence and then the medium was replaced by a DMEM without FBS, followed by incubation for another 24 h in order to stimulate cells to enter in G0 phase. After, the medium was replaced by a DMEM with 10% FBS in the presence of different fucoidans (from 100 to 1000 μg/mL) or absence (control) for 24, 48 or 72 h. At the end of the incubation period, the medium was replaced by a new DMEM without FBS added to 5.0 mg/mL of MTT, followed by incubation for 4 h at 37 °C. The medium was removed and formazan crystals were dissolved with 100 μL of 95% ethanol. After 15 min shaking in a rocking shaker, absorbance was read (570 nm) in a microplate spectrophotometer (Biotek, Winooski, VT, USA). As a negative control, cells were cultivated only with DMEM with 10% FBS. Results were expressed in the percentage of MTT reduction, as in Equation (1).

$$\text{Percentage MTT Reduction} = (\text{Absorbance of sample}/\text{Absorbance of control}) \times 100 \qquad (1)$$

4.8. Adipocyte Differentiation

For adipocyte differentiation the cells were cultured in 24-well plates or 10 mm culture plate containing DMEM medium enriched with 10% FBS and, after reaching 80% confluence, these cells were induced to differentiate by the addition of the adipocyte differentiation cocktail: DMEM, 10% FBS, 1 μM dexamethasone, 0.5 mM 3-isobutyl-1-methylxanthine (IBMX) and 10 μg/mL insulin. After 72 h, the induction medium was replaced by the adipocyte maintenance medium, which consisted of DMEM, 10% FBS and 10 μg/mL insulin. The maintenance medium was changed every 3 days until completing 15 days of differentiation.

4.9. Oil Red O Staining

For oil red O staining, cells were initially induced to differentiate into adipocytes, as previously mentioned, in the absence (control) or presence of fucoidans (200 μg/mL). For this, these samples were added to the differentiation medium. The cells were exposed to fucoidan only in the first three days. After 15 days of differentiation, the cells were washed twice in PBS, fixed with a solution of formaldehyde (3.7%) in PBS for 1 h, washed three times in water, dried and stained with oil red O for 1 h. Excess dye was removed by washing with water. Images of the cells were captured using an optical microscope (TE-Eclipse 300, Nikon, Melville, NY, USA). We performed three different experiments. Subsequently, the dye was eluted from the cells with 100% isopropanol and quantified by measuring the absorbance at 520 nm. The results of the differentiated cells in the presence of the samples were compared with those obtained for the control cells (100% adipocitary differentiation).

4.10. Analysis of the Expression of Adipogenic Markers by Western Blotting

3T3-L1 cells were plated in 100 mm plates and stimulated to differentiate into adipocytes (as described above) in the presence or absence of the 200 µg/mL samples (FF; F0.5; F0.9; F1.1; F2.0). After 15 days of differentiation the cells were suspended in the lysis buffer [50 mM Tris-HCl (pH 7.4); 1% Tween 20; 0.25% sodium deoxycholate; 150 mM NaCl; 1 mM EGTA; 1 mM Na_3VO_4; 1 mM NaF; and protease inhibitors] to obtain the protein extract. The protein content was determined using the Bradford method (1976). The control corresponds to cells that were not exposed to fucoidans. For each sample, 30 µg of protein were subjected to sodium dodecyl sulfate polyacrylamide gel electrophoresis (SDS-PAGE) with subsequent transfer to polyvinylidene difluoride (PVDF) membrane (Millipore, Bedford, MA, USA). The membranes were blocked with skim milk (1%) or albumin (1%) and incubated for 18 h at 4 °C with appropriate primary antibody (β-actin, C/EBPα, C/EBPβ and PPARγ), in a dilution of 1:1000. After incubation with appropriate peroxidase-conjugated (anti-mouse or anti-rabbit) secondary antibody (1:1000 dilution), the detection was performed by chemiluminescence. β-actin was used as an internal control to evaluate the uniformity of protein loading and transfer. The bands were visualized with a ChemiDoc imaging system (Bio-Rad, Hercules, CA, USA) and quantified by ImageJ software ver.1.51k (National Institutes of Health, Bethesda, MD, EUA).

4.11. Statistical Analysis

All data from the experiments were expressed as mean ± standard deviation ($n = 3$) and from three independent assays. The pictures (Figures 1, 3 and 5A) are representative of three separate tests made independently. Statistical analysis between FF and fucoidan´s fraction was done by analysis of variance (ANOVA). The Student-Newman-Keuls post-test (significance was set at $p < 0.05$) was applied to prove some similarities found by ANOVA. All experiments were done in triplicate and data refer to the average of three experiments done independently.

The Pearson correlation coefficient was calculated for the sulfate and the data from the CAT test obtained with fucoidan fractions.

Statistical analysis and Pearson correlation coefficient were performed using GraphPadPrism® software version 5.0, 2014 (GraphPad, La Jolla, CA, USA).

5. Conclusions

In this paper, four different fucoidan-rich fractions (F0.5/F0.9/F1.1/F2.0) of commercial fucoidan from *F. vesiculosus* were obtained using differential precipitation with acetone. Chemical analyzes showed fucose was the major component present in all fractions whereas the relative amounts of other monosaccharides vary according to the fraction. Monosaccharide composition, agarose gel electrophoresis, and antioxidant data showed that each fraction had a different type of fucoidan. F0.5 and F0.9 have an adipogenic effect because they stimulated the lipid accumulation in 3T3-L1 adipocytes through up-regulation of C/EBPα, C/EBPβ, and PPAR gamma. On the other hand, F1.0, and F2.0 have antiadipogenic activity. In addition, all samples had lipolytic action, especially F2.0, which tripled the amount of glycerol in the cellular medium. Among these, F2.0 showed a marked effect on the attenuation of lipid accumulation, antioxidant, and lipolytic activities, and we thus recommend it as a natural antiadipogenic agent for several biotechnological applications.

Author Contributions: R.O. obtained the samples. R.O. and R.C. performed the chemical analysis. R.O., R.C., J.M., R.V., K.M. and M.Q. performed tests with the 3T3-cells. R.O. and Rony Lucas performed the antioxidante tests. R.O., L.F., L.O., and H.R. analyzed the data. R.O., R.L. and H.R. wrote the paper. L.F., L.O. and H.R. revised the paper.

Funding: This research was funded by Coordenação de Aperfeiçoamento Pessoal de Nível Superior-CAPES (Brazil) grants numbers [PROCAD 2965/2014], [Ciências do Mar II—Auxilio 1967/2014].

Acknowledgments: The authors wish to thank Conselho Nacional de Desenvolvimento Científico e Tecnológico-CNPq, CAPES, PROCAD, Ciencias do Mar-CAPES, and the Ministério de Ciência, Tecnologia, Inovação e Comércio-MCTIC (Brazilian Ministry of Science and Technology, loose translation) for the financial support.

Lila Oyama and Hugo Rocha are CNPq fellowship honored researchers. Ruth Medeiros, Rafael Camara, Jessyka Monte, Rony Viana, Karoline Melo and Moacir Queiroz received a scholarship from CAPES. The authors would like to thank the Department of Biochemistry at Universidade Federal do Rio Grande do Norte for letting us to use the cell culture room.

Conflicts of Interest: The authors declare no conflict of interest.

References

1. Skibola, C.F. The effect of *Fucus vesiculosus*, an edible brown seaweed, upon menstrual cycle length and hormonal status in three pre-menopausal women: A case report. *BMC Complement. Altern. Med.* **2004**, *4*, 10. [CrossRef] [PubMed]

2. Moro, C.O.; Basile, G. Obesity and medicinal plants. *Fitoterapia* **2000**, *71*, 73–82. [CrossRef]

3. Schamroth, C.L. The perils of pharmacological treatment for obesity: A case of sibutramine-associated cardiomyopathy and malignant arrhythmias. *Cardiovasc. J. Afr.* **2012**, *23*, 11–12. [CrossRef] [PubMed]

4. Kylin, H. Zur biochemie der Meersalgen. *Physiol. Chem.* **1913**, *83*, 171–197. [CrossRef]

5. McNeely, W. *Fucoidan, Industrial Gums, Polysaccharides and Their Derivatives*, 1st ed.; Whistler, R.L., Bemiller, J.N., Eds.; Academic Press: New York, NY, USA, 1959; Volume 49, pp. 117–125.

6. Patankar, M.S.; Oehninger, S.; Barnett, T.; Williams, R.L.; Clark, G.F. A revised structure for fucoidan may explain some of its biological activities. *J. Biol. Chem.* **1993**, *268*, 21770–21776. Available online: http://www.jbc.org/content/268/29/21770.long (accessed on 13 March 2018). [PubMed]

7. Yokota, T.; Nagashima, M.; Ghazizadeh, M.; Kawanami, O. Increased effect of fucoidan on lipoprotein lipase secretion in adipocytes. *Life Sci.* **2009**, *84*, 523–529. [CrossRef] [PubMed]

8. Park, M.K.; Jung, U.; Roh, C. Fucoidan from marine brown algae inhibits lipid accumulation. *Mar. Drugs* **2011**, *9*, 1359–1367. [CrossRef] [PubMed]

9. Kim, K.J.; Lee, O.H.; Lee, B.Y. Fucoidan, a sulfated polysaccharide, inhibits adipogenesis through the mitogen-activated protein kinase pathway in 3T3-L1 preadipocytes. *Life Sci.* **2010**, *86*, 791–797. [CrossRef] [PubMed]

10. Soeda, S.; Ohmagari, Y.; Shimeno, H.; Nagamatsu, A. Preparation of oversulfated fucoidan fragments and evaluation of their antithrombotic activities. *Thrombos. Res.* **1993**, *72*, 247–256. [CrossRef]

11. Park, K.W.; Halperin, D.S.; Tontonoz, P. Before they were fat: Adipocyte progenitors. *Cell Metab.* **2008**, *8*, 454–457. [CrossRef] [PubMed]

12. Rosen, E.D.; Sarraf, P.; Troy, A.E.; Bradwin, G.; Moore, K.; Milstone, D.S.; Spiegelman, B.M.; Mortensen, R.M. PPAR gamma is required for the differentiation of adipose tissue in vivo and in vitro. *Mol. Cell* **1999**, *4*, 611–617. [CrossRef]

13. Siersbaek, R.; Mandrup, S. Transcriptional networks controlling adipocyte differentiation. In *Cold Spring Harbor Symposia on Quantitative Biology*; Cold Spring Harbor Laboratory Press: Cold Spring Harbor, NY, USA, 2011; Volume 76, pp. 247–255. [CrossRef]

14. Farmer, S.R. Transcriptional control of adipocyte formation. *Cell Metab.* **2006**, *4*, 263–273. [CrossRef] [PubMed]

15. Siersbaek, R.; Nielsen, R.; Mandrupo, S. Transcriptional networks and *Fucus vesiculosus* chromatin remodeling controlling adipogenesis. *Trends Endocrinol. Metab.* **2012**, *23*, 56–64. [CrossRef] [PubMed]

16. Fevè, B. Adipogenesis: Cellular and molecular aspects. *Best Pract. Res. Clin. Endocrinol. Metab.* **2005**, *19*, 483–499. [CrossRef] [PubMed]

17. Nishino, T.; Nishioka, C.; Ura, H.; Nagumo, T. Isolation and partial characterization of a novel amino sugar-containing fucan sulfate from commercial *Fucus vesiculosus* fucoidan. *Carbohydr. Res.* **1994**, *255*, 213–224. [CrossRef]

18. Rocha-Amorim, M.O.; Gomes, D.L.; Dantas, L.A.; Viana, R.L.S.; Chiquetti, S.C.; Almeida-Lima, J.; Silva Costa, L.; Oliveira Rocha, H.A. Fucan-coated silver nanoparticles synthesized by a green method induce human renal adenocarcinoma cell death. *Int. J. Biol. Macromol.* **2016**, *93*, 57–65. [CrossRef] [PubMed]

19. Magalhaes, K.D.; Costa, L.S.; Fidelis, G.P.; Oliveira, R.M.; Nobre, L.T.D.B.; Dantas-Santos, N.; Camara, R.B.G.; Albuquerque, I.R.L.; Cordeiro, S.L.; Sabry, D.A.; et al. Anticoagulant, antioxidant and antitumor activities of heterofucans from the seaweed *Dictyopteris delicatula*. *Int. J. Mol. Sci.* **2011**, *12*, 352–3365. [CrossRef] [PubMed]

20. Albuquerque, I.R.L.; Queiroz, K.C.; Alves, L.G.; Santos, E.A.; Leite, E.L.; Rocha, H.A.O. Heterofucans from *Dictyota menstrualis* have anticoagulant activity. *Braz. J. Med. Biol. Res.* **2004**, *37*, 167–171. [CrossRef] [PubMed]

21. Medeiros, G.F.; Mendes, A.; Castro, R.A.; Baú, E.C.; Nader, H.B.; Dietrich, C.P. Distribution of sulfated glycosaminoglycans in the animal kingdom: Widespread occurrence of heparin-like compounds in invertebrates. *Biochem. Biophys. Acta* **2000**, *1475*, 285–294. [CrossRef]

22. Qi, H.; Zhang, Q.; Zhao, T.; Chen, R.; Zhang, H.; Niu, X.; Li, Z. Antioxidant activity of different sulfate content derivatives of polysaccharide extracted from *Ulva pertusa* (Chlorophyta) in vitro. *Int. J. Biol. Macromol.* **2005**, *4*, 15–37. [CrossRef] [PubMed]

23. Camara, R.B.G.; Costa, L.S.; Fidelis, G.P.; Nobre, L.T.D.B.; Dantas-Santos, N.; Cordeiro, S.L.; Costa, M.S.S.P.; Alves, L.G.; Rocha, H.A.O. Heterofucans from the brown seaweed *Canistrocarpus cervicornis* with anticoagulant and antioxidant activities. *Mar. Drugs* **2011**, *9*, 124–138. [CrossRef] [PubMed]

24. Costa, L.S.; Fidelis, G.P.; Cordeiro, S.L.; Oliveira, R.M.; Sabry, D.A.; Câmara, R.B.; Nobre, L.T.; Costa, M.S.; Almeida-Lima, J.; Farias, E.H.; et al. Biological activities of sulfated polysaccharides from tropical seaweeds. *Biomed. Pharmacother.* **2010**, *1*, 21–28. [CrossRef] [PubMed]

25. Melo, K.R.; Câmara, R.B.; Queiroz, M.F.; Vidal, A.A.; Lima, C.R.; Melo-Silveira, R.F.; Almeida-Lima, J.; Rocha, H.A. Evaluation of sulfated polysaccharides from the brown seaweed *Dictyopteris justii* as antioxidant agents and as inhibitors of the formation of calcium oxalate crystals. *Molecules* **2013**, *25*, 14543–14563. [CrossRef] [PubMed]

26. Kim, M.J.; Chang, U.J.; Lee, J.S. Inhibitory effects of fucoidan in 3T3-L1 adipocyte differentiation. *Mar. Biotechnol.* **2009**, *11*, 557–562. [CrossRef] [PubMed]

27. Langin, D.; Holm, C.; Lafontan, M. Adipocyte hormone sensitive lipase: A major regulator of lipid metabolism. *Proc. Nutr. Soc.* **1996**, *55*, 93–109. [CrossRef] [PubMed]

28. Palatty, P.C.; Saldanha, E. Pharmacotherapy for Weight Management. *J. Assoc. Phys. India* **2012**, *60*, 34–60. Available online: www.japi.org/march_2012/07_ra_pharmacotherapy_for_weight.html (accessed on 14 March 2018).

29. Bays, H.E. Lorcaserin: Drug profile and illustrative model of the regulatory challenges of weight-loss drug development. *Expert Rev. Cardiovasc. Ther.* **2011**, *9*, 265–277. [CrossRef] [PubMed]

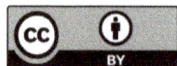

marine drugs

MDPI

Article

Anti-Obesity Effect of Chitosan Oligosaccharide Capsules (COSCs) in Obese Rats by Ameliorating Leptin Resistance and Adipogenesis

Haitao Pan [1,†], Chuhan Fu [2,3,†], Lanlan Huang [4], Yao Jiang [2,3], Xiaoyi Deng [2,3], Jiao Guo [3,*] and Zhengquan Su [2,3,*]

[1]   School of Pharmaceutical Sciences, Sun Yat-Sen University, Guangzhou 510006, China; pangel7835001@163.com

[2]   Guangdong Engineering Research Center of Natural Products and New Drugs, Guangdong Provincial University Engineering Technology Research Center of Natural Products and Drugs, Guangdong Pharmaceutical University, Guangzhou 510006, China; chuhanfu@163.com (C.F.); jiangyaoabcd@163.com (Y.J.); 1500718043DXY@gmail.com(X.D.)

[3]   Guangdong Metabolic Diseases Research Center of Integrated Chinese and Western Medicine, Guangdong Pharmaceutical University, Guangzhou 510006, China

[4]   Guangdong Food and Drug Vocational Technical School, Guangzhou 510663, China; lanlanhuangle@163.com

*   Correspondence: wshxalb@163.com or gyguoyz@163.com (J.G.); suzhq@scnu.edu.cn (Z.S.); Tel.: +86-20-3935-2067 (J.G. & Z.S.)

†   The authors have equally contributed to this work and should be considered co-first authors.

Received: 16 April 2018; Accepted: 1 June 2018; Published: 5 June 2018

Abstract: Obesity is a global disease that causes many metabolic disorders. However, effective agents for the prevention or treatment of obesity remain limited. This study investigated the anti-obesity effect and mechanism of chitosan oligosaccharide capsules (COSCs) on rats suffering from obesity induced by a high-fat diet (HFD). After the eight-week administration of COSCs on obese rats, the body weight gain, fat/body ratio, and related biochemical indices were measured. The hepatic expressions of the leptin signal pathway (JAK2-STAT3) and gene expressions of adipogenesis-related targets were also determined. Our data showed that COSCs can regulate body weight gain, lipids, serum alanine aminotransferase, and aspartate aminotransferase, as well as upregulate the hepatic leptin receptor-b (LepRb) and the phosphorylation of JAK2 and STAT3. Meanwhile, marked increased expressions of liver sterol regulatory element-binding protein-1c, fatty acid synthase, acetyl-CoA carboxylase, 3-hydroxy-3-methylglutaryl-CoA reductase, adiponectin, adipose peroxisome proliferator-activated receptor γ, CCAAT-enhancer binding protein α, adipose differentiation-related protein, and SREBP-1c were observed. The results suggested that COSCs activate the JAK2-STAT3 signaling pathway to alleviate leptin resistance and suppress adipogenesis to reduce lipid accumulation. Thus, they can potentially be used for obesity treatment.

Keywords: chitosan oligosaccharide; obesity; leptin; JAK2-STAT3; adipogenesis

---

1. Introduction

Obesity is a chronically trophic metabolic disease mainly caused by an energy imbalance that leads to excess body fat accumulation. It has caused increasing concern in recent years. Obesity contributes to type 2 diabetes (T2D), hyperlipidemia, hypertension, cerebrovascular incidents, and cancers [1,2]. Recently, several anti-obesity drugs approved by the Food and Drug Administration (FDA) have been withdrawn from the market because of their unexpected adverse effects [3,4]. Currently, Orlistat is the only drug used as an over-the-counter treatment in weight loss aid worldwide, but its adverse effects, including gastrointestinal trauma and greasy feces, should not be ignored [4,5]. Therefore, it is necessary to develop natural products as alternative sources for weight loss agents due to their significant anti-obesity activity, novel structure, and potentially less severe side effects.

Chitosan oligosaccharide ($M_N \leq 1000$ Da, COST) is a small molecular derivative of chitosan (CTS) with 2–10 polymerization degrees [6–8]. Besides non-toxicity to the human body, the absorption rate of COST in the intestinal tract is close to 100% due to its better water-solubility compared to that of CTS, which is slightly soluble in water [9–11]. The biological activities of COST are various, including anti-cancer, anti-inflammatory, hypoglycemic, anti-bacterial, and liver protective effects [11–14]. Additionally, a variety of studies have indicated that COST also exerts effective lipid-lowering and anti-obesity effects on obese animals, which makes it an effective lipid-lowering dietary supplement used in the field of food and nutrition to reduce lipid levels [10,14–16].

Leptin, a 16 kDa polypeptide that is primarily released from white adipose tissue (WAT), is an important hormone for weight management via the homeostatic control of energy equilibrium, thus facilitating the prevention of obesity [17,18]. Leptin exhibits its regulatory effect mainly by binding to the long-form leptin receptor-b (LepRb), which is widely distributed in the bodies of both humans and rodents [19,20]. JAK2-STAT3 (Janus kinase-2-signal transducer and activators of transcription-3) is the most important signaling pathway that mediates the energy balance regulation of leptin, which functions in many organs and tissues, such as the liver, brain, fat, muscle, and pancreas [21]. By binding to the extracellular domain of LepRb, leptin triggers the phosphorylation and activation of JAK2. The activated JAK2 recruits and phosphorylates STAT3 for its activation and translocation to the arcuate nucleus in the hypothalamus, which regulates the expression and neuronal excitability of POMC, AgRP, and NPY, ultimately suppressing appetite, promoting energy expenditure, and reducing body weight [19]. However, most obese patients show high levels of circulating leptin, which is attributed to leptin resistance that has occurred in the body [19]. In consequence, the drugs that improve leptin resistance will present significant anti-obesity effects.

In addition, Inoue et al. [22] revealed a deficiency of STAT3 in mouse liver aggravated steatosis and gluconeogenesis, whereas the overexpression of STAT3 reversed steatosis and suppressed the expression of the gluconeogenic gene. Meanwhile, Shi, et al. [23] showed that a hepatocyte-specific deficiency in JAK2 mice is required for the spontaneous development of steatohepatitis and glucose intolerance. Therefore, the activation of JAK2 or STAT3 in hepatocytes also ameliorates steatosis and improves lipid metabolism, which further contributes to anti-obesity action.

Adiponectin, an endogenous bioactive polypeptide secreted by adipocytes, is associated with the counteracting development of obesity and its related diseases. The gene expression and circulating levels of adiponectin are reported to be inversely correlated with obesity [24–26]. Sterol regulatory element-binding protein-1c (SREBP-1c) regulates de novo lipogenesis mainly in the liver via controlling the expression of its target gene, fatty acid synthase (FAS), a key enzyme for the formation of fatty acids [27,28]. With the increase of SREBP-1c expression, fatty acid metabolism becomes imbalanced, and subsequently the syntheses of hepatic triacylglycerol (TG) and total cholesterol (TC) are increased, which are closely associated with hepatic steatosis [29,30]. Acetyl-CoA is the precursor of fatty acid and cholesterol synthesis, and the reaction that translates acetyl-CoA into fatty acid or cholesterol is regulated by acetyl-CoA carboxylase (ACC), SREBPs, FAS, and so on [31]. In addition, 3-hydroxy-3-methylglutaryl-CoA reductase (HMGCR), the rate-limiting enzyme for hepatic cholesterol synthesis, catalyzes the conversion of HMG-CoA to mevalonate. A decreased expression of HMG-CoA is beneficial for suppressing the synthesis of hepatic cholesterol [32].

The hyperplasia and hypertrophy of adipocytes facilitate the development of obesity and its complications. Therefore, decreasing lipogenesis may benefit obesity prevention or treatment. Peroxisome proliferator-activated receptor γ (PPARγ) and CCAAT-enhancer binding protein α (C/EBPα) are two primary modulators of lipogenesis and regulate the proliferation, differentiation, and fat accumulation of adipocytes in WAT [33,34]. Adipose differentiation-related protein (ADRP), which covers the surface of phospholipid protein lipid droplets and is expressed early during the differentiation of adipose, stimulates fatty acid production and accelerates lipid droplet formation for fatty acid storage [34,35]. Meanwhile, FAS, SREBP-1c, and adiponectin also regulate lipid metabolism in WAT [36].

In this study, COST capsules (COSCs) were first prepared in capsule form due to several advantages, including the enhanced stability of COST manifested through strong hygroscopicity and oxidability, and the accelerated action rate of COST via the rapid dissolution, dispersion, and assimilation of the capsule in the gastrointestinal tract. Also, the capsule form can be easily identified and taken by most people. Subsequently, the anti-obesity effects of COSCs in a rat model exhibiting obesity induced by a high-fat diet (HFD) were investigated. Significantly ameliorated effects of COSCs on the development of obesity and its related complications were observed. To explore the anti-obesity mechanisms, the liver LepRb, JAK2, and STAT3 expressions in the leptin metabolic JAK2-STAT3 signaling pathway were evaluated by Western blotting, which suggested an improved leptin-resistant state via activating the JAK2-STAT3 signaling pathway. Moreover, the lipogenesis-related genes in the liver (including SREBP-1c, FAS, ACC, HMGCR, and adiponectin) and in adipose tissues (including PPARγ, C/EBPα, ADRP, FAS, and SREBP-1c) were also determined using quantitative RT-PCR analysis, indicating the adipogenesis suppression action of COSCs. These studies suggested that COSCs may be a prospective agent for obesity prevention or treatment.

2. Results

2.1. Food Intake, Body Weight, and Body Weight Gain

To evaluate the anti-obesity effects of COSCs, food intake, body weight, and the body weight gain of the rats were measured over an eight-week period, the results of which are shown in Figure 1. For food intake, the high-fat (HF) group was slightly higher than the normal diet group (NF) and treatment groups during the experimental period, but the difference was not significant (Figure 1a), suggesting no influence of COSCs on the appetite of the rats, and the minor decrease of food intake in the treatment groups was attributed to a slight anorectic effect induced by HFD during the long-term HFD intake [10].

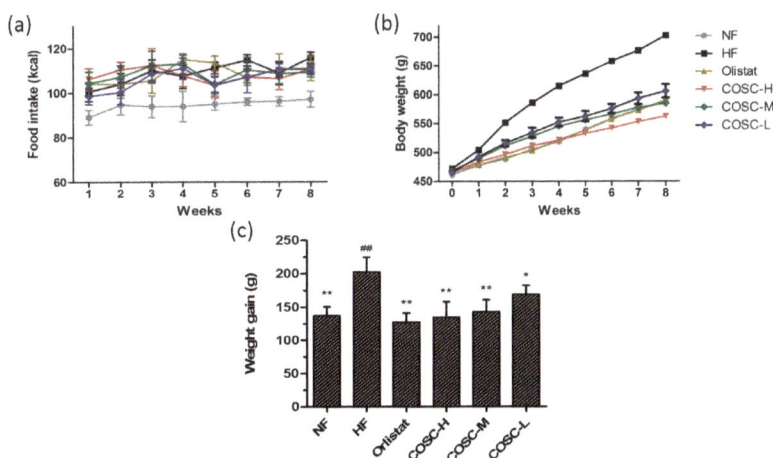

Figure 1. Chitosan oligosaccharide capsules (COSCs) reduced body weight gain of obese rats with no influence on food intake. Changes in the food intake (**a**); body weight (**b**), and body weight gain (**c**) during the eight-week treatment are shown. The data are expressed as means ± SE ($n = 10$). Note: * $p < 0.05$, ** $p < 0.01$ when compared to the high-fat (HF) group; ## $p < 0.01$ when compared to the HF group.

For the body weight gain, the average body weight of the HF group increased by 41.22% after eight weeks of feeding with HFD. Meanwhile, the eight-week administration of Orlistat, high (COSC-H), middle (COSC-M), and low dose of COS (COSC-L) significantly decreased body weight gain by 37.21%, 33.52%, 29.62%, and 16.61%, respectively (Figure 1b,c). Additionally, the effect of COSC-H on reducing weight gain was similar to that of the NF (32.47%) and Orlistat groups, suggesting effective weight loss action in the HFD-induced obese rats.

2.2. Serum Lipids and Leptin

Rat serum lipid levels after the eight-week administration were determined and are displayed in Figure 2. Compared with the NF group, 42.06%, 41.38%, and 29.23% increases of serum total cholesterol (TC), triglyceride (TG), and low-density lipoprotein cholesterol (LDL-C) levels, as well as a 25.20% decrease of serum high-density lipoprotein cholesterol (HDL-C), were shown in the HF group. Orlistat, COSC-H, COSC-M, and COSC-L could markedly lower serum TC by 30.36%, 38.49%, 28.37%, and 17.06% (Figure 2a), as well as TG by 30.88%, 36.41%, 24.42%, and 16.59% (Figure 2b), respectively. Moreover, COSCs, especially COSC-H and COSC-M, significantly ameliorated the increased LDL-C (Figure 2c) and reduced the HDL-C levels (Figure 2d) that were induced by HFD in the obese rats.

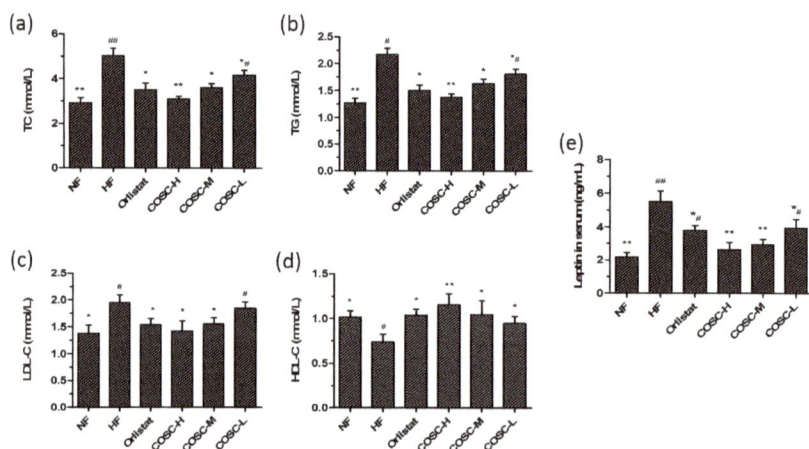

Figure 2. COSCs corrected serum lipid and leptin levels of high-fat diet (HFD)-induced obese rats. Serum TC (**a**); TG (**b**); LDL-C (**c**); HDL-C (**d**); and leptin (**e**) levels after eight weeks of treatment are shown. The data are expressed as means ± SE ($n = 10$). Note: * $p < 0.05$, ** $p < 0.01$ when compared to the HF group; # $p < 0.05$, ## $p < 0.01$ when compared to the HF group.

Various studies have indicated that leptin resistance, manifested by high levels of circulating leptin, is an important characteristic of nutritional obese patients [19]. In the study, the serum leptin of the HF group markedly increased by 60.36% when compared with that of NF group, suggesting that a leptin resistance state was induced by HFD in obese rats. Chitosan oligosaccharide capsule treatment significantly decreased the serum leptin level by 28.01~52.55% when compared to that of the HF group (Figure 2e), and this action was superior to that of Orlistat. All data in Figure 2 indicate that COSCs significantly improve serum lipids and leptin levels, facilitating lipids metabolism and ameliorating leptin resistance, which contribute to the anti-obesity activity of COSCs.

2.3. COSCs Facilitate Hepatoprotective Effects

The liver morphology, lipids, AST, and ALT levels are shown in Figure 3. Compared with the NF group, the average liver weight of rats fed HFD increased by 66.06%, which could be decreased by

13.55~33.12% after the administration of COSCs (Figure 3a). The corresponding results were also shown on the liver index (liver mass/body mass); that of the HF group was 30.50% higher than that of the NF group, although it could be decreased by 13.55~33.12% after the administration of COSCs (Figure 3b). For the liver TC (Figure 3c) and TG (Figure 3d) levels, the significant increases by 67.07% and 71.98% in the HF group were respectively shown when compared with that in the NF group, suggesting an obvious liver lipid accumulation induced by HFD. However, after the administration of Orlistat and the different doses of COSCs, the HFD-induced high levels of TC in the liver were significantly decreased by 29.35% (Orlistat), 46.34% (COSC-H), 35.93% (COSC-M), and 24.13% (COSC-L), and the levels of TG in the liver were also markedly decreased by 37.22% (Orlistat), 51.87% (COSC-H), 31.77% (COSC-M), and 17.63% (COSC-L).

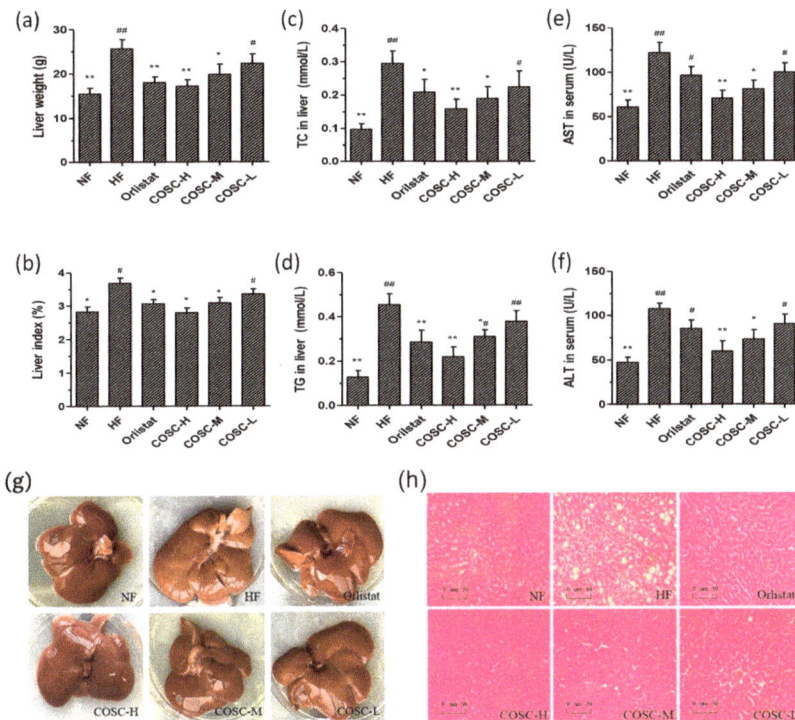

Figure 3. COSCs regulated hepatic lipids and facilitate hepatoprotective effects for obese rats. Liver weight (**a**); liver index (**b**); liver TC (**c**) and TG (**d**); as well as serum AST (**e**) and ALT (**f**) are shown; The whole liver (**g**); and liver histopathological slices (**h**) (200×) in different groups are also presented. Tissue sections were stained with hematoxylin and eosin (H&E). The data are expressed as means ± SE ($n = 10$). Note: compared with rats in the HF group, * $p < 0.05$, ** $p < 0.01$; compared with rats in the NF group, # $p < 0.05$, ## $p < 0.01$.

Meanwhile, the liver morphology (Figure 3g) showed that the whole livers in the NF group were supple, bright red in color, smooth in the tunica of tissues, and characterized by sharp edges and a small volume. However, the livers of the HF group were slightly soft, dull pale in color, characterized by hypertrophic edges, and intumescent and distributed with white fat granules on the surface of the liver, suggesting that the severe fatty-liver-like illnesses had developed. The livers of the animals administered with the different doses of COSCs showed ameliorated hepatic steatosis, a color between bright red and dull pale, and reduced white fat granules. Histopathological slices of rat livers in the different groups were also observed after staining with hematoxylin and eosin (H&E) (Figure 3h). The liver slices revealed that there were no histological abnormalities of hepatocytes in the NF group with fewer fat droplets, whereas the hepatocytes in the HF group possessed serious fat vacuoles, indicating that the rats had developed a high degree of hepatic steatosis induced by HFD. Chitosan oligosaccharide capsules, especially COSC-H, can markedly decrease the fat vacuoles of hepatocytes whose cells are in alignment to varying degrees, similar to those of the NF group.

Liver injury, or hepatotoxicity, is the main relative factor of hyperlipidemia and obesity [37]. To check whether a hepatoprotective effect of COSCs presented, we measured the serum AST and ALT levels (Figure 3e,f). Obviously increased serum AST and ALT were shown in the HF group when compared to that in the NF group. Different doses of COSCs significantly lowered the activities of serum ALT and AST to the normal range. In particular, the effects of COSC-H and COSC-M were superior to those of Orlistat ($p < 0.05$), suggesting that COSCs play an important role in hepatoprotective function.

All data demonstrated that COSCs exert a hepatoprotective effect via decreasing the liver index, enhancing liver function, and relieving fatty liver, which contribute to the anti-obesity effects.

2.4. Fat Pad and Fat/Body Ratio

After the eight-week administration, the epididymal and perirenal WAT weights were measured to calculate the wet weight of the fat pad and fat/body ratio (Figure 4). Compared to the NF rats, the average weights of epididymal (Figure 4a) and perirenal WAT (Figure 4b) in the HF group were markedly increased by 64.38% and 63.19%. Also, COSCs were found to decrease the fat pad (Figure 4c, $p < 0.05$) and fat/body ratio (Figure 4d, $p < 0.05$) of rats dose-dependently to the normal range. Moreover, the inhibiting effects of COSC-H on HFD-induced elevated fat pad and fat/body ratio were slightly superior to that of Orlistat.

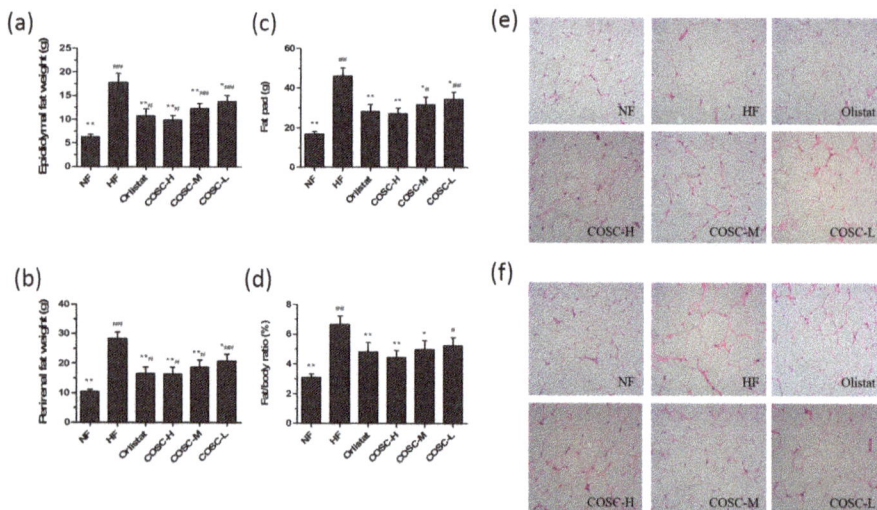

Figure 4. COSCs reduced the fat pad, fat/body ratio, and inhibit the accumulation of adipocytes in white adipose tissue (WAT) of obese rats. The epididymal (**a**) and perirenal (**b**) fat weight, fat pad weight (**c**), and fat/body ratio (**d**) are shown in the figure. The epididymal (**e**) and perirenal adipose tissue (**f**) slices (200×) are also shown. The numbers of epididymal or perirenal adipocytes were calculated in the same field of view. Tissue sections were stained with hematoxylin and eosin (H&E). Note: compared with rats in the HF group, * $p < 0.05$, ** $p < 0.01$; compared with rats in the NF group, # $p < 0.05$, ## $p < 0.01$.

In addition, the histopathological results of epididymal (Figure 4e) and perirenal WAT (Figure 4f) showed that larger and distinctly hypertrophic adipocytes of rats in the HF group (70 epididymal adipocytes and 115 perirenal adipocytes under the 200× visual field) were observed when compared with those in the NF group (26 epididymal adipocytes and 29 perirenal adipocytes under the same field of view). Treatment with Orlistat and the three doses of COSCs inhibited the proliferation and size of adipocytes, as fewer and smaller adipocytes were observed compared to those in the HF group, using the same magnification and field of view. Therefore, COSCs can effectively exert anti-obesity effects by suppressing the growth and accumulation of adipocytes in WAT.

2.5. COSCs Activate Leptin Signaling Transduction

Leptin resistance, characterized by elevated circulating leptin levels and decreased leptin sensitivity, is the central mechanism for the development of obesity. Attenuation of the JAK2-STAT3 signaling transduction pathway can be considered as the crucial risk factor for leptin resistance. Therefore, the improvement of leptin resistance by regulating the JAK2-STAT3 signaling pathway effectively exerts anti-obesity activity [19,38]. In this study, the protein levels of liver LepRb, JAK2, p-JAK2, STAT3, and p-STAT3 in the activation of the JAK2-STAT3 signal pathway were detected using Western blotting, as displayed in Figure 5. The eight-week treatment of COSC-H and COSC-M significantly reversed the lower expression of LepRb in HFD-induced obese rats (Figure 5a,b). The reduced phosphorylation of JAK2 (Figure 5c–e) and STAT3 levels (Figure 5f–h) in the HFD group were also prominently upregulated by COSCs (especially COSC-H and COSC-M), indicating the improvement of the leptin resistance state. Therefore, COSCs can ameliorate leptin resistance via upregulating LepRb and activating the JAK2-STAT3 signaling pathway, contributing to the improvement of obesity.

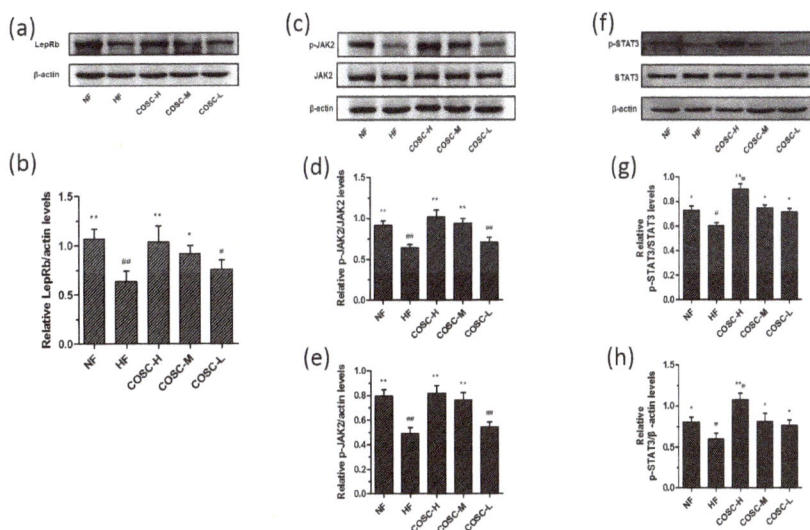

Figure 5. COSCs activated the JAK2-STAT3 signaling transduction of obese rats. Protein expression and quantification of LepRb (**a,b**); phosphorylation of JAK2 (p-JAK2, **c–e**) and phosphorylation of STAT3 (p-STAT3, **f–h**) in liver are shown here. The data are expressed as means ± SE (*n* = 10). Note: compared with rats in the HF group, * $p < 0.05$, ** $p < 0.01$; compared with rats in the NF group, # $p < 0.05$, ## $p < 0.01$.

2.6. COSCs Regulate the Expression of Lipogenesis-Related Genes

The liver lipogenesis-related genes, *SREBP-1c, FAS, ACC*, and *HMGCR*, as well as the WAT lipogenesis-related genes, *adiponectin, PPARγ, C/EBPα, ADRP, FAS*, and *SREBP-1c*, were also measured (Figure 6a–e). Compared with the NF group, the significant upregulation of *SREBP-1c, FAS, ACC*, and *HMGCR* as well as the downregulation of *adiponectin* were observed in the HF group. Chitosan oligosaccharide capsules, especially the high and middle doses, reversed the upregulated expression of *PPARγ, C/EBPα, ADRP, FAS*, and *SREBP-1c*, and the downregulation of *adiponectin* induced by HFD in obese rats, indicating an improved hepatic lipid metabolism by inhibiting lipid synthesis in the liver.

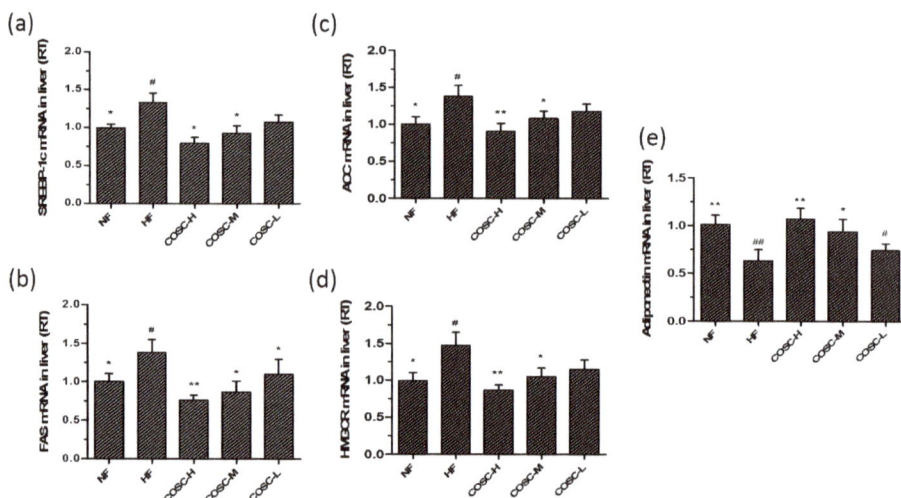

Figure 6. COSCs regulated the expression of liver lipogenesis-related genes in obese rats. The liver mRNA levels of *SREBP-1c* (**a**); *FAS* (**b**); *ACC* (**c**); *HMGCR* (**d**); and *adiponectin* (**e**) were detected by Q-PCR. ΔCt is the average value of 10 samples in the formulation (average mRNA expression of experiment groups/average mRNA expression of the NF group) $= 2^{-\Delta\Delta Ct} = 2^{(-\Delta Ct\ control\ -\Delta Ct\ FF)}$. If $2^{-\Delta\Delta Ct} < 1$, the average mRNA expression of the experiment groups is lower than that in the NF group. If this value is higher than 1, the average mRNA expression of the experiment groups is higher than that in the NF group. The data are expressed as means $\pm$ SE ($n = 10$). Note: compared with rats in the HF group, * $p < 0.05$, ** $p < 0.01$; compared with rats in the NF group, # $p < 0.05$, ## $p < 0.01$.

White adipose tissue is an important tissue for ensuring energy storage and fat mobilization. However, the hyperplasia and hypertrophy of WAT will lead to metabolic syndromes, and the inhibition of adipogenesis can be an effective strategy for obesity treatment [15]. We measured lipogenesis-related genes, including *PPARγ, C/EBPα, ADRP, FAS*, and *SREBP-1c*, in the epididymal adipose tissues (Figure 7). The remarkable downregulation of *PPARγ, C/EBPα, ADRP, FAS*, and *SREBP-1c* were also observed to be correlated with the dose of COSCs.

All of these results suggest that COSCs can inhibit adipogenesis in liver and WAT by regulating the expressions of related genes involved in lipid synthetic metabolism to ameliorate obesity and its related metabolic diseases.

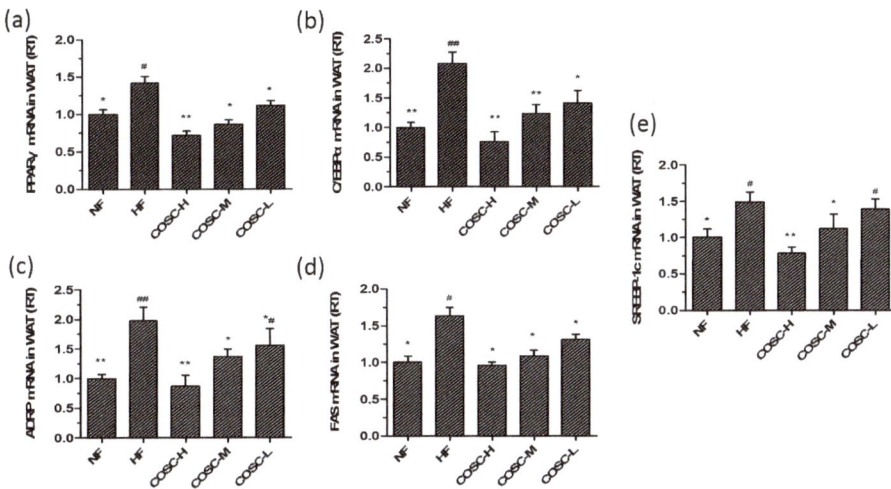

Figure 7. COSCs regulated the expression of lipogenesis-related genes in obese rat WAT. The mRNA levels of *PPARγ* (**a**); *C/EBPα* (**b**); *ADRP* (**c**); *FAS* (**d**); and *SREBP-1c* (**e**) in epididymal adipose tissues were quantified by Q-PCR. The $2^{-\Delta\Delta Ct}$ method was used for the quantification of each mRNA as shown in Figure 6. The data are expressed as means ± SE ($n = 10$). Note: compared with rats in the HF group, * $p < 0.05$, ** $p < 0.01$; compared with rats in the NF group, # $p < 0.05$, ## $p < 0.01$.

3. Discussion

Obesity-related metabolic disorders, including type 2 diabetes, hyperlipidemia, hypertension, cerebrovascular incidents, and cancers, are classified as endocrinology diseases by the World Health Organization (WHO) [1,39]. Obesity, paralleling the acquired immune deficiency syndrome (AIDS), drugs, and alcoholism, is regarded as one of four medical social issues worldwide that are becoming a ponderous burden to public health system [40]. Therefore, it is urgent to develop new types of anti-obesity drugs. Natural products are promising alternative sources due to their effective biological activities and potentially less severe side effects [14].

Several studies by others and our group have demonstrated that COST has anti-obesity effects and is a promising anti-obesity agent [15,16,41]. In the current study, we prepared COST in a capsule form and investigated its anti-obesity effects and molecular mechanisms.

The obese animal model used in the experiment showed obviously increased body weight gain and lipid accumulation as well as elevated organ index, as reported before the anti-obesity treatment [42,43]. The obese rats were treated with COSCs for eight weeks, and the obese evaluation indicators, mainly including body fat pad weight, fat/body ratio, liver and serum lipids, as well as liver and adipose tissue slices, were determined. In agreement with previous experiments [9,10], COSCs showed obvious inhibition of increases in rat body weight (Figure 1c), liver index (Figure 3a,b), body fat (Figure 4c), and the proportion of fat to body weight (Figure 4d) without influence on the appetite, as well as reducing adipocyte hypertrophy and fat accumulation (Figure 4e,f), suggesting significant anti-obesity effects. Simultaneously, COSCs can markedly reverse HFD-induced serum high levels of TC, TG, and LDL-C as well as low HDL-C levels in a dose-dependent manner, which also contribute to its anti-obesity actions (Figure 2).

Hepatic steatosis (fatty liver), induced by excessive lipid accumulation in the liver, is highly relevant to obesity and its related complications [44,45]. In this study, COSCs effectively lowered the high weight and index of the liver, and reversed HFD-induced intumescent, pale, and slightly soft livers as well as diminished fat vacuoles, indicating the ameliorating effect of COSCs on hepatic steatosis mainly achieved by reducing excessive fat accumulation (Figure 3). Meanwhile, the high levels of hepatic TC and TG were also reversed by COSCs, especially COSC-H and COSC-M, indicating that a decrease in excessive hepatic lipids improved liver lipid metabolism (Figure 3), similar to the previous study of COS, which promotes the reverse cholesterol transport (RCT) process for the excretion of liver lipids [10]. Together with the decreased serum AST and ALT of the treatment groups, COSCs exerted liver protective effects.

Leptin resistance, characterized by elevated circulating leptin levels and decreased leptin sensitivity, is the central mechanism for the development of obesity. Attenuation of the JAK2-STAT3 signaling transduction pathway is a crucial risk factor for leptin resistance [19,20]. Chitosan oligosaccharide capsules significantly reduced circulating leptin in obese rats, and improved the leptin resistance state by upregulating the expression of LepRb and the phosphorylation levels of JAK2 and STAT3 (Figures 2e and 5). The activation of the JAK2-STAT3 signaling pathway also contributes to the remissions of steatosis and dyslipidemia of obese rats [22,23]. Therefore, the improvement of leptin resistance by regulating the JAK2-STAT3 signaling pathway is the mechanism by which COSCs exerts effective anti-obesity activity in HFD-induced obese rats.

SREBP-1c, FAS, ACC, and HMGCR are the crucial factors that influence lipid metabolism in the liver. SREBP-1c increases the activity of the key enzyme FAS and regulates the synthesis of TC and TG when free fatty acids are released into hepatocytes [29]. Acetyl-CoA carboxylase catalyzes the conversion of acetyl-CoA to Malonyl-CoA, which regulates the rate of fatty acid synthesis in the first stage [31]. An increase of HMGCR expression led to cholesterol synthesis in the liver due to the fact that HMGCR is a rate-limiting enzyme for hepatic cholesterol synthesis and catalyzes HMG-CoA to be converted to mevalonate [32]. Additionally, adiponectin acts as the negative regulator factor of adipogenesis, counteracting the development of fatty liver and obesity [24,26]. Chitosan oligosaccharide capsules can inhibit hepatic lipid synthesis by prominently regulating the gene expressions of SREBP-1c, FAS, ACC, HMGCR, and adiponectin to improve hepatic steatosis and lipid metabolism disorder, thereby exerting hepatoprotective and anti-obesity effects (Figure 6).

In addition, the expressions of genes involved in WAT were also determined to evaluate the influences of COSCs on adipogenesis in WAT. PPARγ, together with C/EBPα, can promote the proliferation and differentiation of adipocytes and control lipid storage in WAT [33,46]; ADRP can accelerate the formation of fatty acids and lipid droplet accumulation in the early differentiation of adipocytes [34,47]; FAS and SREBP-1c facilitate the synthesis of TC and TG of WAT [48]. Unsurprisingly, the gene expressions of PPARγ, C/EBPα, ADRP, FAS, and SREBP-1c in the epididymal adipose tissues were upregulated after the administration of COSCs, which contribute to the ameliorated effect of hyperplasia or hypertrophy of adipocytes to suppress adipogenesis in WAT (Figure 7).

In summary, COSCs could be used as a drug candidate with a good ability to control obesity. Chitosan oligosaccharide capsules can activate the JAK2-STAT3 signaling pathway to alleviate leptin resistance and inhibit adipogenesis by regulating the relevant adipocytokines. Therefore, COSCs may serve as a natural product prospective agent for obesity prevention and treatment.

4. Materials and Methods

4.1. Materials and Supplies

Chitosan oligosaccharide ($M_N \leq 1000$ g/mol; deacetylation degree, 95.6%) was obtained from Laizhou Haili Biological Products Co. Ltd. Laizhou, Shandong, China. The COSCs used in this work were prepared in our laboratory. The Orlistat capsules were provided by Chongqing Fortune Pharmaceutical Co. Ltd., Chongqing, China. Total cholesterol, TG, HDL-C, LDL-C, AST, and ALT kits were provided by BioSino Biotechnology and Science Inc., Beijing, China. The BCA protein quantified assay kit (Cat. No. P0012) was provided by Beyotime Biotechnology Inc., Shanghai, China. The rabbit polyclonal anti-LepRb (Cat. No. 20966-1-AP), anti-JAK2 (Cat. No. 17670-1-AP), and anti-STAT3 (Cat. No. 10253-2-AP) antibodies were purchased from Proteintech, Inc., Wuhan, China. The rabbit monoclonal anti-JAK2 (Cat. No. ab219728) and anti-STAT3 (Cat. No. ab76315) phosphorylated antibodies were purchased from Abcam Co. Ltd., Cambridge, UK. The rabbit anti-β-actin (Cat. No. bs-0061R) and Goat anti-rabbit IgG/HRP (Cat. No. bs-0295G-HRP) antibodies were purchased from Biosynthesis Biotechnology Co., Ltd., Beijing, China. The reverse transcription kit (PrimeScript™ RT reagent kit with gDNA Eraser (Cat. No. RR047A)) and the PCR kit (SYBR Premix Ex Taq™ kit (Cat. No. RR420A)) were all supplied by TaKaRa Inc. (Otsu, Japan). All of the other reagents were of analytical grade and were used without further purification.

4.2. COSCs Preparation

The COSCs were prepared as shown in Reference [49]. Briefly, COST and 5% povidone (PVP) dissolved in anhydrous ethanol were ground equally in a mortar using the appropriate proportions. Then, the soft materials were made into granules using an oscillating granulator (20 mesh sieves) and desiccation. The dry granules were filled in a 1# hollow capsule shell using a manual capsule filling plate, and the loading amount was 300 mg per capsule.

4.3. Animals and Diets

Ninety-five 5-week-old male specific pathogen free (SPF) Sprague–Dawley (SD) rats (weight, 120~150 g; age, 5 weeks) were provided by the Guangdong Medical Laboratory Animal Center (GMLAC, Guangzhou, China) and were maintained in an SPF room (temperature: 22~25 °C, related humidity: 50~60%, differential pressure: ≥10 Pa, under a constant day-night rhythm). Water was given to rats freely throughout the experiments. The welfare of the animals in the in vivo experiments was handled strictly following "Guidelines on kindly treatments for experimental animals" by the Science and Technology Ministry of China (2006) 398. All protocols were approved by the Institutional Animal Ethics Committee of Guangdong Pharmaceutical University (Approval No. gdpulac 2018092). All animals were fed with the normal diet (Guangdong Pharmaceutical University Laboratory Animal Center, Guangzhou, China) for one week. Subsequently, the 95 rats were divided into two groups: the normal diet group (NF) with 10 rats fed the normal diet, and the HFD group (HF), with 85 animals fed the HFD to obtain the obese model.

The HFD was comprised of 54% basic feed, 15% lard, 15% sucrose, 4% milk powder, 3% peanut, 5% egg yolk powder, 1% sesame oil, 2% salt, 0.6% dicalcium phosphate, and 0.4% mountain flour in SPF packaging (provided by GMLAC (No. 20150925)). After two weeks of feeding with HFD, two thirds of the rats were sorted by body weight gain. The excluded one third of the rats that gained less weight were kept on the HFD for another six weeks. The obese model was regarded as being accomplished when the average weight of the rats fed with HFD surpassed 20% of that of the basic fed rats.

The 50 obesity-sensitive rats were then randomly and equally divided into five groups as follows: (1) HFD group fed with HFD ad libitum only (HF); (2) HFD group treated with Orlistat (75 mg/kg·day) (Orlistat); (3–5) HFD group supplemented with low (150 mg/kg·day, COSC-L), middle (300 mg/kg·day, COSC-M), and high (600 mg/kg·day, COSC-H) dose COSCs. Because the capsules and COST were all water-soluble, the COST capsules were consequently dissolved in distilled water, which formed the COST solution with a constant concentration of 600 mg/mL. The corresponding samples to be tested should be solubilized in distilled water and administered by oral gavage daily with a dose of 1 mL/100 g (the rats' body weight) at the same time for eight weeks until the experiment ended. The rats in the HF and NF groups were simultaneously administered equal amounts of distilled water in the same way as described above. All rats obtained food and water freely during the experimental period, and were sacrificed at the age of 22 weeks.

4.4. Experimental Design

4.4.1. Determination of Food Intake and Weight Gain

The 24-h food intake levels of rats were recorded daily, while body weight, body length, and abdominal girth were determined every week during the animal study.

4.4.2. Determination of Serum Lipid and Leptin Levels

The rats were fasted for 16 h and then subjected to 1% sodium pentobarbital (0.5 mL/100 g body weight) anesthesia, and their blood was collected from the aorta abdominals. The serum was obtained via centrifuging at 3500 rpm for 30 min at 4 °C, and the serum lipid and leptin levels were then measured. The concentrations of TC, TG, HDL-C, LDL-C, AST, and ALT were measured with commercial assay kits using an automated biochemistry analyzer BC200 instrument. The concentration of leptin were measured using an enzyme-linked immunosorbent assay (ELISA) kit (R&D, Systems China Co. Ltd., Shanghai, China), and the absorbance was detected at 450 nm using a multifunctional Berthold Mithras LB940 microplate reader (Berthold Technologies GmbH & Co. KG, Bad Wildbad, Germany).

4.4.3. Determination of Fat Pad, Fat/Body Ratio, and Visceral Index

Rats were subjected to ether anesthesia, sacrificed, and necropsied after serum preparation. Then the liver, epididymal WAT, and perirenal WAT were quickly stripped and weighed by an electronic scale at 4 °C. After a picture was taken of the whole liver from each animal, the total wet weight of liver, epididymal fat, and perirenal fat were used to determine the liver index, fat pad, and fat/body ratio, respectively. The tissues were promptly stored at −80 °C for further analysis following their removal.

4.4.4. Determination of Hepatic Lipids, AST, and ALT

A piece (approximately 0.1 g) of liver tissue was homogenized in 0.9 mL 0.9% sodium chloride, and the supernatant was collected after centrifuging at 2500 rpm for 10 min at 4 °C. The hepatic TC, TG, AST, and ALT levels were measured with commercial assay kits, as was performed for serum lipids previously.

4.5. Histology of the Different Tissues

The liver, white epididymal, and perirenal WAT were cut into 0.6 cm^3, then were rinsed with normal saline and put in a tissue cassette. The cassettes were marked with a pencil and then placed into a 12% formaldehyde solution for 24 h to fix the tissue. After the residual fixative was cleaned with distilled water, the tissues were firstly dehydrated via 30%, 50%, 70%, 80%, 90%, 95%, and 100% ethanol, then embedded in paraffin (BMJ-III embedding machine, Changzhou Electronic Instrument Factory, Jiangsu, China) and lastly cut into 5-μm-thick sections using a Leica RM2235 microtome (Leica, Heidelberg, Germany). The tissues were stained with hematoxylin and eosin (H&E) and observed under a microscope at 200× magnification.

4.6. Western Blotting Assays

Total protein was isolated from the liver tissues (25 mg) with 0.50 mL of cold RIPA Lysis Buffer (50 mM Tris (pH 7.4), 150 mM NaCl, 1% Triton X-100, 1% sodium deoxycholate, 0.1% SDS, and protease and phosphatase inhibitor), followed by centrifugation twice at 12,000 g for 30 min at 4 °C. The protein concentrations were quantified by the Beyotime BCA protein assay kit. The isolated proteins were diluted to the same protein concentrations. An equal amount of each protein lysate (35 μg) was subjected to sodium dodecyl sulfate-polyacrylamide gel electrophoresis (SDS-PAGE) on 10% gels. After electrophoresis, the gels were then transferred to polyvinylidene fluoride membranes (Millipore,

USA). After blocking with 5% bovine serum albumin (BSA) in TBST buffer (25 mM Tris, 150 mM NaCl, 0.05% Tween 20, pH 7.4) for two hours, the membranes were correspondingly incubated for 2 h with primary antibodies, including rabbit polyclonal anti-LepRb, anti-JAK2, and anti-STAT3 antibodies, and rabbit monoclonal anti-JAK2 and anti-STAT3 phosphorylated antibodies, as well as rabbit anti-β-actin antibody, in 5% skim milk. The secondary antibody (Goat anti-rabbit IgG linked HRP) was incubated with the membranes for another 1 h after washing with TBST buffer. The membranes were developed with Pierce's West Pico chemiluminescence substrate (Millipore, Burlington, MA, USA) after washing with TBST buffer. The chemiluminescence imaging system (Sage Creation, Beijing, China) and its Lane 1D gel image software were applied to quantify the grayscale of the protein bands with the value of the β-actin band as an internal reference.

4.7. Reverse Transcription-Polymerase Chain Reaction (RT-PCR) Analysis

Total RNA was isolated from rat livers or white epididymal adipose tissues using the TRIzol reagent (Invitrogen, Inc., Carlsbad, CA, USA). Single-stranded cDNA was generated from 1 μg of total RNA using TaKaRa PrimeScript™ RT reagent kit. The cDNA products were amplified by real-time RT-PCR using TaKaRa SYBR Premix Ex Taq™ kit and the Bio-Rad IQ5 real-time PCR system, and its analysis software (Applied Biosystems, Carlsbad, CA, USA) was used for data collection and analysis. The primer sequences (Table 1) used for PCR were synthesized by Sangon Biotech Co. Ltd. (Shanghai, China). β-actin was used as the internal control (housekeeping gene).

The PCR protocols were performed as follows: 95 °C for 30 s (initial denaturation), followed by 39–40 cycles at 95 °C for 5 s and 60 °C for 30 s, after which the amplified products were heated from 65 °C to 95 °C at 0.5 °C steps for 5 s. The relative quantification of mRNA expression was analyzed using the $2^{-\Delta\Delta Ct}$ method.

Table 1. The primer sequences used for PCR analysis.

Sequence ID	Name	Sequences
NM_144744.3	*Adiponectin*	Forward: TGGAATGACAGGAGCGGAAG Reverse: GCGAATGGGAACATTGGGGA
NM_001276707.1	*SREBP-1c*	Forward: ATCCTGGCCACAGTACCACT Reverse: GGAACGGTAGCGCTTCTCA
NM_017332.1	*FAS*	Forward: TCGACTTCAAAGGACCCAGC Reverse: ACTGCACAGAGGTGTTAGGC
NM_022193.1	*ACC*	Forward: GTACCGAAGTGGCATCCGTG Reverse: TCTCTTCCCGAAGGGCGAAT
NM_013134.2	*HMGCR*	Forward: CCTCCATTGAGATCCGGAGGA Reverse: ACAAAGAGGCCATGCATACGG
NM_001145366.1	*PPARγ*	Forward: TGGGGATGTCTCACAATGCC Reverse: AGACTCTGGGTTCAGCTGGT
NM_001287577.1	*C/EBPα*	Forward: AGGCCAAGAAGTCGGTGGATA Reverse: TCACTGGTCAACTCCAACACC
NM_001007144.1	*ADRP*	Forward: GGCAGGTGACATCTACTCGG Reverse: AAAGGGACCTACCAGCCAGT
NM_031144	*β-actin*	Forward: CACCCGCGAGTACAACCTTC Reverse: CCCATACCCACCATCACACC

4.8. Statistical Analysis

All data are expressed as the means ± standard error (SE) for each group, and the differences between the groups were compared with a two-way ANOVA test using SPSS for Windows, version

19.0 (SPSS Inc., Chicago, IL, USA). The significant differences among the means were determined using Student–Newman–Keuls multiple range tests, and $p < 0.05$ was considered statistically significant.

Author Contributions: H.P. and Z.S. conceived and designed the research study; C.F. and L.H. prepared the COSCs and raised the animals; C.F. and X.D. determined the related biomarkers, and performed the western blotting and PCR analysis; L.H. and Y.J. performed the animal experiments; H.P. and C.F. analyzed the data; J.G. supplied with the experimental platform; H.P. and C.F. wrote the manuscript. All authors read and approved the final manuscript.

Acknowledgments: This work was financially supported by the Industry University Research Collaborative Innovation Major Projects of Guangzhou Science Technology Innovation Commission, China (no. 201604020164); the Science and Technology Planning Project of Yunfu, Guangdong, China (no. 201702-9), and the National Science Foundation of China (no. 81173107).

Conflicts of Interest: The authors declare no conflict of interest.

References

1. Ye, Z.J.; Liu, G.H.; Guo, J.; Su, Z.Q. Hypothalamic endoplasmic reticulum stress as a key mediator of obesity-induced leptin resistance. *Obes. Rev.* **2018**, *19*, 770–785. [CrossRef] [PubMed]
2. Franks, P.W.; McCarthy, M.I. Exposing the exposures responsible for type 2 diabetes and obesity. *Science* **2016**, *354*, 69–73. [CrossRef] [PubMed]
3. Onakpoya, I.J.; Heneghan, C.J.; Aronson, J.K. Post-marketing withdrawal of anti-obesity medicinal products because of adverse drug reactions: A systematic review. *BMC Med.* **2016**, *14*, 191. [CrossRef] [PubMed]
4. Srivastava, G.; Apovian, C. Future pharmacotherapy for obesity: New anti-obesity drugs on the horizon. *Curr. Obes. Rep.* **2018**, *7*, 147–161. [CrossRef] [PubMed]
5. Gallwitz, B. Novel oral anti-obesity agents: New perspectives with lorcaserin? *Drugs* **2013**, *73*, 393–395. [CrossRef] [PubMed]
6. Zhang, H.L.; Zhong, X.B.; Tao, Y.; Wu, S.H.; Su, Z.Q. Effects of chitosan and water-soluble chitosan micro- and nanoparticles in obese rats fed a high-fat diet. *Int. J. Nanomed.* **2012**, *7*, 4069–4076. [CrossRef] [PubMed]
7. Tan, S.R.; Gao, B.; Tao, Y.; Guo, J.; Su, Z.Q. Antiobese effects of capsaicin-chitosan microsphere (CCMS) in obese rats induced by high fat diet. *J. Agric. Food Chem.* **2014**, *62*, 1866–1874. [CrossRef] [PubMed]
8. Zheng, J.; Yuan, X.; Cheng, G.; Jiao, S.; Feng, C.; Zhao, X.; Yin, H.; Du, Y.; Liu, H. Chitosan oligosaccharides improve the disturbance in glucose metabolism and reverse the dysbiosis of gut microbiota in diabetic mice. *Carbohydr. Polym.* **2018**, *190*, 77–86. [CrossRef] [PubMed]
9. Huang, L.L.; Chen, J.; Cao, P.Q.; Pan, H.T.; Ding, C.; Xiao, T.C.; Zhang, P.F.; Guo, J.; Su, Z.Q. Anti-obesity effect of glucosamine and chitosan oligosaccharide in high-fat diet-induced obese rats. *Mar. Drugs* **2015**, *13*, 2732–2756. [CrossRef] [PubMed]
10. Pan, H.T.; Yang, Q.Y.; Huang, G.D.; Ding, C.; Cao, P.Q.; Huang, L.L.; Xiao, T.C.; Guo, J.; Su, Z.Q. Hypolipidemic effects of chitosan and its derivatives in hyperlipidemic rats induced by a high-fat diet. *Food Nutr. Res.* **2016**, *60*, 31137. [CrossRef] [PubMed]
11. Yang, X.; Zhang, J.; Chen, L.; Wu, Q.; Yu, C. Chitosan oligosaccharides enhance lipid droplets via down-regulation of PCSK9 gene expression in HepG2 cells. *Exp. Cell Res.* **2018**, *366*, 152–160. [CrossRef] [PubMed]
12. Fernandes, J.C.; Sereno, J.; Garrido, P.; Parada, B.; Cunha, M.F.X.; Reis, F.; Pintado, M.E.; Santos-Silva, A. Inhibition of bladder tumor growth by chitooligosaccharides in an experimental carcinogenesis model. *Mar. Drugs* **2012**, *10*, 2661–2675. [CrossRef] [PubMed]
13. Muanprasat, C.; Chatsudthipong, V. Chitosan oligosaccharide: Biological activities and potential therapeutic applications. *Pharmacol. Therapeut.* **2017**, *170*, 80–97. [CrossRef] [PubMed]
14. Fu, C.H.; Jiang, Y.; Guo, J.; Su, Z.Q. Natural products with anti-obesity effects and different mechanisms of action. *J. Agric. Food Chem.* **2016**, *64*, 9571–9585. [CrossRef] [PubMed]
15. Fu, C.H.; Guo, J.; Su, Z.Q. The anti-obesity effect of chitosan oligosaccharide capsules in a high-fat diet-induced obese rat model. *Basic Clin. Pharmacol.* **2017**, *121*, 12.
16. Chiu, C.Y.; Feng, S.A.; Liu, S.H.; Chiang, M.T. Functional comparison for lipid metabolism and intestinal and fecal microflora enzyme activities between low molecular weight chitosan and chitosan oligosaccharide in high-fat-diet-fed rats. *Mar. Drugs* **2017**, *15*, 234. [CrossRef] [PubMed]

17. Ruud, J.; Bruning, J.C. METABOLISM Light on leptin link to lipolysis. *Nature* **2015**, *527*, 43–44. [CrossRef] [PubMed]

18. Schneeberger, M.; Dietrich, M.O.; Sebastian, D.; Imbernon, M.; Castano, C.; Garcia, A.; Esteban, Y.; Gonzalez-Franquesa, A.; Rodriguez, I.C.; Bortolozzi, A.; et al. Mitofusin 2 in POMC neurons connects ER stress with leptin resistance and energy imbalance. *Cell* **2013**, *155*, 172–187. [CrossRef] [PubMed]

19. Pan, H.T.; Guo, J.; Su, Z.Q. Advances in understanding the interrelations between leptin resistance and obesity. *Physiol. Behav.* **2014**, *130*, 157–169. [CrossRef] [PubMed]

20. Kwon, O.; Kim, K.W.; Kim, M.S. Leptin signalling pathways in hypothalamic neurons. *Cell. Mol. Life Sci.* **2016**, *73*, 1457–1477. [CrossRef] [PubMed]

21. Peelman, F.; Zabeau, L.; Moharana, K.; Savvides, S.N.; Tavernier, J. 20 YEARS OF LEPTIN Insights into signaling assemblies of the leptin receptor. *J. Endocrinol.* **2014**, *223*, T9–T23. [CrossRef] [PubMed]

22. Inoue, H.; Ogawa, W.; Ozaki, M.; Haga, S.; Matsumoto, M.; Furukawa, K.; Hashimoto, N.; Kido, Y.; Mori, T.; Sakaue, H.; et al. Role of STAT-3 in regulation of hepatic gluconeogenic genes and carbohydrate metabolism in vivo. *Nat. Med.* **2004**, *10*, 168–174. [CrossRef] [PubMed]

23. Shi, S.Y.; Martin, R.G.; Duncan, R.E.; Choi, D.; Lu, S.Y.; Schroer, S.A.; Cai, E.P.; Luk, C.T.; Hopperton, K.E.; Domenichiello, A.F.; et al. Hepatocyte-specific deletion of Janus Kinase 2 (JAK2) Protects against diet-induced steatohepatitis and glucose intolerance. *J. Biol. Chem.* **2012**, *287*, 10277–10288. [CrossRef] [PubMed]

24. Adolph, T.E.; Grander, C.; Grabherr, F.; Tilg, H. Adipokines and non-alcoholic fatty liver disease: Multiple interactions. *Int. J. Mol. Sci.* **2017**, *18*, 1649. [CrossRef] [PubMed]

25. Ghadge, A.A.; Khaire, A.A.; Kuvalekar, A.A. Adiponectin: A potential therapeutic target for metabolic syndrome. *Cytokine Growth Factor Rev.* **2018**, *39*, 151–158. [CrossRef] [PubMed]

26. Polyzos, S.A.; Mantzoros, C.S. Adiponectin as a target for the treatment of nonalcoholic steatohepatitis with thiazolidinediones: A systematic review. *Metabolism* **2016**, *65*, 1297–1306. [CrossRef] [PubMed]

27. Linden, A.G.; Li, S.L.; Choi, H.Y.; Fang, F.; Fukasawa, M.; Uyeda, K.; Hammer, R.E.; Horton, J.D.; Engelking, L.J.; Liang, G.S. Interplay between ChREBP and SREBP-1c coordinates postprandial glycolysis and lipogenesis in livers of mice. *J. Lipid Res.* **2018**, *59*, 475–487. [CrossRef] [PubMed]

28. Ferre, P.; Foufelle, F. Hepatic steatosis: A role for de novo lipogenesis and the transcription factor SREBP-1c. *Diabetes Obes. Metab.* **2010**, *12* (Suppl. 2), 83–92. [CrossRef] [PubMed]

29. Lai, Y.S.; Lee, W.C.; Lin, Y.E.; Ho, C.T.; Lu, K.H.; Lin, S.H.; Panyod, S.; Chu, Y.L.; Sheen, L.Y. Ginger essential oil ameliorates hepatic injury and lipid accumulation in high fat diet-induced nonalcoholic fatty liver disease. *J. Agric. Food Chem.* **2016**, *64*, 2062–2071. [CrossRef] [PubMed]

30. Wang, C.M.; Yuan, R.S.; Zhuang, W.Y.; Sun, J.H.; Wu, J.Y.; Li, H.; Chen, J.G. Schisandra polysaccharide inhibits hepatic lipid accumulation by downregulating expression of SREBPs in NAFLD mice. *Lipids Health Dis.* **2016**, *15*, 195. [CrossRef] [PubMed]

31. Chen, Q.; Wang, T.T.; Li, J.; Wang, S.J.; Qiu, F.; Yu, H.Y.; Zhang, Y.; Wang, T. Effects of natural products on fructose-induced nonalcoholic fatty liver disease (NAFLD). *Nutrients* **2017**, *9*, 96. [CrossRef] [PubMed]

32. Ren, R.D.; Gong, J.J.; Zhao, Y.Y.; Zhuang, X.Y.; Ye, Y.; Lin, W.T. Sulfated polysaccharides from Enteromorpha prolifera suppress SREBP-2 and HMG-CoA reductase expression and attenuate non-alcoholic fatty liver disease induced by a high-fat diet. *Food Funct.* **2017**, *8*, 1899–1904. [CrossRef] [PubMed]

33. Cipolletta, D.; Feuerer, M.; Li, A.; Kamei, N.; Lee, J.; Shoelson, S.E.; Benoist, C.; Mathis, D. PPAR-gamma is a major driver of the accumulation and phenotype of adipose tissue Treg cells. *Nature* **2012**, *486*, 549–553. [CrossRef] [PubMed]

34. Cui, J.X.; Chen, W.; Liu, J.; Xu, T.; Zeng, Y.Q. Study on quantitative expression of PPAR. and ADRP in muscle and its association with intramuscular fat deposition of pig. *Springerplus* **2016**, *5*, 1501. [CrossRef] [PubMed]

35. Imamura, M.; Inoguchi, T.; Ikuyama, S.; Taniguchi, S.; Kobayashi, K.; Nakashima, N.; Nawata, H. ADRP stimulates lipid accumulation and lipid droplet formation in murine fibroblasts. *Am. J. Physiol.-Endocrinol. Metab.* **2002**, *283*, E775–E783. [CrossRef] [PubMed]

36. Scheller, E.L.; Burr, A.A.; MacDougald, O.A.; Cawthorn, W.P. Inside out: Bone marrow adipose tissue as a source of circulating adiponectin. *Adipocyte* **2016**, *5*, 251–269. [CrossRef] [PubMed]

37. Polyzos, S.A.; Kountouras, J.; Mantzoros, C.S. A dipose tissue, obesity and non-alcoholic fatty liver disease. *Minerva Endocrinol.* **2017**, *42*, 92–108. [PubMed]

38. Cui, H.X.; Lopez, M.; Rahmouni, K. The cellular and molecular bases of leptin and ghrelin resistance in obesity. *Nat. Rev. Endocrinol.* **2017**, *13*, 338–351. [CrossRef] [PubMed]

39. Khandekar, M.J.; Cohen, P.; Spiegelman, B.M. Molecular mechanisms of cancer development in obesity. *Nat. Rev. Cancer* **2011**, *11*, 886–895. [CrossRef] [PubMed]
40. Ahima, R.S. Digging deeper into obesity. *J. Clin. Investig.* **2011**, *121*, 2076–2079. [CrossRef] [PubMed]
41. Kumar, S.G.; Rahman, M.A.; Lee, S.H.; Hwang, H.S.; Kim, H.A.; Yun, J.W. Plasma proteome analysis for anti-obesity and anti-diabetic potentials of chitosan oligosaccharides in ob/ob mice. *Proteomics* **2009**, *9*, 2149–2162. [CrossRef] [PubMed]
42. Lijnen, H.R. Murine models of obesity and hormonal therapy. *Thromb. Res.* **2011**, *127*, 17S–20S. [CrossRef]
43. Preston, S.H.; Mehta, N.K.; Stokes, A. Modeling obesity histories in cohort analyses of health and mortality. *Epidemiology* **2013**, *24*, 158–166. [CrossRef] [PubMed]
44. Byrne, C.D.; Perseghin, G. Non-alcoholic fatty liver disease: A risk factor for myocardial dysfunction? *J. Hepatol.* **2018**, *68*, 640–642. [CrossRef] [PubMed]
45. Hsu, C.C.; Ness, E.; Kowdley, K.V. Nutritional approaches to achieve weight loss in nonalcoholic fatty liver disease. *Adv. Nutr.* **2017**, *8*, 253–265. [CrossRef] [PubMed]
46. Rosen, E.D.; Spiegelman, B.M. PPAR gamma: A nuclear regulator of metabolism, differentiation, and cell growth. *J. Biol. Chem.* **2001**, *276*, 37731–37734. [CrossRef] [PubMed]
47. Lin, L.C.; Gao, A.C.; Lai, C.H.; Hsieh, J.T.; Lin, H. Induction of neuroendocrine differentiation in castration resistant prostate cancer cells by adipocyte differentiation-related protein (ADRP) delivered by exosomes. *Cancer Lett.* **2017**, *391*, 74–82. [CrossRef] [PubMed]
48. Zhao, Y.; Li, H.; Zhang, Y.Y.; Li, L.L.; Fang, R.P.; Li, Y.H.; Liu, Q.; Zhang, W.Y.; Qiu, L.Y.; Liu, F.B.; et al. Oncoprotein HBXIP modulates abnormal lipid metabolism and growth of breast cancer cells by activating the LXRs/SREBP-1c/FAS signaling cascade. *Cancer Res.* **2016**, *76*, 4696–4707. [CrossRef] [PubMed]
49. Huang, L. *Preparation of Chitosan Oligosaccharide Capsules, Chitosan Capsules and Assessment of Their Weight Control Function*; Guangdong Pharmaceutical University: Guangzhou, China, 2016.

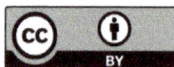

marine drugs

MDPI

Article

Anti-Obesity Effects of Collagen Peptide Derived from Skate (*Raja kenojei*) Skin Through Regulation of Lipid Metabolism

Minji Woo [1], Yeong Ok Song [1], Keon-Hee Kang [2] and Jeong Sook Noh [3,*]

[1]   Department of Food Science and Nutrition and Kimchi Research Institute, Pusan National University,
    Busan 46241, Korea; woo07140@pusan.ac.kr (M.W.); yosong@pusan.ac.kr (Y.O.S.)
[2]   Yeongsan Skate Co., Ltd., Busan 48520, Korea; skate1438@naver.com
[3]   Department of Food Science & Nutrition, Tongmyong University, Busan 48520, Korea
*   Correspondence: jsnoh2013@tu.ac.kr; Tel.: +82-51-629-1716

Received: 1 August 2018; Accepted: 28 August 2018; Published: 30 August 2018

Abstract: This study investigated the anti-obesity effects of collagen peptide derived from skate skin on lipid metabolism in high-fat diet (HFD)-fed mice. All C57BL6/J male mice were fed a HFD with 60% kcal fat except for mice in the normal group which were fed a chow diet. The collagen-fed groups received collagen peptide (1050 Da) orally (100, 200, or 300 mg/kg body weight per day) by gavage, whereas the normal and control groups were given water ($n = 9$ per group). The body weight gain and visceral adipose tissue weight were lower in the collagen-fed groups than in the control group ($p < 0.05$). Plasma and hepatic lipid levels were significantly reduced by downregulating the hepatic protein expression levels for fatty acid synthesis (sterol regulatory element binding protein-1 (SREBP-1), fatty acid synthase (FAS), and acetyl-CoA carboxylase (ACC)) and cholesterol synthesis (SREBP-2 and 3-hydroxy-3-methylglutaryl-CoA reductase (HMGCR)) and upregulating those for β-oxidation (peroxisome proliferator-activated receptor alpha (PPAR-α) and carnitine palmitoyltransferase 1 (CPT1)) and synthesis of bile acid (cytochrome P450 family 7 subfamily A member 1 (CYP7A1)) ($p < 0.05$). In the collagen-fed groups, the hepatic protein expression level of phosphorylated 5′ adenosine monophosphate-activated protein kinase (p-AMPK) and plasma adiponectin levels were higher, and the leptin level was lower ($p < 0.05$). Histological analysis revealed that collagen treatment suppressed hepatic lipid accumulation and reduced the lipid droplet size in the adipose tissue. These effects were increased in a dose-dependent manner. The findings indicated that skate collagen peptide has anti-obesity effects through suppression of fat accumulation and regulation of lipid metabolism.

Keywords: collagen peptide; skate skin; high fat diet; fatty acid metabolism; cholesterol metabolism

---

1. Introduction

Obesity is characterized by an abnormal accumulation of body fat that contributes to the etiologies of various metabolic disorders including dyslipidemia, hepatic steatosis, insulin resistance, and type 2 diabetes mellitus [1]. Obese individuals have high central adiposity due to the accumulation of visceral adipose tissue, which may be linked to a significantly increased risk of hepatic steatosis. The increased flux of non-esterified free fatty acid (NEFA) from the visceral fat to the liver is one of the suggested underlying mechanisms [2]. In addition, hyperlipidemia is induced by the dysregulation of hepatic lipid metabolism, which upregulates the synthesis of triglyceride (TG) and cholesterol and downregulates fatty acid oxidation [1]. These metabolic reactions could accelerate fat accumulation in the liver and exacerbate hepatic steatosis. Therefore, dietary approaches for attenuating hyperlipidemia, reducing free fatty acid levels, and inhibiting hepatic lipid synthesis and fat accumulation have attracted interest in obesity prevention or treatment.

Collagen, a fibrous protein composed of amino acid sequence glycine (Gly)-proline (Pro)-X and Gly-hydroxyproline (Hyp)-X, plays a vital role in the maintenance of the structure of various tissues and organs in the body [3]. Collagen has been widely used as a material in the food, cosmetic, and pharmaceutical industries due to its biological and functional properties [4]. Recently, marine collagen has been preferred over cattle or porcine collagen, because of bovine spongiform encephalopathy and transmissible spongiform encephalopathy, or religious reasons [5]. The skin, scale, cartilage and bone of marine fish are good sources of collagen [6]. These parts are by-products obtained during the processing of marine fish, which are considered as disposed waste [7]. Several studies have focused on the development of a technique to utilize marine collagen peptides to reduce pollution. Marine collagen has various beneficial properties such as antioxidative [8–10], anti-skin aging [11], antihypertensive [12,13], anti-ulcer [14], and bone integrity maintenance [15] effects. Especially as a biomaterial in tissue engineering, marine collagen has less cross-linking and higher solubility than bovine collagen, and exerts anti-ageing and anti-wrinkling effects [16].

To extract collagen peptides, several marine species have been used including red snapper [3], tuna [4], jelly fish [8], tilapia [10], salmon [17], cuttlefish [18], flatfish [19], pufferfish [20], bamboo shark [21], cod [22], carp [23], catfish [24], paper nautilus [25], marine sponges [26] and skate [27]. In particular, skate (*Raja kenojei*) is a popular food consumed in South Korea. As a result, large amounts of skate skin are disposed of as waste. Our recent study showed the lipid-lowering effect of skate skin-derived collagen peptide in genetic obese mice [28]. However, there is limited information on the effects of marine collagen in a diet-induced obese animal model. In this study, the anti-obesity effects of skate collagen peptide on improving lipid metabolism in high-fat diet (HFD)-induced obese mice were investigated. In addition, three different doses were used to examine the dose-dependent effects. Also, to elucidate the mechanism of its action with regard to synthesis and oxidation of fatty acid, adenosine monophosphate-activated protein kinase (AMPK) activation was investigated in the liver.

2. Results

2.1. Effect of Skate Collagen Peptide on Body Weight Gain and Changes in Adipose Tissue Weight and Size

As shown in Figure 1A, there were no significant differences in the initial body weight among the experimental groups. However, HFD intake for eight weeks significantly increased body weight ($p < 0.05$). As a result, the final body weight was the highest in the control group (CON, 36.6 ± 1.0 g) followed by the 100 mg/kg collagen-fed group (CL100, 34.2 ± 0.8 g), 200 mg/kg collagen-fed group (CL200, 33.6 ± 1.1 g), 300 mg/kg collagen-fed group (CL300, 33.3 ± 1.0 g), and normal group (NOR, 26.0 ± 0.4 g) ($p < 0.05$). Among HFD-fed mice groups, collagen intake did not affect the amount of daily food intake (Figure 1B). The increased liver weight following HFD intake was reduced by collagen treatment; however, the decrease was not significant (Figure 1C). Adipose tissue weights were higher in the HFD-fed groups (Figure 1D–F). The weights of liver, visceral and subcutaneous adipose tissue in the collagen-fed groups were significantly lower compared with that in the CON group ($p < 0.05$). However, the epididymis adipose tissue was not significantly different among the HFD-fed groups. Histological analysis of the adipose tissue revealed that HFD intake facilitated the differentiation and enlargement of adipocytes. The lipid droplet size was smaller in the collagen fed-groups than in the CON group.

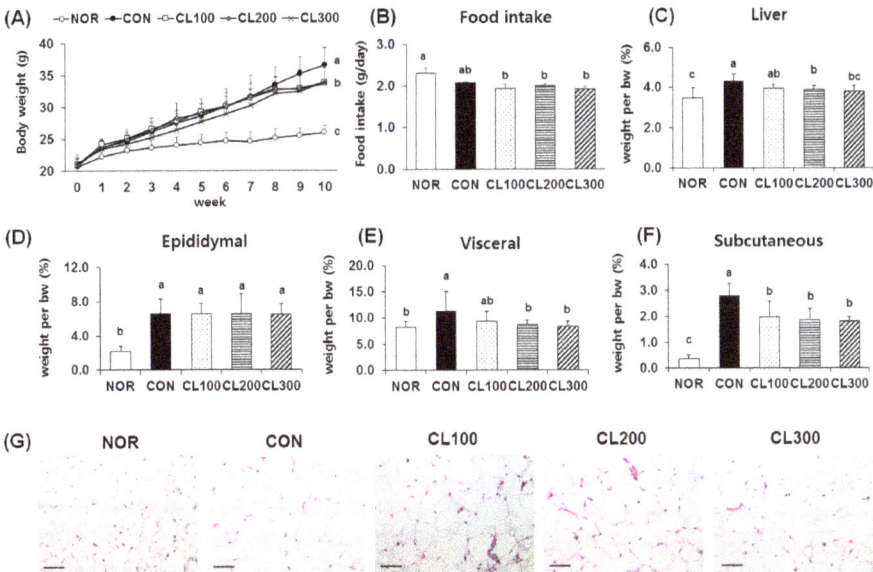

Figure 1. Effects of skate collagen peptide on body weight, food intake, and organ weight and histological analysis of adipose tissue in high-fat diet-fed C57BL6/J mice for eight weeks. Data are mean ± standard deviation (SD) (*n* = 9 per group). Normal (NOR) C57BL/6J mice fed a chow diet with water; control (CON) C57BL/6J mice fed a high fat diet (HFD) with water; collagen 100 (CL100), collagen 200 (CL200), and collagen 300 (CL300) C57BL/6J mice fed a HFD with oral administration of skate collagen peptide at a concentration of 100, 200, and 300 mg/kg body weight per day, respectively. [a–c] Different letters mean significant differences to one-way analysis of variance (ANOVA), followed by Duncan's multiple-range test at *p* < 0.05. (**A**) change in body weight (bw) for 10 week; (**B**) food intake; (**C**) liver weight per bw; (**D**) epididymal adipose tissue weight per bw; (**E**) visceral adipose tissue weight per bw; (**F**) subcutaneous adipose tissue weight per bw; (**G**) hematoxylin and eosin staining, magnification: 200×, bar: 50 μm.

2.2. Effect of Skate Collagen Peptide on Lipid Levels in the Plasma and Hepatic Tissue

Plasma lipid levels were higher in HFD-fed groups and were reduced by collagen intake (Figure 2A–E). Plasma TG (Figure 2A) and NEFA (Figure 2B) levels were significantly lower in the CL200 (30% and 30%, respectively) and CL300 (30% and 31%, respectively) groups compared with the levels in the CON group (*p* < 0.05). Plasma total cholesterol (TC) level was also lower; however, there was no significant difference in the HFD-fed groups (Figure 2C). Plasma low-density lipoprotein cholesterol (LDL-C) level was significantly lower in the CL200 and CL300 groups by 20% and 42%, respectively (Figure 2D, *p* < 0.05). In contrast, plasma high-density lipoprotein cholesterol (HDL-C) level was higher in the CL100, CL200, and CL300 groups by 245%, 276%, and 320%, respectively (Figure 2E, *p* < 0.05). Hepatic TG and TC levels were higher in the HFD-fed groups and were reduced by collagen intake (Figure 2F,G). In comparison with hepatic TG level in the CON group, the level was significantly lower in the CL200 and CL300 groups by 22% and 25%, respectively (Figure 2(F), *p* < 0.05). However, hepatic TC level was not significantly different between the CON and collagen-fed groups (Figure 2G). Histological analysis of the liver tissue revealed that lipid accumulation was increased by HFD intake and was suppressed by collagen intake. In particular, the degree of lipid accumulation in the CL200 and CL300 groups was similar to that in the NOR group. The histological results were in agreement with the changes in plasma and hepatic TG levels.

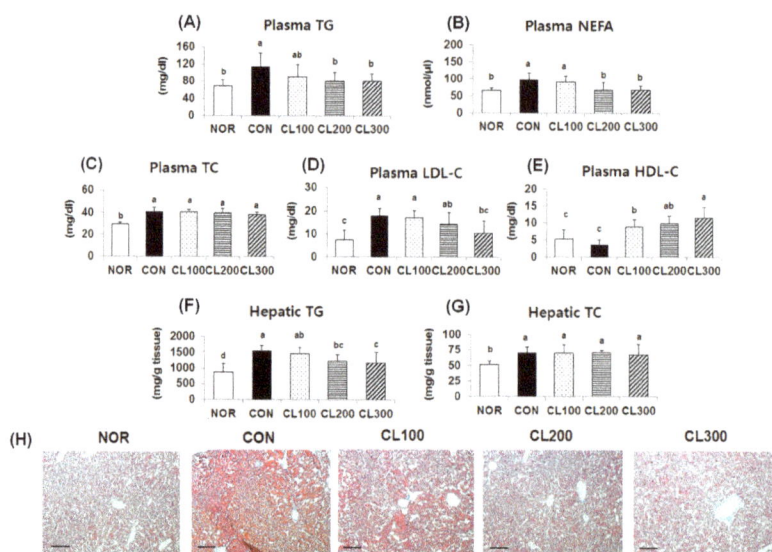

Figure 2. Effects of skate collagen peptide on plasma and hepatic lipid levels and histological analysis of liver tissue in high-fat diet-fed C57BL6/J mice for eight weeks. Data are mean ± SD (*n* = 9 per group). See the legend of Figure 1 for experimental groups in detail. [a–d] Different letters mean significant differences according to one-way ANOVA, followed by Duncan's multiple-range test at *p* < 0.05. (**A**) plasma TG (triacylglycerol); (**B**) plasma NEFA (non-esterified free fatty acid); (**C**) plasma TC (total cholesterol); (**D**) plasma LDL-C (low-density lipoprotein cholesterol); (**E**) plasma HDL-C (high-density lipoprotein cholesterol); (**F**) hepatic TG; (**G**) hepatic TC; (**H**) Oil red O staining, magnification: 100×, bar: 100 μm.

2.3. Effect of Skate Collagen Peptide on β-Oxidation in the Liver

The protein expression levels of peroxisome proliferator-activated receptor alpha (PPAR-α) and carnitine palmitoyltransferase 1 (CPT1) (proteins involved in β-oxidation) were significantly higher in the CL200 (159% and 163%, respectively) and CL300 (146% and 151%, respectively) groups compared with their expression levels in the CON group (*p* < 0.05) (Figure 3).

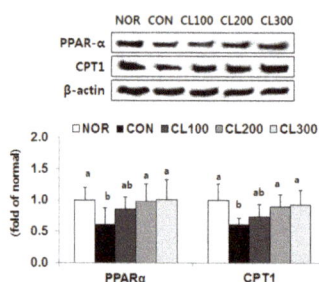

Figure 3. Effects of skate collagen peptide on hepatic protein expression for β-oxidation in high-fat diet-fed C57BL6/J mice for eight weeks. Data are mean ± SD (*n* = 9 per group). See the legend of Figure 1 for experimental groups in detail. [a,b] Different letters mean significant differences according to one-way ANOVA, followed by Duncan's multiple-range test at *p* < 0.05. PPARα, peroxisome proliferator-activated receptor alpha; CPT1, carnitine palmitoyltransferase 1.

2.4. Effect of Skate Collagen Peptide on Fatty Acid Synthesis in the Liver

The protein expression level of sterol regulatory element binding protein-1 (SREBP-1) (mature/precursor), a transcription factor for fatty acid synthesis, was significantly reduced in the CL100, CL200, and CL300 groups by 13%, 18%, and 18%, respectively, compared with its expression level in the CON group (Figure 4, $p < 0.05$). The protein expression level of fatty acid synthase (FAS) was significantly lower in the CL200 and CL300 groups by 28% and 29%, respectively ($p < 0.05$). In addition, the protein expression level of acetyl-CoA carboxylase (ACC) was significantly reduced in the CL300 group by 39% ($p < 0.05$).

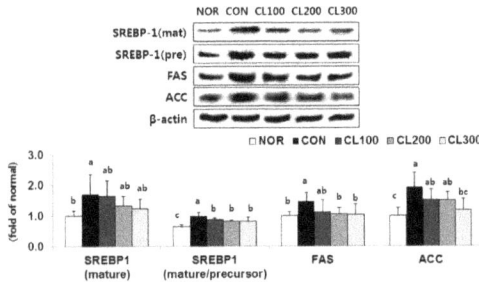

Figure 4. Effects of skate collagen peptide on hepatic protein expression for fatty acid synthesis in high-fat diet-fed C57BL6/J mice for eight weeks. Data are mean ± SD ($n = 9$ per group). See the legend of Figure 1 for experimental groups in detail. [a–c] Different letters mean significant differences according to one-way ANOVA, followed by Duncan's multiple-range test at $p < 0.05$. SREBP-1, sterol regulatory element binding protein-1; FAS, fatty acid synthase; ACC, acetyl-CoA carboxylase.

2.5. Effect of Skate Collagen Peptide on Cholesterol Metabolism in the Liver

The protein expression level of SREBP-2 (mature/precursor), a transcription factor for cholesterol synthesis, was significantly reduced in the CL200 and CL300 groups by 12% and 13%, respectively, compared with its expression level in the CON group (Figure 5, $p < 0.05$). The protein expression level of 3-hydroxy-3-methylglutaryl-CoA reductase (HMGCR) was significantly lower in the CL300 group by 32% ($p < 0.05$). On the other hand, the protein expression level of cytochrome P450 family 7 subfamily A member 1 (CYP7A1) was significantly reduced in the CL200 and CL300 groups by 161% and 176%, respectively ($p < 0.05$).

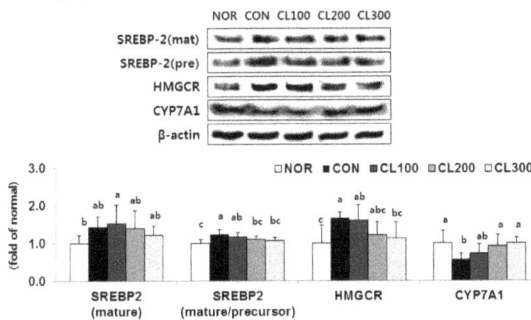

Figure 5. Effects of skate collagen peptide on hepatic protein expression for cholesterol synthesis and export in high-fat diet-fed C57BL6/J mice for eight weeks. Data are mean ± SD ($n = 9$ per group). See the legend of Figure 1 for experimental groups in detail. [a–c] Different letters mean significant differences according to one-way ANOVA, followed by Duncan's multiple-range test at $p < 0.05$. SREBP-2, sterol regulatory element binding protein-2; HMGCR, 3-hydroxy-3-methylglutaryl-CoA reductase; CYP7A1, cytochrome P450 family 7 subfamily A member 1.

2.6. Effect of Skate Collagen Peptide on AMPK in the Liver

In comparison with the protein expression level of phosphorylated 5′ adenosine monophosphate-activated protein kinase (p-AMPK) in the CON group, its expression level was significantly higher in the collagen-fed groups. In the CL300 group, it was significantly higher by 156% (Figure 6, $p < 0.05$).

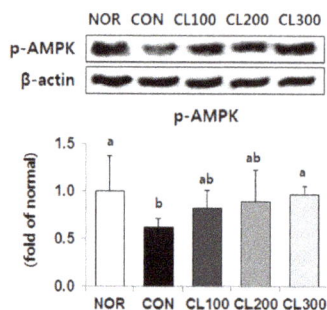

Figure 6. Effects of skate collagen peptide on hepatic protein expression of p-AMPK in high-fat diet-fed C57BL6/J mice for eight weeks. Data are mean ± SD ($n = 9$ per group). See the legend of Figure 1 for experimental groups in detail. [a,b] Different letters mean significant differences according to one-way ANOVA, followed by Duncan's multiple-range test at $p < 0.05$. p-AMPK, phosphorylated 5′ adenosine monophosphate-activated protein kinase.

2.7. Effect of Skate Collagen Peptide on Adiponectin and Leptin Levels

Collagen intake reduced leptin levels and increased adiponectin levels in the collagen-fed groups compared with the levels in the CON group (Table 1). The adiponectin level in the CL100, CL200, and CL300 groups was higher by 110%, 123%, and 131%, respectively ($p < 0.05$). In contrast, the leptin level in the CL300 group was significantly reduced by 23% ($p < 0.05$).

Table 1. Changes in leptin and adiponectin levels of high-fat diet-fed C57BL6/J mice for eight weeks.

Group [(1)]	Leptin	Adiponectin
NOR	54.6 ± 5.0 [c]	198.6 ± 14.1 [d]
CON	122.6 ± 34.9 [a]	214.4 ± 46.3 [c,d]
CL100	98.0 ± 24.6 [a,b]	236.3 ± 21.5 [b,c]
CL200	97.0 ± 22.9 [a,b]	263.8 ± 35.3 [a,b]
CL300	94.0 ± 15.2 [b]	281.1 ± 17.9 [a]

Data are mean ± SD ($n = 9$ per group). [(1)] See the legend of Figure 1 for experimental groups in detail. [a–d] Different letters mean significant differences according to one-way ANOVA, followed by Duncan's multiple-range test at $p < 0.05$.

3. Discussion

Owing to overnutrition and lifestyle changes, the prevalence of obesity has greatly increased worldwide. Researches have attempted to identify food materials or agents that can ameliorate obesity. A HFD-induced obese animal is pathophysiologically similar to an obese person [29]. As a result of the high caloric density, the consumption of a HFD causes obesity by increasing lipid levels and the adipocyte number and size [30]. Marine-derived nutrients and bioactive components have excellent potential as functional food ingredients due to their beneficial health effects [31]. Marine collagen peptides rich in glycine, glutamic acid, proline, and hydroxyproline are produced by the enzymatic hydrolysis of collagen. Among several amino acids in collagen peptides, the lipid-lowering effect of glycine has been reported [32,33]. In this study, the anti-obesity effects of collagen peptide derived from skate skin were evaluated and were found to be mediated through the regulation of hepatic lipid metabolism-related transcription factors and enzymes.

In an obese state, hyperlipidemia is closely associated with fat accumulation in major organs such as the liver and adipose tissue. In the present study, the HFD-fed groups had higher plasma TG, NFFA, and LDL-C levels and lower plasma HDL-C levels; these effects were reversed following collagen peptide administration. However, a change in TC level was not observed. The decrease in the lipid levels of collagen-fed groups might be attributed to the reduction in body weight gain and visceral and subcutaneous adipose tissue weights. Additionally, the collagen-fed groups had a lower level of hepatic TG, which was consistent with liver histological results. The TG-lowering effect of collagen suppressed adipose tissue differentiation, as demonstrated by the histological analysis of the adipose tissue. In comparison with CON mice, collagen-fed mice had smaller adipocytes. Our results were consistent with those of a previous study, in which the concentration of TG, TC, and LDL-C in HFD-fed rats was reduced by supplementation with marine collagen peptides [34]. Similarly, the intake of collagen derived from salmon [35], flathead mullet [36], and skate [28] could decrease plasma lipid levels in animals. Lipid-lowering effects were also observed in a human study showing that marine collagen peptides reduced the level of TG, free fatty acid, TC, and LDL-C, and increased that of HDL-C [37]. The intake of gelatin, a mixture of water-soluble protein derived from collagen, was reported to markedly reduce serum TG and TC levels in mice [38]. These effects might be associated with the properties of amino acid-rich collagen. A previous study found a negative correlation between plasma TG and the levels of hydroxyproline, glycine, and proline in collagen [35]. In particular, glycine intake was reported to decrease plasma free fatty acid and adipose cell size in sucrose-fed rats [32]. These results suggest that collagen peptides rich in glycine may exert hypolipidemic effects in the plasma and liver.

Abnormal fat accumulation is caused by an imbalance between lipid synthesis (lipogenesis) and breakdown (lipolysis or β-oxidation). Lipogenesis is transcriptionally regulated by SREBP-1, which controls the lipogenic enzymes FAS and ACC [39]. On one hand, PPAR-α is a transcription factor that facilitates fatty acid oxidation by upregulating target genes such as CPT1 [40]. In the current study, the hepatic protein expression levels of SREBP-1, ACC, and FAS (involved in fatty acid synthesis) in the collagen-fed groups were suppressed compared with those in the CON group. On the other hand, β-oxidation was enhanced in the collagen-fed groups by upregulating the PPAR-α and CPT1 levels. These results were consistent with those of a previous study showing that the intake of collagen peptide decreased fatty acid synthesis and increased β-oxidation in the liver of *db/db* mice [28]. Similarly, tuna-derived peptide was found to decrease the expression levels of SREBP-1, FAS, and ACC in differentiated 3T3-L1 adipocytes [41]. It is possible that glycine-rich collagen has a regulatory effect on some factors related to storage and energy burning, such as PPAR-α, -γ, -δ, and uncoupling protein type 2 [33]. Our results suggested that supplementation with skate collagen peptide effectively attenuated hepatic fat accumulation by improving fatty acid metabolism through the inhibition of fatty acid synthesis and facilitation of β-oxidation in the liver of HFD-fed mice.

AMPK has emerged as a regulator of energy balance that affects whole-body fuel utilization. AMPK can induce fatty acid oxidation and inhibit the synthesis of hepatic fatty acid, cholesterol and adipocyte differentiation [42]. A previous study showed that AMPK activation could ameliorate lipogenesis in the liver of mice by suppressing SREBP-1 and -2, inhibiting their target enzyme expression [43]. In contrast, the inhibition of AMPK could increase the accumulation of hepatocellular lipids in hepatocytes [44]. Moreover, AMPK is involved in the regulation of adipokines such as adiponectin and leptin, which can stimulate the phosphorylation of AMPK [45]. In obesity-induced animals, decreased adiponectin levels and increased leptin levels in the plasma have been observed [46]. However, after weight reduction, these effects were reversed with the augmentation of AMPK activation. AMPK is an important metabolic regulator; thus, it is recognized as a key target for obesity prevention. In the present study, the intake of collagen peptide increased the hepatic protein expression of p-AMPK. Furthermore, adiponectin and leptin levels were increased and decreased, respectively, in the plasma. In a previous study, the serum adiponectin level of patients with type 2 diabetes was increased following treatment with marine collagen peptides for three months compared with that of healthy control patients [37]. Furthermore, glycine treatment was reported to decrease leptin and increase adiponectin in 3T3-L1 adipocytes [33,47]. Therefore, AMPK activation and adipokine regulation by skate collagen peptide might reduce lipid accumulation through the inhibition of lipid synthesis and activation of energy production in the liver.

The reduction in plasma lipid level following the intake of fish collagen peptides is closely associated with the amino acids in the peptides. According to a previous study, the peptides in protein hydrolysates have different biological effects and physicochemical properties depending on the molecular weight or structure of the amino acids [35]. The structure and molecular weight of collagen peptides vary according to the type, source, and preparation method of the collagen [35]. The production of low molecular weight fragments is easier using collagen from marine sources than from land vertebrates [48]. Nevertheless, further research is required to study the health benefits of marine collagens with different molecular weights obtained via ultrafiltration. In conclusion, our findings revealed that the intake of collagen peptide of skate skin might exert anti-obesity activities through reduction of body weight gain and visceral adipose tissue, and improve the dyslipidemia via regulation of hepatic lipid metabolism and activation of AMPK, as well as its targeted adiponectin.

4. Materials and Methods

4.1. Animals and Diets

Male C57BL6/J mice (5 weeks old) were purchased from Orient, Inc. (Seongnam, Korea). The mice were raised under controlled temperature (23 $\pm$ 1 °C) and humidity (50 $\pm$ 5%) conditions with a 12 h light-dark cycle. After a 1 week acclimation period, the mice were divided into five groups (n = 9 per group) based on body weight as follows; (1) normal group (NOR), given AIN-76A chow diet and water as vehicle by gavage; (2) control group (CON), given HFD and water as vehicle by gavage; (3) CL100, given HFD and 100 mg/kg body weight (bw)/day of skate collagen peptide by gavage; (4) CL200, given HFD and 200 mg/kg bw/day of skate collagen peptide by gavage; CL300, given HFD and 300 mg/kg bw/day of skate collagen peptide by gavage. The dosage given to the mice was converted from a human equivalent dosage: assuming the human equivalent dose for 1.0 g/60 kg/day $\times$ 12.3 = 0.2 g/kg/day. A conversion coefficient of 2.3 was used to account for differences between mice and humans [49]. To examine the dose-dependent effects, three different doses were determined for oral administration based on a previous study [30]. HFD with 60% kcal fat was provided from Central Lab Animal Inc. (Seoul, Korea) which has been commonly used for the development of obesity in experimental rodent models [50]. Skate collagen peptide was dissolved in water and orally administered to mice. The collagen peptide was obtained from Yeongsan Skate Co., Ltd. (Jeollanam-do, Korea) with an average molecular weight of 1050 Da. The amino acid composition of the collagen sample used in this study was as follows: glycine 22.09%, glutamate 10.78%, proline 9.02%, alanine 7.66%, arginine 7.84%, aspartate 7.11%, hydroxyproline 6.85%, serine 5.71%, lysine 3.49%, leucine 3.67%, threonine 3.42%, valine 3.34%, isoleucine 2.45%, phenylalanine 2.23%, methionine 2.15%, histidine 1.38%, and others 0.81%. The mice had free access to the diet and water. The dietary intake was checked daily and body weight was measured every week. After 8 weeks, all mice were fasted for 12 h and sacrificed after CO_2 anesthetization. Blood was obtained using heparin tubes from the heart and the organs were collected after perfusion with ice-cold phosphate-buffered saline (PBS, 10 mM, pH 7.2). Epididymis adipose tissue was derived from the fat attached to the two testicles of the mice. Visceral adipose tissue was excised from the perirenal fat depot. Subcutaneous adipose tissue was collected from the fat located beneath the skin of the legs. The organs were stored at -80 °C until use. The study was approved by the Pusan National University Institutional Animal Care and Use Committee (Approval number: PNU-2016-1640).

4.2. Plasma Lipid, Aminotransferase, and Adipokines Levels

The levels of plasma TG, TC, and HDL-C were measured using commercially available kits (AM157S-K, AM202-K, and AM203-K; Asan Pharmaceutical Co., Seoul, Korea). NEFA was determined using commercial kits (ab65341; Abcam Inc., Cambridge, MA, USA). Plasma LDL-C level was calculated using a previously reported method [51] In addition, commercial kits were used to evaluate adipokines such as leptin (#ADI-900-019A; Enzo Life Sciences AG, Lausen, Switzerland) and adiponectin (LF-EK0239; AbFrontier, Seoul, Korea).

4.3. Hepatic Lipid Concentration

The hepatic lipids of the liver homogenate were extracted according to a modified method [52]. In brief, liver tissue was homogenized in PBS and extracted using chloroform and methanol (2:1, v/v). The extracts were vortexed for 2 h, filtered, and dried. Hepatic TG and TC levels were measured with the same commercial kit used for measuring plasma lipid levels.

4.4. Western Blot Analysis

Quantitation of protein was carried out by Western blot assay as previously described [53]. In brief, protein was separated by sodium dodecylsulfate polyacrylamide gel and transferred to a nitrocellulose membrane (Amersham Biosciences, Uppsla, Sweden). The targeted protein band was detected using CAS-400 (Core Bio, Seoul, Korea). The calculation was performed using ImageJ software (National Institutes of Health, Bethesda, MD, USA). Protein expression was normalized to that of β-actin. The primary antibodies used in this study were β-actin (ab8227) and FAS (ab22759), which were purchased from Abcam Inc. (Cambridge, UK). Phospho-AMPKα (p-AMPK, #2535) was obtained from Cell Signaling Technology (Beverly, MA, USA). SREBP-1 (sc-8984), ACC (sc-26817), PPAR-α (sc-9000), CPT1 (sc-139482), SREBP-2 (sc-5603), HMGCR (sc-33827), and CYP7A1 (sc-25536) were purchased from Santa Cruz Biotechnology (Santa Cruz, CA, USA). The secondary horseradish peroxidase-conjugated antibodies (from Abcam Inc.) were donkey anti-rabbit IgG H&L (ab6802), rabbit anti-goat IgG H&L (ab6741), and rabbit anti-mouse IgG H&L (ab6728).

4.5. Histological Analysis

The liver and adipose tissue were fixed in 4% formalin for preparation of frozen and paraffin blocks, respectively. Sections of the frozen-blocked liver tissues were cut at a thickness of 3 μm using a microtome (CM1510S-3; Leica, Wetzlar, Germany) and stained with Oil Red O. Sections of the paraffin-blocked adipose tissue were cut using a microtome at a thickness of 3 μm (Microm HM 325; Thermo Fisher Scientific, Waltham, MA, USA) and stained with hematoxylin and eosin. The slides were examined under an optical microscope (Nikon ECLIPSE Ti; Nikon Corp., Tokyo, Japan).

4.6. Statistical Analysis

Data are presented as the mean ± SD. Statistical analysis was performed using SPSS version 23 (SPSS Inc., Chicago, IL, USA). The significance of differences were determined by one-way analysis of variance (ANOVA) followed by Duncan's multiple-range test. Differences with $p < 0.05$ were considered significant.

Author Contributions: J.S.N., Y.O.S., and K.-H.K. conceived and designed the research; M.W. and J.S.N. performed the experiments, analyzed the data, and wrote the paper; Y.O.S. and K.-H.K. provided materials and analysis tools.

Funding: This research received no external funding.

Acknowledgments: This work was supported by the Technological Innovation R&D Program (S2409860) funded by the Small and Medium Business Administration (SMBA, Korea) and supported by the Basic Science Research Program through the National Research Foundation of Korea (NRF) funded by the Ministry of Education (NRF-2017R1D1A3B03034845).

Conflicts of Interest: The authors declare no conflict of interest.

References

1. Savage, D.B.; Petersen, K.F.; Shulman, G.I. Disordered lipid metabolism and the pathogenesis of insulin resistance. *Physiol. Rev.* **2007**, *87*, 507–520. [CrossRef] [PubMed]
2. Viljanen, A.P.; Iozzo, P.; Borra, R.; Kankaanpää, M.; Karmi, A.; Lautamäki, R.; Järvisalo, M.; Parkkola, R.; Ronnemaa, T.; Guiducci, L. Effect of weight loss on liver free fatty acid uptake and hepatic insulin resistance. *J. Clin. Endocrinol. Metab.* **2009**, *94*, 50–55. [CrossRef] [PubMed]
3. Jongjareonrak, A.; Benjakul, S.; Visessanguan, W.; Nagai, T.; Tanaka, M. Isolation and characterisation of acid and pepsin-solubilised collagens from the skin of brownstripe red snapper (*Lutjanus vitta*). *Food Chem.* **2005**, *93*, 475–484. [CrossRef]
4. Han, S.-H.; Uzawa, Y.; Moriyama, T.; Kawamura, Y. Effect of collagen and collagen peptides from bluefin tuna abdominal skin on cancer cells. *Health* **2011**, *3*, 129–134. [CrossRef]
5. Gómez-Guillén, M.C.; Giménez, B.; López-Caballero, M.E.; Montero, M.P. Functional and bioactive properties of collagen and gelatin from alternative sources: A review. *Food Hydrocoll.* **2011**, *25*, 1813–1827. [CrossRef]
6. Ri, S.X.; Hideyuki, K.; Koretaro, T. Characterization of molecular species of collagen in scallop mantle. *Food Chem.* **2007**, *102*, 1187–1191.
7. Park, S.-H.; Lee, J.-K.; Jeon, J.-K.; Byun, H.-G. Characterization of a collagenase-1 inhibitory peptide purified from skate dipturus chilensis skin. *Korean J. Fish. Aquat. Sci.* **2011**, *44*, 456–463. [CrossRef]
8. Zhuang, Y.; Sun, L.; Zhao, X.; Wang, J.; Hou, H.; Li, B. Antioxidant and melanogenesis-inhibitory activities of collagen peptide from jellyfish (*Rhopilema esculentum*). *J. Sci. Food Agric.* **2009**, *89*, 1722–1727. [CrossRef]
9. Mendis, E.; Rajapakse, N.; Kim, S.-K. Antioxidant properties of a radical-scavenging peptide purified from enzymatically prepared fish skin gelatin hydrolysate. *J. Agric. Food Chem.* **2005**, *53*, 581–587. [CrossRef] [PubMed]
10. Lai, C.; Wu, P.; Wu, C.; Shiau, C. Studies on antioxidative activities of hydrolysates from fish scales collagen of tilapia. *J. Taiwan Fish. Res* **2008**, *15*, 99–108.
11. Tanaka, M.; Koyama, Y.-I.; Nomura, Y. Effects of collagen peptide ingestion on UV-B-induced skin damage. *Biosci. Biotechnol. Biochem.* **2009**, *73*, 930–932. [CrossRef] [PubMed]
12. Fahmi, A.; Morimura, S.; Guo, H.-C.; Shigematsu, T.; Kida, K.; Uemura, Y. Production of angiotensin I converting enzyme inhibitory peptides from sea bream scales. *Process Biochem.* **2004**, *39*, 1195–1200. [CrossRef]
13. Zhang, F.; Wang, Z.; Xu, S. Macroporous resin purification of grass carp fish (*Ctenopharyngodon idella*) scale peptides with in vitro angiotensin-I converting enzyme (ACE) inhibitory ability. *Food Chem.* **2009**, *117*, 387–392. [CrossRef]
14. Zolotarev, Y.A.; Badmaeva, K.; Bakaeva, Z.; Samonina, G.; Kopylova, G.; Dadayan, A.; Zverkov, Y.B.; Garanin, S.; Vaskovsky, B.; Ashmarin, I. Short peptide fragments with antiulcer activity from a collagen hydrolysate. *Russ. J. Bioorg. Chem.* **2006**, *32*, 174–178. [CrossRef]
15. Bello, A.E.; Oesser, S. Collagen hydrolysate for the treatment of osteoarthritis and other joint disorders: A review of the literature. *Curr. Med. Res. Opin.* **2006**, *22*, 2221–2232. [CrossRef] [PubMed]
16. Berillis, P. Marine collagen: Extraction and applications. In *Research Trends in Biochemistry, Molecular Biology and Microbiology*; Madhukar, S., Ed.; SM Group: Dover, DE, USA, 2015; pp. 1–13.
17. Liang, J.; Pei, X.-R.; Wang, N.; Zhang, Z.-F.; Wang, J.-B.; Li, Y. Marine collagen peptides prepared from chum salmon (*Oncorhynchus keta*) skin extend the life span and inhibit spontaneous tumor incidence in sprague-dawley rats. *J. Med. Food* **2010**, *13*, 757–770. [CrossRef] [PubMed]
18. Nagai, T.; Yamashita, E.; Taniguchi, K.; Kanamori, N.; Suzuki, N. Isolation and characterisation of collagen from the outer skin waste material of cuttlefish (*Sepia lycidas*). *Food Chem.* **2001**, *72*, 425–429. [CrossRef]
19. Heu, M.S.; Lee, J.H.; Kim, H.J.; Jee, S.J.; Lee, J.S.; Jeon, Y.-J.; Shahidi, F.; Kim, J.-S. Characterization of acid-and pepsin-soluble collagens from flatfish skin. *Food Sci. Biotechnol.* **2010**, *19*, 27–33. [CrossRef]
20. Nagai, T.; Araki, Y.; Suzuki, N. Collagen of the skin of ocellate puffer fish (*Takifugu rubripes*). *Food Chem.* **2002**, *78*, 173–177. [CrossRef]
21. Kittiphattanabawon, P.; Benjakul, S.; Visessanguan, W.; Kishimura, H.; Shahidi, F. Isolation and characterisation of collagen from the skin of brownbanded bamboo shark (*Chiloscyllium punctatum*). *Food Chem.* **2010**, *119*, 1519–1526. [CrossRef]

22. Sadowska, M.; Kołodziejska, I.; Niecikowska, C. Isolation of collagen from the skins of Baltic cod (*Gadus morhua*). *Food Chem.* **2003**, *81*, 257–262. [CrossRef]

23. Duan, R.; Zhang, J.; Du, X.; Yao, X.; Konno, K. Properties of collagen from skin, scale and bone of carp (*Cyprinus carpio*). *Food Chem.* **2009**, *112*, 702–706. [CrossRef]

24. Singh, P.; Benjakul, S.; Maqsood, S.; Kishimura, H. Isolation and characterisation of collagen extracted from the skin of striped catfish (*Pangasianodon hypophthalmus*). *Food Chem.* **2011**, *124*, 97–105. [CrossRef]

25. Nagai, T.; Suzuki, N. Preparation and partial characterization of collagen from paper nautilus (*Argonauta argo*, Linnaeus) outer skin. *Food Chem.* **2002**, *76*, 149–153. [CrossRef]

26. Tziveleka, L.A.; Ioannou, E.; Tsiourvas, D.; Berillis, P.; Foufa, E.; Roussis, V. Collagen from the marine sponges *Axinella cannabina* and *Suberites carnosus*: Isolation and morphological, biochemical, and biophysical characterization. *Mar. Drugs* **2017**, *15*, 152. [CrossRef] [PubMed]

27. Baek, J.M.; Kang, K.H.; Kim, S.H.; Noh, J.S.; Jeong, K.S. Development of high functional collagen peptide materials using skate skins. *J. Environ. Sci. Int.* **2016**, *25*, 579–588. [CrossRef]

28. Lee, H.J.; Woo, M.; Song, Y.O.; Noh, J.S. Inhibitory effect of skate skin collagen on hepatic lipid accumulation through regulation of lipid metabolism. *J. Korean Soc. Food Sci. Nutr.* **2018**, *47*, 235–242. [CrossRef]

29. Kim, J.H.; Kim, O.-K.; Yoon, H.-G.; Park, J.; You, Y.; Kim, K.; Lee, Y.-H.; Choi, K.-C.; Lee, J.; Jun, W. Anti-obesity effect of extract from fermented *Curcuma longa* L. through regulation of adipogenesis and lipolysis pathway in high-fat diet-induced obese rats. *Food Nutr. Res.* **2016**, *60*, 30428. [CrossRef] [PubMed]

30. Bray, G.A.; Popkin, B.M. Dietary fat intake does affect obesity! *Am. J. Clin. Nutr.* **1998**, *68*, 1157–1173. [CrossRef] [PubMed]

31. Lordan, S.; Ross, R.P.; Stanton, C. Marine bioactives as functional food ingredients: Potential to reduce the incidence of chronic diseases. *Mar. Drugs* **2011**, *9*, 1056–1100. [CrossRef] [PubMed]

32. Hafidi, M.E.; Pérez, I.; Zamora, J.; Soto, V.; Carvajal-Sandoval, G.; Banos, G. Glycine intake decreases plasma free fatty acids, adipose cell size, and blood pressure in sucrose-fed rats. *Am. J. Physiol. Regul. Integr. Comp. Physiol.* **2004**, *287*, R1387–R1393. [CrossRef] [PubMed]

33. Almanza-Perez, J.; Alarcon-Aguilar, F.; Blancas-Flores, G.; Campos-Sepulveda, A.; Roman-Ramos, R.; Garcia-Macedo, R.; Cruz, M. Glycine regulates inflammatory markers modifying the energetic balance through PPAR and UCP-2. *Biomed. Pharmacother.* **2010**, *64*, 534–540. [CrossRef] [PubMed]

34. Wang, J.; Xie, Y.; Pei, X.; Yang, R.; Zhang, Z.; Li, Y. The lipid-lowering and antioxidative effects of marine collagen peptides. *Chin. J. Prev. Med.* **2008**, *42*, 226–230.

35. Saito, M.; Kiyose, C.; Higuchi, T.; Uchida, N.; Suzuki, H. Effect of collagen hydrolysates from salmon and trout skins on the lipid profile in rats. *J. Agric. Food Chem.* **2009**, *57*, 10477–10482. [CrossRef] [PubMed]

36. Kim, H.S.; Seong, J.H.; Lee, Y.G.; Xie, C.L.; Choi, W.S.; Kim, S.H.; Yoon, H.D. Effect of low-molecular-weight collagen peptide extract isolated from scales of the flathead mullet (*Mugil cephalus*) on lipid metabolism in hyperlipidemic rats. *Korean J. Food Preserv.* **2009**, *16*, 938–945.

37. Zhu, C.-F.; Li, G.-Z.; Peng, H.-B.; Zhang, F.; Chen, Y.; Li, Y. Treatment with marine collagen peptides modulates glucose and lipid metabolism in Chinese patients with type 2 diabetes mellitus. *Appl. Physiol. Nutr. Metab.* **2010**, *35*, 797–804. [CrossRef] [PubMed]

38. Oliveira, D.R.; Portugal, L.R.; Cara, D.C.; Vieira, E.C.; Alvarez-Leite, J.I. Gelatin intake increases the atheroma formation in apoE knock out mice. *Atherosclerosis* **2001**, *154*, 71–77. [CrossRef]

39. Strable, M.S.; Ntambi, J.M. Genetic control of de novo lipogenesis: Role in diet-induced obesity. *Crit. Rev. Biochem. Mol. Biol.* **2010**, *45*, 199–214. [CrossRef] [PubMed]

40. Reddy, J.K.; Hashimoto, T. Peroxisomal β-oxidation and peroxisome proliferator–activated receptor α: An adaptive metabolic system. *Annu. Rev. Nutr.* **2001**, *21*, 193–230. [CrossRef] [PubMed]

41. Kim, Y.M.; Kim, I.H.; Choi, J.W.; Lee, M.K.; Nam, T.J. The anti-obesity effects of a tuna peptide on 3T3-L1 adipocytes are mediated by the inhibition of the expression of lipogenic and adipogenic genes and by the activation of the Wnt/β-catenin signaling pathway. *Int. J. Mol. Med.* **2015**, *36*, 327–334. [CrossRef] [PubMed]

42. Lage, R.; Diéguez, C.; Vidal-Puig, A.; López, M. AMPK: A metabolic gauge regulating whole-body energy homeostasis. *Trends Mol. Med.* **2008**, *14*, 539–549. [CrossRef] [PubMed]

43. Li, Y.; Xu, S.; Mihaylova, M.M.; Zheng, B.; Hou, X.; Jiang, B.; Park, O.; Luo, Z.; Lefai, E.; Shyy, J.Y.-J. AMPK phosphorylates and inhibits SREBP activity to attenuate hepatic steatosis and atherosclerosis in diet-induced insulin-resistant mice. *Cell Metab.* **2011**, *13*, 376–388. [CrossRef] [PubMed]

44. Zang, M.; Xu, S.; Maitland-Toolan, K.A.; Zuccollo, A.; Hou, X.; Jiang, B.; Wierzbicki, M.; Verbeuren, T.J.; Cohen, R.A. Polyphenols stimulate AMP-activated protein kinase, lower lipids, and inhibit accelerated atherosclerosis in diabetic LDL receptor–deficient mice. *Diabetes* **2006**, *55*, 2180–2191. [CrossRef] [PubMed]

45. Da Costa Guerra, J.F.; Maciel, P.S.; de Abreu, I.C.M.E.; Pereira, R.R.; Silva, M.; de Morais Cardoso, L.; Pinheiro-Sant'Ana, H.M.; de Lima, W.G.; Silva, M.E.; Pedrosa, M.L. Dietary açai attenuates hepatic steatosis via adiponectin-mediated effects on lipid metabolism in high-fat diet mice. *J. Funct. Foods* **2015**, *14*, 192–202. [CrossRef]

46. Park, K.-G.; Park, K.S.; Kim, M.-J.; Kim, H.-S.; Suh, Y.-S.; Ahn, J.D.; Park, K.-K.; Chang, Y.-C.; Lee, I.-K. Relationship between serum adiponectin and leptin concentrations and body fat distribution. *Diabetes Res. Clin. Pract.* **2004**, *63*, 135–142. [CrossRef] [PubMed]

47. Garcia-Macedo, R.; Sanchez-Muñoz, F.; Almanza-Perez, J.C.; Duran-Reyes, G.; Alarcon-Aguilar, F.; Cruz, M. Glycine increases mRNA adiponectin and diminishes pro-inflammatory adipokines expression in 3T3-L1 cells. *Eur. J. Pharmacol.* **2008**, *587*, 317–321. [CrossRef] [PubMed]

48. Nomura, Y.; Sakai, H.; Ishii, Y.; Shirai, K. Preparation and some properties of type I collagen from fish scales. *Biosci. Biotechnol. Biochem.* **1996**, *60*, 2092–2094. [CrossRef] [PubMed]

49. USFDA. Guidance for industry. In *Estimating the Maximum Safe Starting Dose in Adult Healthy Volunteer*; US Food and Drug Administration: Rockville, MD, USA, 2005.

50. Hariri, N.; Thibault, L. High-fat diet-induced obesity in animal models. *Nutr. Res. Rev.* **2010**, *23*, 270–299. [CrossRef] [PubMed]

51. Friedewald, W.T.; Levy, R.I.; Fredrickson, D.S. Estimation of the concentration of low-density lipoprotein cholesterol in plasma, without use of the preparative ultracentrifuge. *Clin. Chem.* **1972**, *18*, 499–502. [PubMed]

52. Folch, J.; Lees, M.; Sloane-Stanley, G. A simple method for the isolation and purification of total lipids from animal tissues. *J. Biol. Chem.* **1957**, *226*, 497–509. [PubMed]

53. Jung, K.; Hong, S.H.; Kim, M.; Han, J.-S.; Jang, M.-S.; Song, Y.O. Antiatherogenic effects of Korean cabbage kimchi with added short arm octopus. *Food Sci. Biotechnol.* **2015**, *24*, 249–255. [CrossRef]

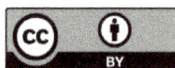

marine drugs

MDPI

Article

Chitosan Oligosaccharides Improve Glucolipid Metabolism Disorder in Liver by Suppression of Obesity-Related Inflammation and Restoration of Peroxisome Proliferator-Activated Receptor Gamma (PPARγ)

Yibo Bai [1,2], Junping Zheng [2,3], Xubing Yuan [2], Siming Jiao [2], Cui Feng [2], Yuguang Du [2,*], Hongtao Liu [2,3,*] and Lanyan Zheng [1,*]

1   Department of Pathogen Biology, College of Basic Medical Sciences, China Medical University, No. 77 Puhe Road, Shenyang North New Area, Shenyang 110122, China; YiboBaicmu@163.com
2   State Key Laboratory of Biochemical Engineering and Key Laboratory of Biopharmaceutical Production & Formulation Engineering, PLA, Institute of Process Engineering, Chinese Academy of Sciences, Beijing 100190, China; junpingzheng2013@163.com (J.Z.); xbyuan@ipe.ac.cn (X.Y.); smjiao@ipe.ac.cn (S.J.); cfeng@ipe.ac.cn (C.F.)
3   Zhengzhou Institute of Emerging Industrial Technology, Zhengzhou 450000, China
*   Correspondence: ygdu@ipe.ac.cn (Y.D.); liuhongtao@ipe.ac.cn (H.L.); lyzheng@cmu.edu.cn (L.Z.)

Received: 10 October 2018; Accepted: 16 November 2018; Published: 19 November 2018

Abstract: Chitosan oligosaccharides (COS) display various biological activities. In this study, we aimed to explore the preventive effects of COS on glucolipid metabolism disorder using palmitic acid (PA)-induced HepG2 cells and high-fat diet (HFD)-fed C57BL/6J mice as experimental models in vitro and in vivo, respectively. The results showed that COS pretreatment for 12 h significantly ameliorated lipid accumulation in HepG2 cells exposed to PA for 24 h, accompanied by a reversing of the upregulated mRNA expression of proinflammatory cytokines (IL-6, MCP-1, TNF-α) and glucolipid metabolism-related regulators (SCD-1, ACC1, PCK1-α). In addition, COS treatment alleviated glucolipid metabolism disorder in mice fed with HFD for five months, including reduction in body weight and fasting glucose, restoration of intraperitoneal glucose tolerance, and suppression of overexpression of proinflammatory cytokines and glucolipid metabolism-related regulators. Furthermore, our study found that COS pretreatment significantly reversed the downregulation of PPARγ at transcriptional and translational levels in both PA-induced HepG2 cells and liver tissues of HFD-fed mice. In summary, the study suggests that COS can improve glucolipid metabolism disorder by suppressing inflammation and upregulating PPARγ expression. This indicates a novel application of COS in preventing and treating glucolipid metabolism-related diseases.

Keywords: chitosan oligosaccharide; glucolipid metabolism disorder; high-fat diet; inflammation; peroxisome proliferator-activated receptor gamma

---

1. Introduction

Data shows that over 30% of adults and 16.9% of children in the US are obese or overweight, and the figures are 14.3% and 12.8% in China, respectively [1,2]. Obesity is usually accompanied by numerous complications, such as metabolic syndrome, nonalcoholic fatty liver diseases (NAFLDs), cardiocerebrovascular diseases, and cancers [3]. At present, lifestyle intervention, drug treatment, and surgical operation are the main therapies used for obesity, but the safety and effectiveness of these methods are unsatisfactory [4,5]. Thus, an efficient preventive strategy is necessary to improve glucolipid metabolism disorder without being confined to search for effective treatments.

Chitosan oligosaccharides (COS) are a kind of multifunctional oligosaccharides. COS are produced from chitosan, a polysaccharide constituent of crustaceans such as shrimps, crabs, lobsters, and prawns, by enzymatic degradation or acidic hydrolysis [6]. COS are known to display various bioactivities, such as anti-inflammation, anticancer, and antioxidation [7–9]. In addition, studies have shown that both chitosan and COS could improve overweight and dyslipidemia in rats [10–12]. Regretfully, the preventive effect of COS on metabolism disorder and the underlying molecular mechanism have failed to be fully elucidated. Recently, chitosan was reported to decrease the number of *Firmicutes* and *Lactobacillus* spp. in the caecum and colon but increase the population of *Bifidobacteria* in caecum of pigs [13], indicating that chitosan might be a kind of prebiotics. Unlike chitosan, COS are totally deacetylated polymers of *N*-acetylglucosamine, which have shorter chain length and lower molecular weights [6]. Compared to chitosan, COS have been shown to have higher solubility, lower viscosity, and higher absorption rate in both in vitro and in vivo transport experiments [14]. Based on the above, COS should be easily transported across the gastrointestinal tract and absorbed into the blood flow, where they display biologic effects on metabolic diseases.

So far, several functional polysaccharides have been proven to reverse glucose and lipid metabolism disorders by upregulating the activity of nuclear receptor peroxisome proliferator-activated receptor gamma (PPARγ) [15–17]. PPARγ is an important member of the nuclear receptor super family of transcription factors, standing at the crossroads of controlling metabolic disorders, including obesity, insulin resistance, and cardiovascular diseases [18]. PPARγ was first found to be responsible for adipocyte differentiation [19]. In recent years, it has been reported that PPARγ can improve lipid metabolism and insulin sensitivity through regulation of inflammatory mediators and plentiful enzymes involved in lipid synthesis, uptake, and release [20,21]. Studies have also shown that activation of PPARγ alleviates liver injury and liver fibrosis [22,23]. PPARγ was also found to prevent the progression of hepatic steatosis in mouse models [24,25]. Therefore, PPARγ has been regarded as a drug target against metabolic diseases [18,26].

The purpose of this study was to determine whether COS administrated in advance could alleviate obesity-associated liver lipid metabolic disorder, both in vitro and in vivo, and if so, to determine the mechanism involved. Because of the critical role of PPARγ in the regulation of lipid metabolism, we specifically examined the effect of COS on PPARγ in palmitic acid (PA)-induced HepG2 cells and high-fat diet (HFD)-induced mice.

2. Result

2.1. Effect of COS and PA Treatment on HepG2 Cells Viability

We first evaluated the effect of COS and PA on HepG2 cells viability by the 3-(4,5-dimethylthiazol-2-yl)-2,5-diphenyltetrazolium bromide (MTT) assay. As shown in Figure 1A, PA at 100 µM had no effect on HepG2 cells viability after treatment for 24 h, while higher concentrations of PA (200,400 µM) resulted in significant decrease in the viability of HepG2 cells ($p < 0.01$, vs. the control group). On the other hand, the incubation of COS (100 µg/mL) for 12 h or pretreatment with 25, 50, and 100 µg/mL COS for 12 h and then exposure to 100 µM of PA for 24 h both caused no toxicity to HepG2 cells (Figure 1B). Therefore, 100 µM of PA and 25–100 µg/mL of COS were chosen for further experiments.

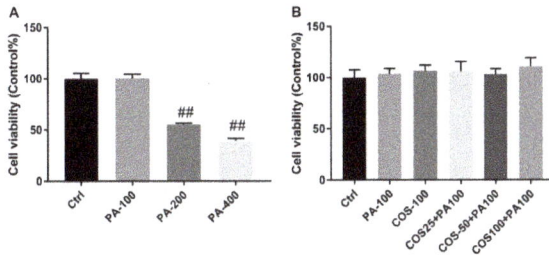

Figure 1. Effect of palmitic acid (PA) and chitosan oligosaccharides (COS) on viability of HepG2 cells. (**A**) HepG2 cells were treated with PA (100–400 μM) for 24 h. (**B**) HepG2 cells were treated with COS (100 μg/mL) for 12 h or pretreated with COS (25–100 μg/mL) for 12 h and then exposed to PA (100 μM) for 24 h. After that, the cell viability was determined by MTT assay. The data presented are averages and standard deviations of three independent experiments, quintuplicate in each experiment. ## $p < 0.01$, compared to the control group.

2.2. COS Ameliorated PA-Induced Lipid Accumulation in HepG2 Cells

To investigate whether COS could alleviate PA-induced lipid accumulation, HepG2 cells were pretreated with COS (25–100 μg/mL) for 12 h and then exposed to PA (100 μM) for 24 h. The results by oil red O staining showed that PA induced a considerable lipid accumulation in HepG2 cells, which was suppressed by COS pretreatment in a concentration-dependent manner (Figure 2).

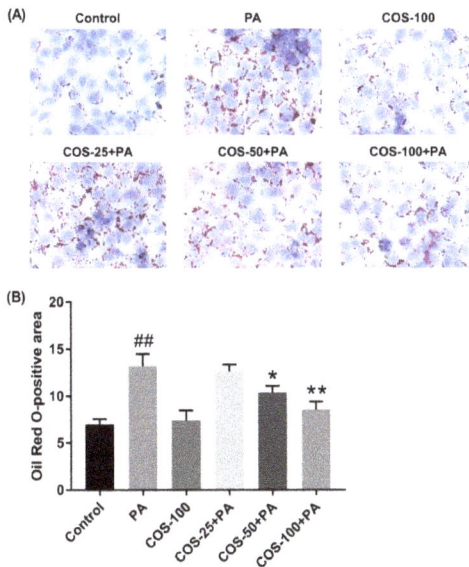

Figure 2. Effects of COS on PA-induced lipid deposition in HepG2 cells. (**A**) Cells were pretreated with COS (25–100 μg/mL) for 12 h and then exposed to PA (100 μM) for 24 h. Finally, cells were stained with oil red O, and the visualized red oil droplets were observed using a Leica light microscope. The photographs are representative of three independent experiments with similar results, triplicate in each experiment. (**B**) Quantitative data for the percentage of lipid droplets in HepG2 cells (oil red O-positive areas) shown as a histogram. The data presented are averages and standard deviations of three independent experiments. ## $p < 0.01$, compared to the control group; * $p < 0.05$ or ** $p < 0.01$ compared to the PA group.

2.3. COS Reversed the upregulation of Proinflammatory Cytokines and Glucolipid Metabolism-Related Regulators at mRNA Level in PA-Induced HepG2 Cells

Considering that obesity is associated with low-grade chronic inflammation [3], we next detected the transcriptional levels of inflammatory cytokines in HepG2 cells with PA or PA plus COS treatment by RT-PCR.

As shown in Figure 3A–C, PA (100 µM) treatment for 24 h obviously activated the mRNA expression of IL-6, MCP-1, and TNF-α ($p < 0.01$, vs. the control group) in HepG2 cells. In contrast, the PA-induced inflammation was remarkably suppressed by COS (100 µg/mL) pretreatment for 12 h ($p < 0.01$, vs. the PA group).

On the other hand, PA treatment (100 µM) for 24 h significantly increased the mRNA levels of fatty acid synthesis-related regulators (stearoyl-CoA desaturase, SCD-1, and acetyl-CoA carboxylase, ACC1) and glucogenesis-associated regulator PCK1-α ($p < 0.01$, vs. the control group) in HepG2 cells, which were evidently inhibited by COS (100 µg/mL) pretreatment for 12 h (Figure 3D–F).

When these factors in PA plus COS treatment group were compared with the control group, no significant differences were observed (Figure 3A–D) except for the ACC-1 (Figure 3E) and PCK1-α (Figure 3F). To exclude unexpected accidents, we repeated these experiments more than three times independently and got consistent results. A review of the literature shows that analogous results were generated by other groups [12,27]. For example, in one study, COS treatment initiated less expression of proinflammatory cytokines in LPS-treated endothelial cells compared to the control group [27]. Another study found COS stimulated stronger leptin signaling transduction in obese rats [12]. Unfortunately, there is no plausible explanation about the mechanism involved thus far. Although this matter is out of the scope of this study, it deserves further investigation in the future.

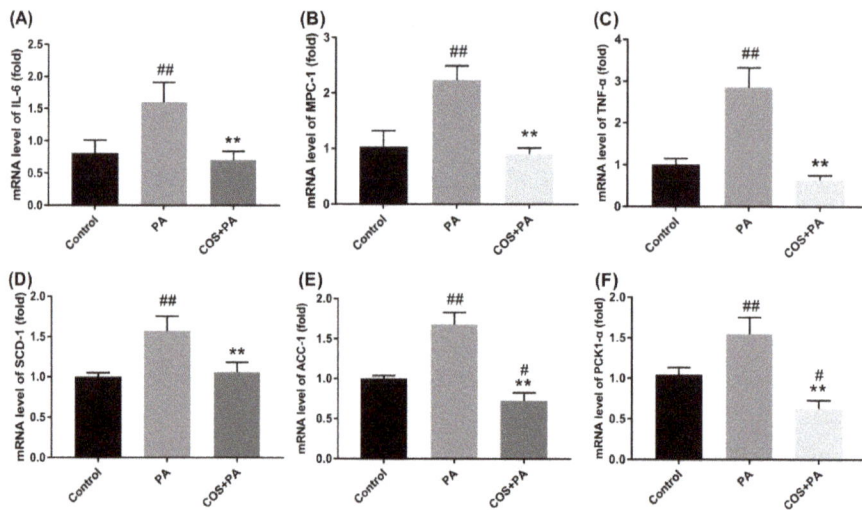

Figure 3. Effects of COS on PA-induced proinflammatory cytokines and fatty acid metabolism-related regulators in HepG2 cells. Cells were pretreated with COS (100 µg/mL) for 12 h and then exposed to PA (100 µM) for 24 h. After that, the mRNA levels of (**A**) IL-6, (**B**) MCP-1, (**C**) TNF-α, (**D**) SCD-1, (**E**) ACC-1, and (**F**) PKC1-α were determined by RT-PCR. The data presented are averages and standard deviations of three independent experiments with similar results, triplicate in each experiment. # $p < 0.05$ or ## $p < 0.01$, compared to the control group; ** $p < 0.01$ compared to the PA group.

2.4. COS Reversed the downregulation of PPARγ at Both mRNA and Protein Levels in PA-Induced HepG2 Cells

To explore the potential molecular mechanism by which COS prevent PA-induced inflammation and glucolipid metabolism disorder, we measured the expression changes of PPARγ in PA-induced HepG2 cells, which plays a key role in the regulation of lipid metabolism. The results in Figure 4 shows that PA (100 μM) exposure for 24 h led to a distinct reduction in PPARγ at both mRNA and protein levels in HepG2 cells ($p < 0.05$ or 0.01, vs. the control group). However, after COS pretreatment (100 μg/mL) for 12 h, the decreased expressions of PPARγ were statistically reversed in PA-induced HepG2 cells.

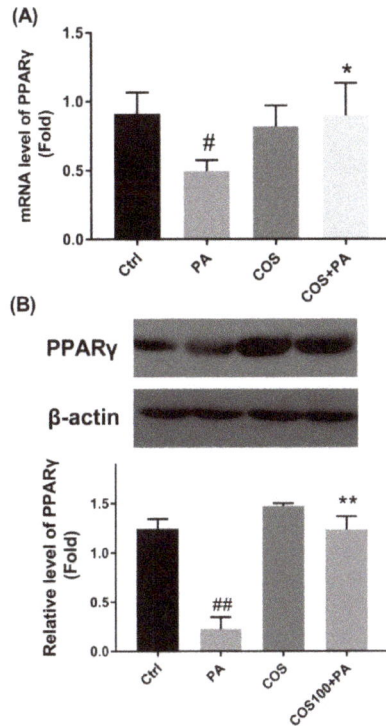

Figure 4. Effects of COS on PA-induced downregulation of PPARγ in HepG2 cells. Cells were pretreated with COS (100 μg/mL) for 12 h and then exposed to PA (100 μM) for 24 h. (**A**) The mRNA level of PPARγ as determined by RT-PCR. (**B**) The protein level of PPARγ as measured by western blot (WB) analysis. The data presented are representative images of three independent experiments with similar results. Data are represented as the mean ± SD ($n = 3$). # $p < 0.05$ or ## $p < 0.01$, compared to the control group; * $p < 0.05$ or ** $p < 0.01$ compared to the PA group.

2.5. COS Alleviated Glucose Intolerance in HFD-Fed Mice

To study the effects of COS on glucolipid metabolism disorder in vivo, C57BL/6J mice were fed with control diet (CD), HFD, CD plus COS (1 mg/mL in drinking water), or HFD plus COS for five months. The results showed that COS significantly lowered HFD-induced increase in body weight ($p < 0.05$, vs. the HFD group) (Figure 5A) and fasting glucose level ($p < 0.01$, vs. the HFD group) (Figure 5B). In addition, intraperitoneal glucose tolerance test (IGTT) suggested that the mice in HFD group displayed poorer behavior in terms of glucose tolerance compared to the CD group, while COS treatment remarkably alleviated glucose intolerance in HFD-fed mice (Figure 5C).

Furthermore, the area under curve (AUC) of glucose in the IGTT was found to be much higher in the HFD group than the control group ($p < 0.01$), while COS treatment obviously reduced the AUC in HFD-fed mice, which was almost comparable to the CD group (Figure 5D).

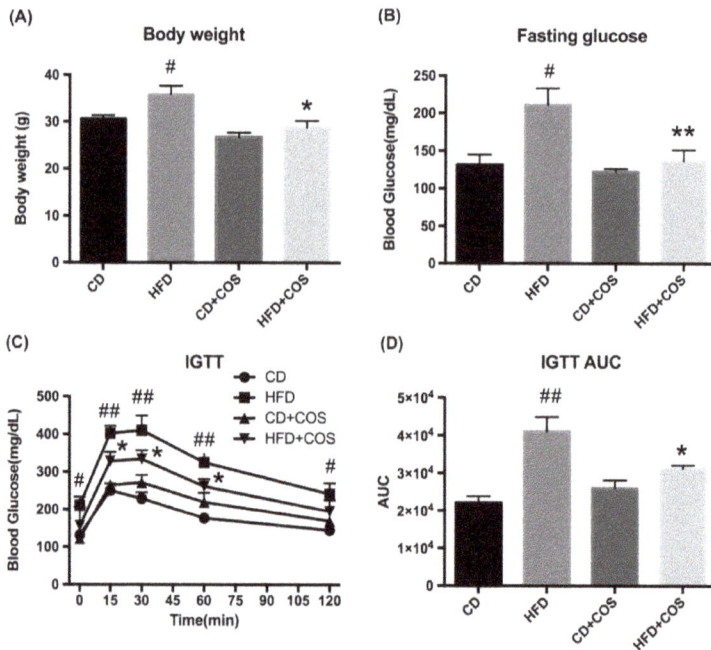

Figure 5. Effects of COS on body weight, fasting glucose, intraperitoneal glucose tolerance test (IGTT), and area under curve (AUC) of IGTT in HFD-fed mice. C57BL/6J mice were fed with control diet (CD), high-fat diet (HFD), CD plus COS (1 mg/mL in drinking water), or HFD plus COS for five months. After the treatment, the (**A**) body weight and (**B**) fasting glucose were monitored. (**C**) The IGTT was also measured, and (**D**) the AUC of IGTT was calculated. Data are represented as the mean ± SD ($n = 5$). # $p < 0.05$ or ## $p < 0.01$, compared to the CD group; * $p < 0.05$ or ** $p < 0.01$ compared to the HFD group.

2.6. COS Treatment Ameliorated Glucolipid Metabolism Disorder in HFD-Fed Mice

To explore the effect of COS on hepatic steatosis, the lipid accumulation in all groups was measured using oil red O staining. As indicated in Figure 6A, a mass of lipid droplets were observed after staining in the hepatocytes of liver tissues of HFD-fed mice, and the lipid accumulation was hampered in HFD-fed mice with COS treatment.

Next, the effect of COS on inflammatory responses in HFD-fed mice was assessed. As shown in Figure 6B, HFD feeding caused significant increase in mRNA expression of three proinflammatory cytokines (IL-6, MCP-1, and TNF-α) in liver tissues ($p < 0.05$ or 0.01, vs. the CD group), which was reversed by COS treatment ($p < 0.05$ or 0.01, vs. the HFD group). Likewise, COS treatment led to evident transcriptional inhibition of glucolipid metabolism-related regulators (SCD-1, ACC1, and PCK1-α) in liver tissues of HFD-fed mice ($p < 0.01$) (Figure 6C).

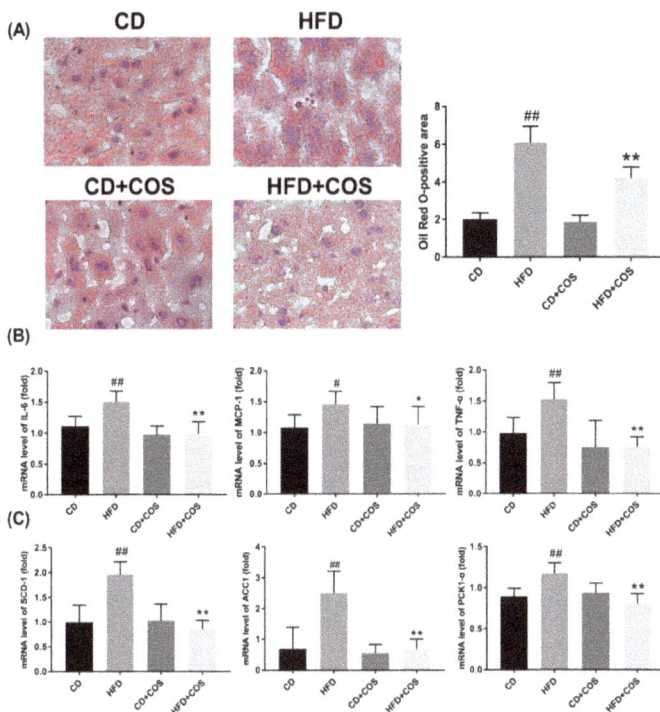

Figure 6. Improvement in lipid metabolism disorder by COS in HFD-fed mice. C57BL/6J mice were fed with CD, HFD, CD plus COS (1 mg/mL in drinking water), or HFD plus COS for five months. After the treatment, all mice were sacrificed and the liver tissues were collected. Next, the lipid deposits in hepatocytes were observed by oil red O staining (**A**). Quantitative data for the percentage of oil deposits in the liver (oil red O-positive areas) as calculated by Image j. (**B**) The mRNA levels of proinflammatory cytokines (IL-6, MCP-1, TNF-α) and (**C**) fatty acid metabolism-related regulators (SCD-1, ACC-1, PKC1-α) in liver as determined by RT-PCR. Data are represented as the mean ± SD ($n = 5$). # $p < 0.05$ or ## $p < 0.01$, compared to the CD group; * $p < 0.05$ or ** $p < 0.01$ compared to the HFD group.

Finally, to further confirm the role of PPARγ in COS-mediated improvement of glucolipid metabolism disorder in HFD-fed mice, we measured the variation of PPARγ in liver tissues of all experimental groups. As shown in Figure 7, both the transcription and the translation of PPARγ were significantly downregulated in liver tissues of HFD-fed mice compared to the CD group ($p < 0.01$). However, COS treatment obviously reversed the reduction of PPARγ expression (Figure 7).

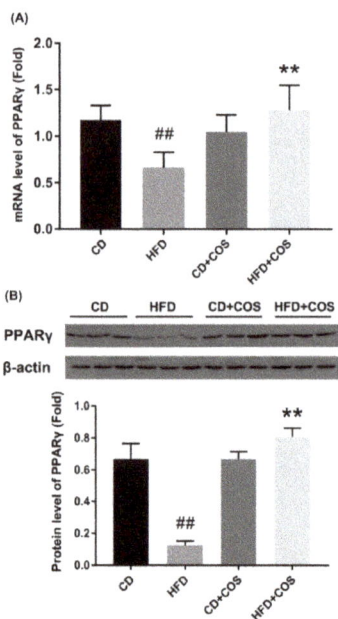

Figure 7. Reversal of downregulated PPARγ by COS in liver tissues of HFD-fed mice. C57BL/6J mice were fed with CD, HFD, CD plus COS (1 mg/mL in drinking water), or HFD plus COS for five months. After the treatment, all mice were sacrificed and the liver tissues were collected. The expressions of PPARγ (**A**) at transcriptional level as determined by RT-PCR, and (**B**) at translational level as determined by WB analysis. Data are represented as the mean ± SD (*n* = 5). ## *p* < 0.01, compared to the CD group; ** *p* < 0.01 compared to the HFD group.

3. Discussion

Obesity associated with NAFLD, diabetes, and cancer has become a major global health challenge [3]. Currently, the main therapies against obesity include lifestyle intervention, drug treatment, and surgical operation [4,5]. However, the efficacy and safety of these methods are of concern. Thus, it is urgently necessary to identify alternative therapeutic methods to curb the increasing incidence of obesity. Recently, a series of polysaccharides or oligosaccharides as prebiotics were found to alleviate glucolipid metabolism disorders, and good results were obtained [13,28,29]. Among them, COS were reported to display excellent antioxidative and anti-inflammatory effects [7,30]. Additionally, COS were shown to have antiobese effect in HFD-feed rats [10–12]. However, the preventive effect of COS on metabolism disorder and the molecular mechanism remain obscure. As COS can be easily absorbed into the blood flow [14], we speculated that COS might directly initiate the regulatory effect on glucolipid metabolism. In this study, we found that COS improved HFD-induced glucose intolerance and dyslipidemia by restoring the downregulated PPARγ in PA-induced HepG2 cells or HFD-fed mice.

In this study, we used PA-induced HepG2 cells as in vitro model to investigate the preventive function of COS on lipid stress. Besides the biosynthetic capacity of plasma proteins and inflammatory mediators, HepG2 cells can express most of the cellular surface receptors of normal hepatocytes and are more stable than the latter in vitro [31]. Therefore, HepG2 cells are usually chosen to study liver-related metabolism diseases instead of primary hepatocytes. In addition, as the most abundant nonesterified fatty acids in plasma, PA is the most widely used inducer in the investigation of lipid metabolism [32]. In line with the published results [32,33], our studies showed that PA not only led to lipid droplet deposition and activation of the inflammatory response, but it also dramatically affected the expression of glucolipid metabolism-related regulators in HepG2 cells.

Liver plays an important role in lipid metabolism by which excessive dietary lipids are stored in hepatocytes [34]. This further impairs the metabolism of glucose and fatty acids, even leading to the occurrence of insulin resistance. In the present study, both HepG2 cells exposed to PA and mice chronically subjected to HFD exhibited evident lipid droplet accumulation, suggesting the formation of dyslipidemia (Figures 2 and 6). On the contrary, the imbalance of lipid metabolism in both HepG2 cells and liver tissues of HFD-fed mice was reversed by COS treatment (Figures 2 and 6). In particular, COS displayed significantly inhibitory effect on glucose intolerance in mice with HFD feeding (Figure 5C,D). These results are parallel to our previous study in which chitin oligosaccharides, the acetylated form of COS, was proven to ameliorate HFD-induced dyslipidemia in mice [35]. Based on the above, it is suggested that COS could attenuate the metabolism syndrome associated with obesity.

Glucolipid metabolism disorder related to systemically upregulated chronic inflammatory responses and obesity is also characterized by increasing systemic inflammation and insulin resistance [36]. Thus, attempts have been made to repress metabolic diseases through the blockade of inflammatory responses. It has been reported that PA overload activates inflammatory signaling to produce cytokines, such as IL-6, MCP-1, and TNF-α [37,38]. Our results showed that COS significantly downregulated the overexpression of IL-6, MCP-1, and TNF-α in PA-induced HepG2 cells as well as in liver tissues of HFD-fed mice at the mRNA level (Figure 3A–C and Figure 6B). Considering that the increased influx of hepatic free fatty acids impairs insulin signaling, stimulates hepatic gluconeogenesis, and activates the de novo lipogenesis [39], we next investigated whether COS treatment could affect the expression of glucolipid metabolism-related regulators, i.e., PCK1-α, SCD-1, and ACC-1. PCK1-α is one of the key gluconeogenic enzymes, while SCD-1 is a microsomal enzyme required for the synthesis of oleate and palmitoleate, and ACC-1 is a major enzyme in de novo fatty acid biosynthetic pathway [40–42]. Our results indicated that overexpression of the three regulators was drastically inhibited by COS treatment at the mRNA level both in vitro and in vivo (Figure 3D–F and Figure 6C), indicating the suppressive effect of COS on gluconeogenesis and free fatty acid synthesis in hepatocytes and liver tissues with overflowing fatty acids. Based on the above, we propose that COS improve glucolipid disorder in obesity mice, perhaps by suppressing inflammation.

PPARγ is an important transcription factor responsible for lipid metabolism and inflammatory responses [18], which has been proven to regulate the expression of various metabolic enzymes involved in lipid synthesis and fatty acid β-oxidation [20]. A previous study demonstrated that hepatic PPARγ mRNA and protein expression level decreased in NAFLD rats compared to the controls [43]. In livers of diabetic nephropathy rat and db/db mice, the protein level of PPARγ was shown to decrease, and restoring PPARγ gene expression to baseline could improve metabolic disorders [15,44]. Therefore, a balanced level of PPARγ in liver tissues may be important for homeostasis. In addition, PPARγ activation has been reported to inhibit the expression of inflammatory mediators by blocking the NF-κB [45–47]. Here, we explored whether PPARγ was critical to COS-mediated improvement of glucolipid metabolic disorder. Our study showed that PA induced a significant decrease in the expression of PPARγ at both mRNA and protein levels in HepG2 cells, which was almost totally reversed by COS treatment (Figure 4). Similar results were identified in the liver tissues of HFD-fed mice (Figure 7). These results are in line with findings from other groups, which demonstrated that some polysaccharides or their derivatives prevented the occurrence of metabolic diseases by upregulating the expression of PPARγ [15–17]. From the above, we speculate that PPARγ may be a potential molecular target, with COS initiating the protective effect on glucolipid metabolism disorder. In conclusion, we proved that COS displayed strong improvement on glucolipid metabolism disorder in PA-induced HepG2 cells as well as liver tissues of HFD-fed mice. This molecular mechanism might be associated with the reversal effect of COS on reduced PPARγ production, which subsequently downregulated the overexpression of proinflammatory cytokines and inhibited the activation of gluconeogenesis and lipogenesis in hepatocytes with overflowing fatty acids. This study suggests a novel application of COS to prevent and treat glucolipid metabolism-related diseases.

4. Materials and Methods

4.1. Chemicals and Reagents

HepG2 cells were supplied by the Chinese Academy of Sciences Cell Bank (Shanghai, China). COS were prepared in our laboratory [48]. PA was purchased from Thermo Fisher Scientific (Waltham, MA, USA). Minimum essential medium (MEM), penicillin/streptomycin, and nonessential amino acids (NEAA) were obtained from Gibco (Grand Island, NY, USA). Fetal bovine serum (FBS) was purchased from Kang Yuan biology company (Beijing, China). Anti-PPARγ, anti-β-actin, horseradish peroxidase (HRP)-conjugated goat anti-rabbit IgG, and HRP-conjugated goat anti-mouse IgG were obtained from Cell Signaling Biotechnology (Beverly, MA, USA).

4.2. Cell Culture and Drug Treatment

HepG2 cells were maintained in MEM containing 10% FBS and 1% NEAA, 1% penicillin–streptomycin at 37 °C in humidified atmosphere with 5% CO_2. After reaching subconfluence, cells were incubated with 0, 25, 50, 100 μg/mL COS for 12 h and then exposed to 100 μM of PA diluted in culture medium for 24 h at 37 °C for further assay.

4.3. Cell Viability Assay

HepG2 cells were plated at density of 1×10^4 cells/well in 96-well plates for 24 h. After treatment with PA at concentrations of 100 μM, 200 μM, and 400 μM or COS (100 μg/mL) for 24 h, the toxic effects of PA or COS alone on cell viability were determined. To assess the effect of COS plus PA on cell viability, the HepG2 cells were separately pretreated with 25, 50, and 100 μg/mL COS for 12 h and then exposed to 100 μM of PA for 24 h. After that, the cells were washed with PBS and incubated with MTT (5 mg/mL) in culture medium for 3 h at 37 °C. Next, the medium was discarded, and the formazan blue, which formed inside the cells, was dissolved using 100 μL dimethyl sulfoxide (DMSO). The optical density at 490 nm was determined with a Sunrise Remote Microplate Reader (Grodig, Austria). The experiments were repeated 3 times independently, and 5 replicates were involved in each sample. The cell viability of each well was presented as the percentage of control level.

4.4. Animal Experiment

C57BL/6J wild-type male mice were obtained from Vital River Laboratory Animal Technology Co., Ltd. (Beijing China) and kept in a room with a 12 h light/dark cycle, a temperature of 22 ± 2 °C, and a relative humidity of 50 ± 5% during the whole experiment period. Mice were fed with a control diet for two weeks for adaptation. Then, all mice were randomly divided into four groups ($n = 5$): CD group, HFD group, CD + COS (1 mg/mL in drinking water, about 200 mg/kg/d) group, and HFD + COS group. The HFD was composed of 60% basic feed, 10% lard, 10% egg yolk powder, 2.5% cholesterol, 0.5% bile salts, 5% sucrose, 5% peanut, 5% milk powder, and 2% salt. Both diets used in this study were bought from Aoke Xieli Co., Ltd. (Beijing, China). After the treatment for five months, the body weight and fasting glucose level of each mouse were detected. Then the mice were sacrificed, and liver tissues were collected. All samples were stored at −80 °C for further experiments.

All the experimental procedures were approved by the Institutional Animal Care and Use Committee of Animal Center, Institute of Process Engineering, Chinese Academy of Sciences (Beijing, China) and in accordance with the guidelines of the National Act on Use of Experimental Animals (China).

4.5. Intraperitoneal Glucose Tolerance Test (IGTT)

An IGTT was conducted after the COS and HFD treatment for five months. Before the test, mice of each group (*n* = 5) were fasted for 12 h and then given an intraperitoneal (i.p.) injection of glucose at a dose of 500 mg/kg body weight. Blood was collected from the tail vein at 0, 15, 30, 60, and 120 min, and the glucose levels were determined using a blood glucometer (Roche Diagnostics, Basel, Switzerland).

4.6. Oil Red O Staining

Liver tissues of each group (*n* = 5) were fixed overnight in 4% paraformaldehyde, embedded in paraffin, and made into 4 μm sections. After the deparaffinization and rehydration, the sections were stained with haematoxylin–eosin (HE) for 1 min and then with 0.5% oil red O solution for 30 min at room temperature. The visualized red oil droplets staining in the slides were observed using a Leica DMI4000 B light microscope (Wetzlar, Germany).

For HepG2 cells staining, the cells were treated as before, washed with PBS, and fixed with 4% paraformaldehyde for 60 min. Then, cells were stained with 0.5% oil red O solution and photographed as mentioned above. The experiments were repeated 3 times independently, and 3 replicates were involved in each sample.

4.7. RNA Extraction, cDNA Synthesis, and Quantitative Real-Time (qRT)-PCR

Total RNA was extracted from HepG2 cells and liver tissues using TRIzol reagent (Invitrogen, Carlsbad, CA, USA) following the manufacturer's instructions. Isolated RNA (1 μg) was reverse transcribed into cDNA using a HifiScript cDNA synthesis kit (Takara Bio Inc., Otsu, Shiga, Japan). For qRT-PCR, the reaction was performed using a 7500 Fast Real-Time PCR System (Applied Biosystems, Foster City, CA, USA) with the thermal cycle condition as follows: 95 °C for 2 min; 40 cycles of amplification (95 °C for 15 s, 60 °C for 60 s, 72 °C for 1 min). The experiments were repeated 3 times independently, and 3 replicates were involved in each sample in vitro. Five replicates were involved in each group in vivo. The primer sequences used in this study are listed in Table 1, and β-actin was used as reference gene for calculation of the relative target gene expression using the $2^{-\Delta\Delta CT}$ method.

Table 1. List of the primer sequences used in RT-PCR analysis.

Gene	Forward Primer (5′-3′)	Reverse Primer (5′-3′)
β-Actin	AGGTGACAGCATTGCTTCTG	GCTGCCTCAACACCTCAAC
IL-6	GGCACTGGCAGAAAACAACC	GCAAGTCTCCTCATTGAATCC
MCP-1	GGGATCATCTTGCTGGTGAA	AGGTCCCTGTCATGCTTCTG
TNF-α	AGGGTCTGGGCCATAGAACT	CCACCACGCTCTTCTGTCTAC
PCK1	CTGCATAACGGTCTGGACTTC	CAGCAACTGCCCGTACTCC
SCD-1	ATACCACCACCACCACCATT	CATACAGGGCTCCCAAGTGT
ACC1	CTGCCATCCCATGTGCTAAT	AGCAGTCGTTCCCCTTCATT
PPARγ	TCGCTGATGCCTGCCTATG	GGAGCACCTTGGCGAACA

4.8. Western Blot Analysis

HepG2 cells and liver tissues were homogenized using radio-immunoprecipitation assay (RIPA) buffer (Cell Signaling, Danvers, MA, USA) supplemented with protease inhibitor cocktail (Merck, Darmstadt, Germany). The sample homogenate was centrifuged at 15,000× *g* for 15 min at 4 °C, and the supernatant was collected. The protein concentration was determined using a bicinchoninic acid (BCA protein assay kit (Beyotime, Shanghai, China). The lysate samples (40 μg/lane) were separated by sodium dodecyl sulfate polyacrylamide gel electrophoresis (SDS-PAGE) and transferred to a polyvinylidene fluoride (PVDF) membrane. The membranes were blocked with 5% fat-free milk in Tris-buffered saline with 0.1% Tween-20 (TBST) buffer (10 mM Tris, 150 mM NaCl, 0.1% Tween

20, pH 7.6) for 1 h at room temperature and then incubated with primary antibodies against PPARγ overnight at 4 °C. Next, the membranes were incubated with HRP-conjugated secondary antibodies for 1 h. The protein bands were captured by enhanced chemiluminescence (ECL) (Cell Signaling Technology, Beverly, MA, USA), and the densitometry analysis was performed using an Image J2x software (National Institute of Health, Bethesda, MD, USA). The protein level of PPARγ of each sample was measured 3 times independently in vitro, and 5 samples expressing PPARγ protein of each group in vivo were assessed.

4.9. Statistics

Statistical analysis was carried out using SPSS 10.0 package (SPSS Inc, Chicago, IL, USA). Data are presented as means ± SD. Differences between groups were assessed with one-way analysis variance (ANOVA), along with the Tukey–Kramer test. $p < 0.05$ was regarded as statistically significant.

Author Contributions: H.L. and L.Z. designed the study. Y.B., J.Z., X.Y., S.J., and F.C. were responsible for the acquisition of data. Y.B. and Y.D. analyzed the experimental data. H.L. and Y.B. were the major contributors in drafting and revising the manuscript. All authors read and approved the final manuscript.

Funding: This research was funded by National Natural Science Foundation of China, grant number 31570801 and 31500747, and the National Programs for High Technology Research and Development, grant number 863 Programs, 2014AA093604.

Conflicts of Interest: The authors declare that there is no conflict of interest.

Abbreviations

NAFLDs	nonalcoholic fatty liver diseases
COS	chitosan oligosaccharides
PA	palmitic acid
HFD	high-fat diet
CD	chow diet
IL-6	interleukin-6
MCP-1	monocyte chemoattractant protein 1
TNF-α	tumor necrosis factor-alpha
PCK1	phosphoenolpyruvate carboxykinase-1
SCD-1	stearoyl-CoA desaturase
ACC1	acetyl-CoA carboxylase

References

1. Ogden, C.L.; Carroll, M.D.; Kit, B.K.; Flegal, K.M. Prevalence of obesity in the United States, 2009–2010. *NCHS Data Brief* **2012**, *82*, 1–8.
2. Yu, Z.; Han, S.; Chu, J.; Xu, Z.; Zhu, C.; Guo, X. Trends in overweight and obesity among children and adolescents in China from 1981 to 2010: A meta-analysis. *PLoS ONE* **2012**, *7*, e51949. [CrossRef] [PubMed]
3. Hotamisligil, G.S. Inflammation and metabolic disorders. *Nature* **2006**, *444*, 860–867. [CrossRef] [PubMed]
4. Kissane, N.A.; Pratt, J.S. Medical and surgical treatment of obesity. *Best Pract. Res. Clin. Anaesthesiol.* **2011**, *25*, 11–25. [CrossRef] [PubMed]
5. Baretic, M. Obesity drug therapy. *Minerva Endocrinol.* **2013**, *38*, 245–254. [PubMed]
6. Zou, P.; Yang, X.; Wang, J.; Li, Y.; Yu, H.; Zhang, Y.; Liu, G. Advances in characterisation and biological activities of chitosan and chitosan oligosaccharides. *Food Chem.* **2016**, *190*, 1174–1181. [CrossRef] [PubMed]
7. Kunanusornchai, W.; Witoonpanich, B.; Tawonsawatruk, T.; Pichyangkura, R.; Chatsudthipong, V.; Muanprasat, C. Chitosan oligosaccharide suppresses synovial inflammation via AMPK activation: An in vitro and in vivo study. *Pharmacol. Res.* **2016**, *113 Pt A*, 458–467. [CrossRef]
8. Zhao, D.; Wang, J.; Tan, L.; Sun, C.; Dong, J. Synthesis of N-furoyl chitosan and chito-oligosaccharides and evaluation of their antioxidant activity in vitro. *Int. J. Biol. Macromol.* **2013**, *59*, 391–395. [CrossRef] [PubMed]
9. Azuma, K.; Osaki, T.; Minami, S.; Okamoto, Y. Anticancer and anti-inflammatory properties of chitin and chitosan oligosaccharides. *J. Funct. Biomater.* **2015**, *6*, 33–49. [CrossRef] [PubMed]

10. Pan, H.; Yang, Q.; Huang, G.; Ding, C.; Cao, P.; Huang, L.; Xiao, T.; Guo, J.; Su, Z. Hypolipidemic effects of chitosan and its derivatives in hyperlipidemic rats induced by a high-fat diet. *Food Nutr. Res.* **2016**, *60*, 31137. [CrossRef] [PubMed]

11. Huang, L.; Chen, J.; Cao, P.; Pan, H.; Ding, C.; Xiao, T.; Zhang, P.; Guo, J.; Su, Z. Anti-obese effect of glucosamine and chitosan oligosaccharide in high-fat diet-induced obese rats. *Mar. Drugs* **2015**, *13*, 2732–2756. [CrossRef] [PubMed]

12. Pan, H.; Fu, C.; Huang, L.; Jiang, Y.; Deng, X.; Guo, J.; Su, Z. Anti-Obesity Effect of Chitosan Oligosaccharide Capsules (COSCs) in Obese Rats by Ameliorating Leptin Resistance and Adipogenesis. *Mar. Drugs* **2018**, *16*, 198. [CrossRef] [PubMed]

13. Egan, A.M.; Sweeney, T.; Hayes, M.; O'Doherty, J.V. Prawn Shell Chitosan Has Anti-Obesogenic Properties, Influencing Both Nutrient Digestibility and Microbial Populations in a Pig Model. *PLoS ONE* **2015**, *10*, e0144127. [CrossRef] [PubMed]

14. Chae, S.Y.; Jang, M.K.; Nah, J.W. Influence of molecular weight on oral absorption of water soluble chitosans. *J. Control. Release* **2005**, *102*, 383–394. [CrossRef] [PubMed]

15. Ge, J.; Miao, J.J.; Sun, X.Y.; Yu, J.Y. Huangkui capsule, an extract from *Abelmoschus manihot* (L.) medic, improves diabetic nephropathy via activating peroxisome proliferator-activated receptor (PPAR)-alpha/gamma and attenuating endoplasmic reticulum stress in rats. *J. Ethnopharmacol.* **2016**, *189*, 238–249. [CrossRef] [PubMed]

16. Lee, H.; Kang, R.; Kim, Y.S.; Chung, S.I.; Yoon, Y. Platycodin D inhibits adipogenesis of 3T3-L1 cells by modulating Kruppel-like factor 2 and peroxisome proliferator-activated receptor gamma. *Phytother. Res.* **2010**, *24* (Suppl. 2), 161–167. [CrossRef] [PubMed]

17. Sakamoto, Y.; Naka, A.; Ohara, N.; Kondo, K.; Iida, K. Daidzein regulates proinflammatory adipokines thereby improving obesity-related inflammation through PPARgamma. *Mol. Nutr. Food Res.* **2014**, *58*, 718–726. [CrossRef] [PubMed]

18. Lehrke, M.; Lazar, M.A. The many faces of PPARgamma. *Cell* **2005**, *123*, 993–999. [CrossRef] [PubMed]

19. Barak, Y.; Nelson, M.C.; Ong, E.S.; Jones, Y.Z.; Ruiz-Lozano, P.; Chien, K.R.; Koder, A.; Evans, R.M. PPAR gamma is required for placental, cardiac, and adipose tissue development. *Mol. Cell* **1999**, *4*, 585–595. [CrossRef]

20. Virtue, S.; Masoodi, M.; Velagapudi, V.; Tan, C.Y.; Dale, M.; Suorti, T.; Slawik, M.; Blount, M.; Burling, K.; Campbell, M.; et al. Lipocalin prostaglandin D synthase and PPARgamma2 coordinate to regulate carbohydrate and lipid metabolism in vivo. *PLoS ONE* **2012**, *7*, e39512. [CrossRef] [PubMed]

21. Tontonoz, P.; Spiegelman, B.M. Fat and beyond: The diverse biology of PPARgamma. *Annu. Rev. Biochem.* **2008**, *77*, 289–312. [CrossRef] [PubMed]

22. Alqahtani, S.; Mahmoud, A.M. Gamma-Glutamylcysteine Ethyl Ester Protects against Cyclophosphamide-Induced Liver Injury and Hematologic Alterations via Upregulation of PPARgamma and Attenuation of Oxidative Stress, Inflammation, and Apoptosis. *Oxid. Med. Cell. Longev.* **2016**, *2016*, 4016209. [CrossRef] [PubMed]

23. Yang, L.; Stimpson, S.A.; Chen, L.; Harrington, W.W.; Rockey, D.C. Effectiveness of the PPARgamma agonist, GW570, in liver fibrosis. *Inflamm. Res.* **2010**, *59*, 1061–1071. [CrossRef] [PubMed]

24. Nan, Y.M.; Han, F.; Kong, L.B.; Zhao, S.X.; Wang, R.Q.; Wu, W.J.; Yu, J. Adenovirus-mediated peroxisome proliferator activated receptor gamma overexpression prevents nutritional fibrotic steatohepatitis in mice. *Scand. J. Gastroenterol.* **2011**, *46*, 358–369. [CrossRef] [PubMed]

25. Huang, Y.Y.; Gusdon, A.M.; Qu, S. Nonalcoholic fatty liver disease: Molecular pathways and therapeutic strategies. *Lipids Health. Dis.* **2013**, *12*, 171. [CrossRef] [PubMed]

26. Ferre, P. The biology of peroxisome proliferator-activated receptors: Relationship with lipid metabolism and insulin sensitivity. *Diabetes* **2004**, *53* (Suppl. 1), 43–50. [CrossRef]

27. Liu, H.T.; Li, W.M.; Li, X.Y.; Xu, Q.S.; Liu, Q.S.; Bai, X.F.; Yu, C.; Du, Y.G. Chitosan oligosaccharides inhibit the expression of interleukin-6 in lipopolysaccharide-induced human umbilical vein endothelial cells through p38 and ERK1/2 protein kinases. *Basic Clin. Pharmacol. Toxicol.* **2010**, *106*, 362–371. [CrossRef] [PubMed]

28. Shi, L.L.; Li, Y.; Wang, Y.; Feng, Y. MDG-1, an Ophiopogon polysaccharide, regulate gut microbiota in high-fat diet-induced obese C57BL/6 mice. *Int. J. Biol. Macromol.* **2015**, *81*, 576–583. [CrossRef] [PubMed]

29. Kong, X.F.; Zhou, X.L.; Lian, G.Q.; Blachier, F.; Liu, G.; Tan, B.E.; Nyachoti, C.M.; Yin, Y.L. Dietary supplementation with chitooligosaccharides alters gut microbiota and modifies intestinal luminal metabolites in weaned Huanjiang mini-piglets. *Livest. Sci.* **2014**, *160*, 97–101. [CrossRef]

30. Qiao, Y.; Bai, X.F.; Du, Y.G. Chitosan oligosaccharides protect mice from LPS challenge by attenuation of inflammation and oxidative stress. *Int. Immunopharmacol.* **2011**, *11*, 121–127. [CrossRef] [PubMed]

31. Sauer, M.; Doss, S.; Ehler, J.; Mencke, T.; Wagner, N.M. Procalcitonin Impairs Liver Cell Viability and Function in vitro: A Potential New Mechanism of Liver Dysfunction and Failure during Sepsis? *BioMed Res. Int.* **2017**, *2017*, 6130725. [CrossRef] [PubMed]

32. Ishiyama, J.; Taguchi, R.; Yamamoto, A.; Murakami, K. Palmitic acid enhances lectin-like oxidized LDL receptor (LOX-1) expression and promotes uptake of oxidized LDL in macrophage cells. *Atherosclerosis* **2010**, *209*, 118–124. [CrossRef] [PubMed]

33. Kim, S.K.; Seo, G.; Oh, E.; Jin, S.-H.; Chae, G.T.; Lee, S.-B. Palmitate induces RIP1-dependent necrosis in RAW 264.7 cells. *Atherosclerosis* **2012**, *225*, 315–321. [CrossRef] [PubMed]

34. Benoit, B.; Plaisancié, P.; Géloën, A.; Estienne, M.; Debard, C.; Meugnier, E.; Loizon, E.; Daira, P.; Bodennec, J.; Cousin, O.; et al. Pasture v. standard dairy cream in high-fat diet-fed mice: Improved metabolic outcomes and stronger intestinal barrier. *Br. J. Nutr.* **2014**, *112*, 520–535. [CrossRef] [PubMed]

35. Zheng, J.; Cheng, G.; Li, Q.; Jiao, S.; Feng, C.; Zhao, X.; Yin, H.; Du, Y.; Liu, H. Chitin Oligosaccharide Modulates Gut Microbiota and Attenuates High-Fat-Diet-Induced Metabolic Syndrome in Mice. *Mar. Drugs* **2018**, *16*, 66. [CrossRef] [PubMed]

36. Caesar, R.; Fåk, F.; Bäckhed, F. Effects of gut microbiota on obesity and atherosclerosis via modulation of inflammation and lipid metabolism. *J. Intern. Med.* **2010**, *268*, 320–328. [CrossRef] [PubMed]

37. Li, W.; Fang, Q.; Zhong, P.; Chen, L.; Wang, L.; Zhang, Y.; Wang, J.; Li, X.; Wang, Y.; Wang, J.; et al. EGFR Inhibition Blocks Palmitic Acid-induced inflammation in cardiomyocytes and Prevents Hyperlipidemia-induced Cardiac Injury in Mice. *Sci. Rep.* **2016**, *6*, 24580. [CrossRef] [PubMed]

38. Zhou, B.R.; Zhang, J.A.; Zhang, Q.; Permatasari, F.; Xu, Y.; Wu, D.; Yin, Z.Q.; Luo, D. Palmitic acid induces production of proinflammatory cytokines interleukin-6, interleukin-1beta, and tumor necrosis factor-alpha via a NF-kappaB-dependent mechanism in HaCaT keratinocytes. *Mediat. Inflamm.* **2013**, *2013*, 530429. [CrossRef] [PubMed]

39. Lai, C.S.; Liao, S.N.; Tsai, M.L.; Kalyanam, N.; Majeed, M.; Majeed, A.; Ho, C.T.; Pan, M.H. Calebin-A inhibits adipogenesis and hepatic steatosis in high-fat diet-induced obesity via activation of AMPK signaling. *Mol. Nutr. Food Res.* **2015**, *59*, 1883–1895. [CrossRef] [PubMed]

40. Hwang, J.S.; Park, J.W.; Nam, M.S.; Cho, H.; Han, I.O. Glucosamine enhances body weight gain and reduces insulin response in mice fed chow diet but mitigates obesity, insulin resistance and impaired glucose tolerance in mice high-fat diet. *Metabolism* **2015**, *64*, 368–379. [CrossRef] [PubMed]

41. Poloni, S.; Blom, H.J.; Schwartz, I.V. Stearoyl-CoA Desaturase-1: Is It the Link between Sulfur Amino Acids and Lipid Metabolism? *Biology* **2015**, *4*, 383–396. [CrossRef] [PubMed]

42. Berod, L.; Friedrich, C.; Nandan, A.; Freitag, J.; Hagemann, S.; Harmrolfs, K.; Sandouk, A.; Hesse, C.; Castro, C.N.; Bahre, H.; et al. De novo fatty acid synthesis controls the fate between regulatory T and T helper 17 cells. *Nat. Med.* **2014**, *20*, 1327–1333. [CrossRef] [PubMed]

43. Schmilovitz-Weiss, H.; Hochhauser, E.; Cohen, M.; Chepurko, Y.; Yitzhaki, S.; Grossman, E.; Leibowitz, A.; Ackerman, Z.; Ben-Ari, Z. Rosiglitazone and bezafibrate modulate gene expression in a rat model of non-alcoholic fatty liver disease—A historical prospective. *Lipids Health. Dis.* **2013**, *12*, 41. [CrossRef] [PubMed]

44. Jimenez-Flores, L.M.; Lopez-Briones, S.; Macias-Cervantes, M.H.; Ramirez-Emiliano, J.; Perez-Vazquez, V. A PPARgamma, NF-kappaB and AMPK-dependent mechanism may be involved in the beneficial effects of curcumin in the diabetic db/db mice liver. *Molecules* **2014**, *19*, 8289–8302. [CrossRef] [PubMed]

45. Pascual, G.; Fong, A.L.; Ogawa, S.; Gamliel, A.; Li, A.C.; Perissi, V.; Rose, D.W.; Willson, T.M.; Rosenfeld, M.G.; Glass, C.K. A SUMOylation-dependent pathway mediates transrepression of inflammatory response genes by PPAR-gamma. *Nature* **2005**, *437*, 759–763. [CrossRef] [PubMed]

46. Kaplan, J.; Nowell, M.; Chima, R.; Zingarelli, B. Pioglitazone reduces inflammation through inhibition of NF-kappaB in polymicrobial sepsis. *Innate Immun.* **2014**, *20*, 519–528. [CrossRef] [PubMed]

47. Li, C.C.; Yang, H.T.; Hou, Y.C.; Chiu, Y.S.; Chiu, W.C. Dietary fish oil reduces systemic inflammation and ameliorates sepsis-induced liver injury by up-regulating the peroxisome proliferator-activated receptor gamma-mediated pathway in septic mice. *J. Nutr. Biochem.* **2014**, *25*, 19–25. [CrossRef] [PubMed]

48. Zhang, H.; Du, Y.; Yu, X.; Mitsutomi, M.; Aiba, S. Preparation of chitooligosaccharides from chitosan by a complex enzyme. *Carbohydr. Res.* **1999**, *320*, 257–260. [CrossRef]

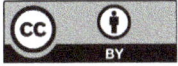

marine drugs

MDPI

Article

Reduced Number of Adipose Lineage and Endothelial Cells in Epididymal fat in Response to Omega-3 PUFA in Mice Fed High-Fat Diet

Katerina Adamcova [†], Olga Horakova [†], Kristina Bardova [†], Petra Janovska, Marie Brezinova, Ondrej Kuda, Martin Rossmeisl and Jan Kopecky *

Department of Adipose Tissue Biology, Institute of Physiology of the Czech Academy of Sciences, Videnska 1083, 142 20 Prague, Czech Republic; katerina.adamcova@fgu.cas.cz (K.A.); olga.horakova@fgu.cas.cz (O.H.); kristina.bardova@fgu.cas.cz (K.B.); petra.janovska@fgu.cas.cz (P.J.); marie.brezinova@fgu.cas.cz (M.B.); ondrej.kuda@fgu.cas.cz (O.K.); martin.rossmeisl@fgu.cas.cz (M.R.)
* Correspondence: kopecky@biomed.cas.cz; Tel.: +(00420) 241-062-554
† These authors contributed equally to this work.

Received: 29 November 2018; Accepted: 14 December 2018; Published: 18 December 2018

Abstract: We found previously that white adipose tissue (WAT) hyperplasia in obese mice was limited by dietary omega-3 polyunsaturated fatty acids (omega-3 PUFA). Here we aimed to characterize the underlying mechanism. C57BL/6N mice were fed a high-fat diet supplemented or not with omega-3 PUFA for one week or eight weeks; mice fed a standard chow diet were also used. In epididymal WAT (eWAT), DNA content was quantified, immunohistochemical analysis was used to reveal the size of adipocytes and macrophage content, and lipidomic analysis and a gene expression screen were performed to assess inflammatory status. The stromal-vascular fraction of eWAT, which contained most of the eWAT cells, except for adipocytes, was characterized using flow cytometry. Omega-3 PUFA supplementation limited the high-fat diet-induced increase in eWAT weight, cell number (DNA content), inflammation, and adipocyte growth. eWAT hyperplasia was compromised due to the limited increase in the number of preadipocytes and a decrease in the number of endothelial cells. The number of leukocytes and macrophages was unaffected, but a shift in macrophage polarization towards a less inflammatory phenotype was observed. Our results document that the counteraction of eWAT hyperplasia by omega-3 PUFA in dietary-obese mice reflects an effect on the number of adipose lineage and endothelial cells.

Keywords: cellularity; adipocyte; obesity; nutrition; fat; proliferation; white adipose tissue

---

1. Introduction

An unhealthy lifestyle, including overnutrition, is the main driving force behind the recent pandemic of obesity and associated diseases. Obesity is defined as an excessive accumulation of body fat, namely in the form of white adipose tissue (WAT; [1]). This tissue is characterized by extreme plasticity, and fat depot-specific functional and structural heterogeneity (reviewed in [2–4]). The main function of WAT is to store energy in triglycerides that are located within lipid droplets in adipocytes. During exercise, fasting, or cold exposure, fatty acids are released and serve as an energy source. Sufficient capacity for WAT expansion is essential to prevent a spillover of fatty acids and lipotoxic damage of insulin signalling in other tissues [5]. Therefore, both an insufficient amount of WAT as well as hypertrophic WAT can lead to harmful systemic metabolic consequences.

The growth of WAT can occur by both increasing the number of adipocytes ("hyperplasia") and by enlarging the size of existing adipocytes ("hypertrophy"). WAT can represent 5% to 60% of total body weight [4,6]. Fat mass reflects the energy balance. However, the adipocyte number is very static in adult humans and independent of fluctuations in body weight, even in response to a massive weight loss. Furthermore, adipocyte number is set during childhood and adolescence [6] and approximately only 10% of fat cells are renewed annually in adult humans [7]. New adipocytes arise from adipogenic progenitor cells, as mature adipocytes are postmitotic [8]. Adipocyte progenitors are CD24+ cells, which lose their CD24 expression as they become further committed to the adipocyte lineage. The CD24− preadipocytes represent the next distinct cell type over the course of adipose cell differentiation into mature adipocytes in vivo [9]. Adipose tissue expansion also involves coordinated development of the tissue vascular network and coupled angiogenesis is essential for adipogenesis in obesity [10,11]. In adult humans, obesity is predominantly associated with the hypertrophy of fat cells. However, an increase in fat cell number was also observed in morbidly obese subjects (reviewed in [6,7,12]). In contrast, in laboratory rodents WAT hyperplasia could be induced independent of age, e.g., in response to obesogenic high-fat diets. In particular, the epididymal WAT (eWAT) in the abdomen, the typical WAT depot in rodents (regarding its growth in response to high fat diet [13], negligible capacity for *Ucp1* expression [14] and its frequent analysis in the rodent studies focused on obesity [15]), has a high potential for hyperplastic growth [13,16–18].

WAT is composed of several cell types including adipocytes, preadipocytes (see above), and endothelial cells as well as fibroblasts, stem cells, and almost the full spectrum of immune cells defining a unique adipose-resident immune system [19]. Macrophages accumulate in the hypertrophied WAT of both obese individuals and mice, and divert from the pro-resolving (M2) to the pro-inflammatory phenotype (M1), which contribute to a low-grade adipose tissue inflammation and insulin resistance in obesity [20]. Mutual interactions between adipocytes and immune cells in WAT, mediated by lipokines and cytokines/adipokines and metabolites, are essential for the healthy functioning of WAT ([21–24]; reviewed in [25,26]). Also, the proliferation and differentiation of stem cells and preadipocytes depends on the local niche provided by both the endothelial mural cell compartment [11,27] and macrophages [28]. Also these processes are mainly coordinated by the autocrine and paracrine effects of the WAT-borne signalling molecules and metabolites [29,30]. Therefore, the immunometabolism [31] of WAT, i.e., the cross talk between cells of the immune system contained in the tissue and the tissue metabolism (see above and [26]) contributes to either a lean or obese phenotype. These opposite systemic effects reflect either enhancing or lowering the capacity of WAT for buffering circulating fatty acids. Hence, both the amount of WAT and its immunometabolic properties represent a therapeutic target for the treatment of obesity and associated diseases (reviewed in [25,26,32]).

Our previous studies have shown that the induction of obesity and deterioration of the immunometabolism of WAT in mice fed an obesogenic high-fat diet could be ameliorated in response to dietary supplementation with long-chain polyunsaturated fatty acids of the n-3 series (omega-3 PUFA; reviewed in [26,32]), namely eicosapentaenoic acid (EPA; 20:5 ω-3) and docosahexaenoic acid (DHA; 22:6 ω-3). The effects of omega-3 PUFA were even more pronounced when a combined intervention with either calorie restriction [33] or antidiabetic drugs was used [34]. The multiple beneficial effects on health, exerted by omega-3 PUFA, are mediated by these PUFA themselves, related lipid mediators, and multiple intracellular signalling pathways (reviewed by us in [25,26,32,35]).

Our previous results also indicated that, in addition to modulating the immunometabolic properties of WAT, the reduced accumulation of body fat due to omega-3 PUFA supplementation in mice fed a high-fat diet was in part due to a prevention of the increase in tissue cell number [36,37]. Therefore, the main goal of this study was to characterize in detail the cell types involved the abolishment of hyperplastic growth of WAT in mice fed a high-fat diet in response to the omega-3 PUFA supplementation.

2. Results

2.1. Effect of Omega-3 PUFA on Body Weight and eWAT

C57BL/6N male mice were fed either a standard (STD) or high-fat (HFD) diet or a high-fat diet supplemented with omega-3 PUFA (HFF) for one or eight weeks starting at 13 weeks of age. Both the HFD and HFF diet increased the body weight and eWAT weight at both Week 1 and Week 8 compared to the STD diet, with no impact of omega-3 PUFA on body weight compared to HFD (Table 1). However, eWAT weight tended to be lower after Week 1 and was reduced by 20% at Week 8 in the HFF compared to the HFD fed mice (Table 1).

Table 1. Effects of eicosapentaenoic acid (EPA)/docosahexaenoic acid (DHA) on body weight, epididymal white adipose tissue (eWAT) weight, and DNA content.

	Week 1			Week 8		
	STD	**HFD**	**HFF**	**STD**	**HFD**	**HFF**
BW initial (g)	29.3 ± 1.9	29.6 ± 1.4	30.0 ± 2.4	28.1 ± 1.8 [a]	28.1 ± 1.9 [a]	28.2 ± 1.7 [a]
BW dissection (g)	29.9 ± 1.9	33.9 ± 2.1 [c]	33.9 ± 2.8 [c]	34.0 ± 3.4 [a]	48.8 ± 4.6 [a,c]	47.0 ± 3.4 [a,c]
BW gain (g)	0.7 ± 0.7	4.4 ± 0.8 [c]	3.9 ± 1.1 [c]	5.9 ± 2.9 [a]	20.6 ± 3.8 [a,c]	18.9 ± 3.1 [a,c]
eWAT weight (mg)	509 ± 175	1084 ± 207 [c]	1006 ± 284 [c]	877 ± 365 [a]	2310 ± 301 [a,c]	1816 ± 254 [a,b,c]
eWAT DNA (µg/depot)	194 ± 18	267 ± 47 [c]	192 ± 30 [b]	440 ± 98 [a]	1313 ± 328 [a,c]	1094 ± 183 [a,b,c]
Adipocytes DNA (µg/depot)	n.d.	n.d.	n.d.	274 ± 67	541 ± 140 [c]	445 ± 126

Mice were fed by standard (STD), high-fat diet (HFD), or a high-fat diet supplemented with omega-3 PUFA (HFF) and sacrificed at Week 1 or Week 8. Initial body weight (BW), BW at dissection, BW gain and weight of eWAT were evaluated. DNA was quantified in eWAT. Data are means ± SD; *n* = 8 for Week 1, *n* = 16–26 for Week 8. DNA content was also determined in collagenase-liberated adipocytes from eWAT at Week 8 (*n* = 8). [a] Significantly different from Week 1 between mice given same diet; [b] significantly different from the HFD group for the same period of dietary intervention; [c] significantly different from the STD group for the same period of dietary intervention; n.d., not determined.

The DNA content of eWAT, a surrogate marker of cell number in the tissue, was higher at Week 8 than Week 1. It increased much faster in the mice fed the high-fat diet, resulting in a 3.0-fold and 2.5-fold higher DNA content in the HFD and HFF mice, respectively, compared to the STD mice at Week 8 (Table 1). Thus, omega-3 PUFA supplementation abolished in part the increase in eWAT cell number in the mice fed a high-fat diet, with a significant effect (1.2-fold difference between the HFD and HFF mice) at Week 8. The trend for this effect was already apparent at Week 1 (Table 1). The differences in eWAT DNA content at Week 8 were mirrored by those in the total DNA content of the fraction of collagenase-liberated adipocytes from eWAT. However, in this case, only a trend to reduce DNA content by omega-3 PUFA was observed (Table 1).

Histological examination and morphometry of adipocytes in eWAT revealed that adipocyte size increased between Week 1 and Week 8 in both the HFD and HFF mice. This increase was less pronounced in the HFF mice (Figure 1A–D). In the STD mice, adipocyte size also increased between Week 1 and Week 8, however, this increase was very small (see Supplementary Figure S1A–C for the hematoxylin and eosin staining of eWAT sections at Week 1). At Week 8 in both the HFD (Figure 1F) and HFF (Figure 1G) mice, but not in the STD mice (Figure 1E), the immunostaining of eWAT revealed crown-like structures (CLS) that are formed by macrophages aggregated around dying adipocytes [38]. However, the abundance of CLS was not influenced by omega-3 PUFA supplementation (Figure 1F,G,H). At Week 1, no CLS were detected in any of the dietary groups (Supplementary Figure S1D–F). Also the proliferation of macrophages within CLS, assessed immunohistochemically using Ki67 staining (Ki67 is a commonly used marker of proliferating nuclei, which was shown to control heterochromatin organisation, see [39,40]) did not differ between the dietary groups (HFD: 19 ± 3% vs. HFF: 16 ± 1% of all CLS-contained nuclei; Figure 1I,J). Interestingly, multinucleated giant cells (MGCs) were only observed in the HFF mice (Figure 1K), suggesting macrophage fusion [41,42].

These results documented that the increase in eWAT weight in response to the high-fat diet emerged from both tissue hypertrophy and hyperplasia, and that both these processes could be partially counteracted by omega-3 PUFA supplementation. Moreover, the results suggested that the effect of omega-3 PUFA on tissue cell number probably does not include changes in tissue macrophage content.

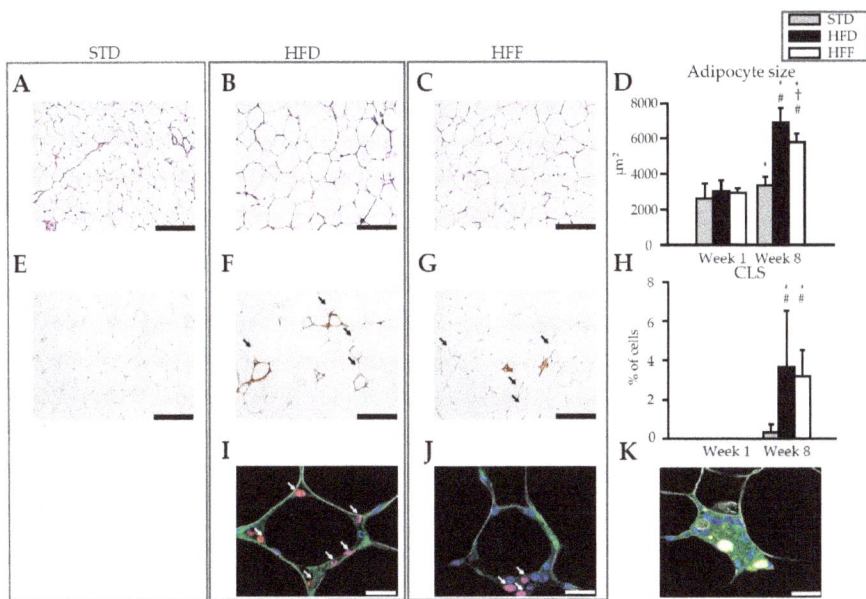

Figure 1. Morphology and immunohistochemistry of eWAT. Representative histological sections of eWAT from mice fed STD (**A,E**), HFD (**B, F, I**) or HFF (**C,G,J,K**) diet at Week 8. Hematoxylin and eosin staining for morphometry of adipocytes (**A,B,C**), as evaluated in (**D**). Immunohistochemical staining using macrophage marker MAC2 for quantification of CLS (**E,F,G**; arrows), as evaluated in (**H**). Representative sections showing the detection of macrophage proliferation within CLS based on immunofluorescence staining (**I,J**; nuclei by DAPI, blue; macrophages by anti-F4/80, green; surface of lipid droplets by anti-perilipin 1, white; proliferating nuclei by anti-Ki67, red; proliferating macrophages are indicated with arrows). Representative section showing multinucleated giant cells (**K**). Data are means ± SD; n = 6–8. * Significant difference from Week 1 between mice on same diets; † significant difference from HFD for the same period of dietary intervention; # significant difference from STD for the same period of dietary intervention. Bar represents 200 μm (**A,B,C,E,F,G**) or 20 μm (**I,J,K**). For morphology and immunohistochemistry of eWAT at Week 1, see Supplementary Figure S1.

2.2. Anti-Inflammatory Effects of Omega-3 PUFA in eWAT in Mice Fed High-Fat Diet

The lack of effect of omega-3 PUFA on the CLS macrophages content in eWAT, despite the decrease in eWAT cell number, prompted us to verify the expected anti-inflammatory effect of omega-3 PUFA in this tissue. First, we addressed the effect on the formation of related lipid mediators [25,43] in eWAT. In the HFD and HFF mice, in total 33 metabolites of arachidonoic acid (AA), α-linolenic acid (ALA), dihomo-γ-linolenic acid (DGLA), DHA, EPA, and linoleic acid (LA) were evaluated at both Week 1 and Week 8 (see Supplementary Table S1). Principal component analysis (PCA) of the data was used to obtain a global view on the effects of the diet and the duration of the dietary intervention. Separation of the dietary groups was evident at both time points, and it was more robust at Week 8 (Figure 2A,B). Among the most discriminating analytes were: hydroxyderivatives of AA, prostaglandins, thromboxane, and hydroxyderivatives of EPA (Figure 2C). As for the levels of individual fatty acid metabolites (Supplementary Table S1), either at Week 1 or Week 8, AA-, ALA-, DGLA-, and LA-derived metabolites were mostly lower in the HFF mice than in the HFD mice, while the levels of EPA-derived lipid mediators in the HFF mice were relatively high. In contrast, the levels of DHA-derived lipid mediators were similar in both dietary groups at both Week 1 and Week 8. Therefore, the pattern of changes in lipid mediators showed an expected shift from the AA-derived pro-inflammatory toward the EPA-derived anti-inflammatory mediators in response to omega-3 PUFA supplementation.

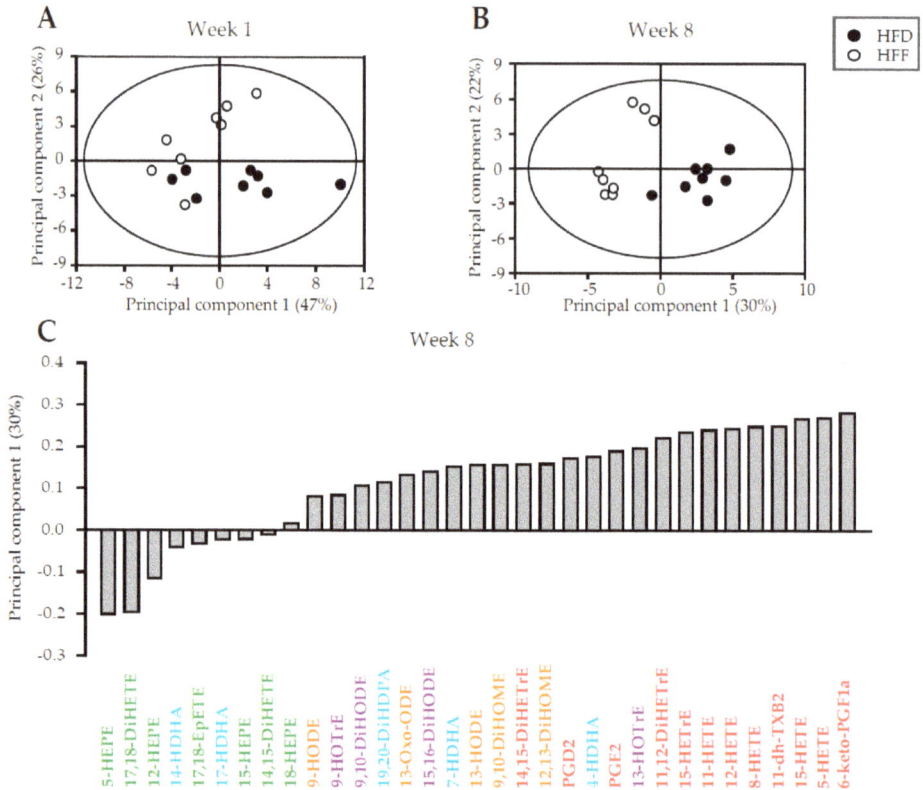

Figure 2. Principal component analysis of the lipidomic data from eWAT of the HFD and HFF mice. Score plots of the principal components 1 and 2 were generated using the lipid mediator profiles at Week 1 (**A**) and Week 8 (**B**). At Week 8 (**C**), results were expressed as a contribution score plot showing one bar per variable, indicating which species differ most between the groups and in which direction. Lipids derived from AA (red), LA (orange), ALA (purple), DHA (blue), and EPA (green) are discerned by colors. For the source data and the abbreviations, see Supplementary Table S1.

Since the hydroxyderivatives of AA and EPA are metabolic products of lipoxygenases (LOX), the expression of the genes for various types of LOX (*Alox5*, *Alox12*, and *Alox15*) was quantified using real-time quantitative PCR (qPCR). However, no differences in the expression of the above genes between the dietary groups were observed in the whole eWAT nor in the subfractions of cells isolated from eWAT, with no dependence on the duration of the dietary intervention (Supplementary Table S2). Tissue levels of lipid mediators are not only influenced by the rate of synthesis, but also by the rate of degradation of these mediators. Importantly, down-regulation of the expression of 15-hydroxyprostaglandin dehydrogenase (*15-Pgdh*) in response to omega-3 PUFA supplementation was detected in both the stromal-vascular fraction (SVF) and adipocyte fraction isolated from eWAT at Week 8 (Supplementary Table S2). This enzyme is responsible for the inactivation of selected prostaglandins, leukotrienes, and several hydroxy-eicosatetraenoic acid species (HETEs; reviewed in [44]).

Subsequently, inflammatory gene expression profiles in eWAT of the HFD and HFF mice were compared. This analysis did not reveal any differences between the dietary groups, neither at Week 1 nor at Week 8 (Figure 3A). Therefore, the analysis was repeated using both SVF and adipocytes isolated from eWAT at Week 8 (Figure 3B). Expression of most of the evaluated inflammatory markers, such as tumor necrosis factor (*Tnfa*), nitric oxide synthase 2 (*Nos2*), C-C chemokine receptor type 2 (*Ccr2*), interleukin 1 beta (*Il1b*), and interferon gamma (*Ifng*) as well as transforming growth factor beta (*Tgfb*; regulator of inflammatory processes), was (or tended to be) lower in the SVF of the HFF mice. In the adipocyte fraction, expression of the above genes was not affected by the omega-3 PUFA supplementation, while the expression of chemokine (C-C motif) ligand 2 (*Ccl2*), another inflammatory marker, was the only one to be down-regulated by omega-3 PUFA in the adipocyte fraction (Figure 3B). The expression of the anti-inflammatory marker arginase (*Arg1*) did not differ between the dietary groups, either in eWAT (Figure 3A) or in the isolated cells (Figure 3B). Thus, mRNA analysis confirmed the lower pro-inflammatory profile of SVF cells within eWAT in HFF compared to the HFD mice.

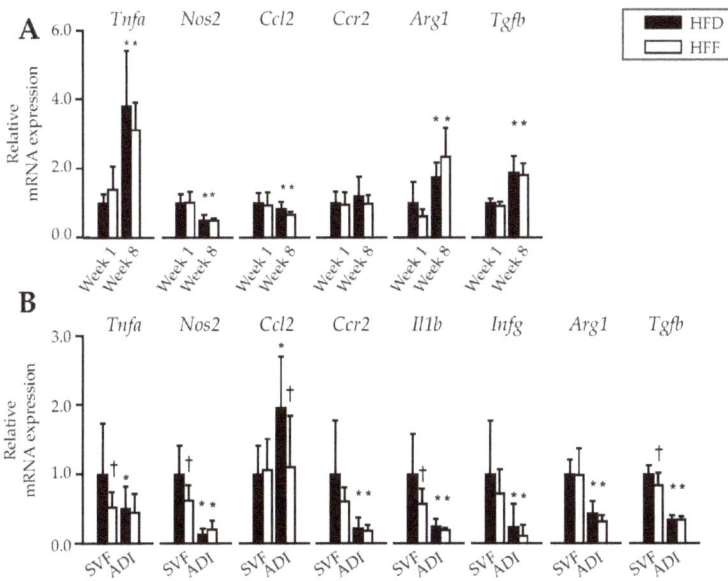

Figure 3. Gene expression of pro- and anti-inflammatory markers in eWAT of mice fed HFD or HFF diet for 1 or 8 weeks (**A**), or in stromal-vascular fraction (SVF) cells or adipocytes (ADI) isolated from eWAT of mice fed the respective diets for 8 weeks (**B**). Data were normalized to the geometrical mean of two reference genes, *Hprt* and *EF1α* in (**A**), and *EF1α* and *Rn18s* in (**B**), and expressed relative to the HFD mice at Week 1 for whole eWAT depot (**A**) or to SVF of HFD group (Week 8) for SVF and ADI (**B**). Data are means ± SD; $n = 6$–8. * Significant difference from Week 1 between mice with the same diet; † significant difference for the same period of dietary intervention.

2.3. Changes in Immune Cell Abundance Cannot Explain the Effect of Omega-3 PUFA on eWAT Cell Number in Mice Fed High-Fat Diet

The above results documented the anti-inflammatory effect of omega-3 PUFA in eWAT and prompted us to characterize in detail the immune cells in the tissue. Flow cytometry was performed using SVF cells isolated from eWAT (Figure 4A–F; for illustrative flow cytometry plots and gating strategy—see Figure 4G) and the appropriate panel of antibodies (Supplementary Tables S3 and S4). The number of leukocytes in the whole eWAT depot (CD45+ cell population containing the majority of the WAT immune cells [45]) increased 5.6- and 5.7-fold in the HFD and HFF mice, respectively, between Week 1 and Week 8. It was similar in both dietary groups at any given time (Figure 4A).

The corresponding increases in the number of eWAT macrophages (i.e., a subfraction of the leukocyte population characterized as $CD45^+/F4/80^+/CD11b^+$ cells) was ~7.4- (HFD) and ~5.3-fold (HFF); again, the cell number was not significantly affected by the diet (Figure 4B). However, the omega-3 PUFA supplementation tended to limit the high-fat diet induced increase in eWAT macrophage content (Figure 4B).

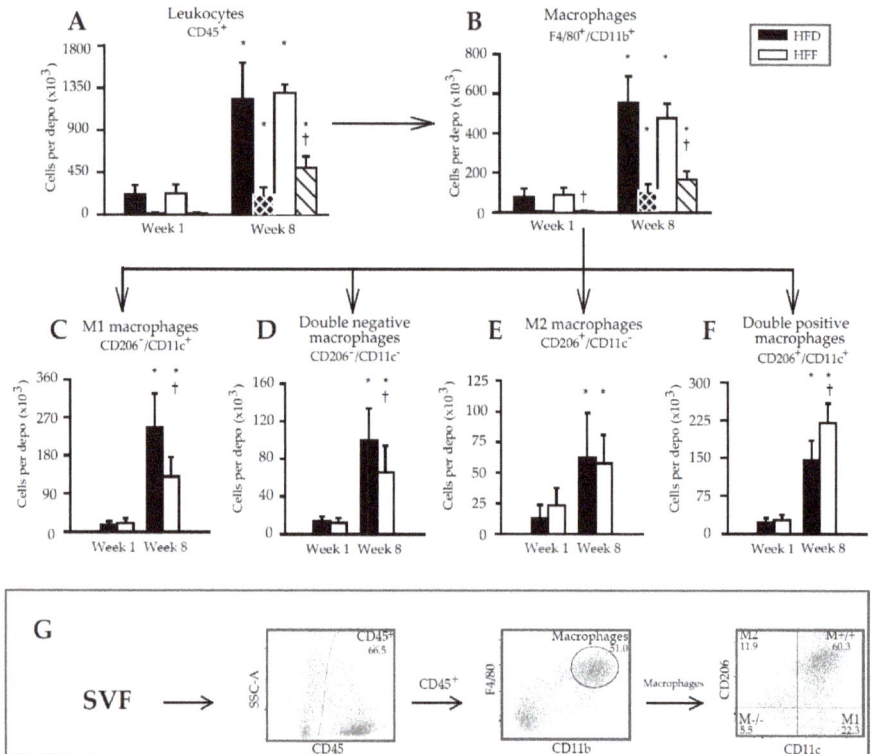

Figure 4. Flow cytometry analysis of immune cell subsets in SVF isolated from eWAT. Numbers of cells are calculated per depot. Arrows indicate the gating strategy used. Cells were first gated on size and singularity for further analysis. Single cells were gated based on the expression of CD45 to identify leukocytes (**A**). Leukocytes were then gated on the co-expression of CD11b and F4/80 to identify macrophages (**B**). Finally, macrophages were further subdivided based on the expression of CD206 and CD11c into: M1 macrophages ($CD206^-/CD11c^+$; **C**), double-negative macrophages ($CD206^-/CD11c^-$; **D**), M2 macrophages ($CD206^+/CD11c^-$; **E**) and double-positive macrophages ($CD206^+/CD11c^+$; **F**). Striped columns (black with white stripes, HFD; white with black stripes, HFF) show the amount of proliferating cells per depot, which were detected using antibodies specific for the Ki67 proliferation marker. Illustrative flow cytometry plots and gating strategy are also shown (**G**). Data are means ± SD.; $n = 6$–8. * Significant difference compared to Week 1 with the same diets; † significant difference between the diets for the same period of dietary intervention.

The proliferation of both leukocytes and macrophages in the SVF, assessed using Ki67 antibodies (Figure 4A,B; striped columns), was negligible at Week 1 but it was relatively high at Week 8. This induction was stronger in the HFF than the HFD mice, resulting in a significantly higher fraction of the proliferating cells in the total population of leukocytes and macrophages at Week 8 (Supplementary Figure S2).

Further subfractionation of the macrophage population was performed using the CD206 and CD11c markers, resulting in the detection of four different macrophage subtypes (Figure 4C–F). At Week 1, no differences between the dietary groups were found. At Week 8, the eWAT content of both CD206$^-$/CD11c$^+$ (M1; Figure 4C) and CD206$^-$/CD11c$^-$ (double negative; Figure 4D) macrophages was relatively low in the HFF mice. The eWAT content of CD206$^+$/CD11c$^-$ (M2; Figure 4E) macrophages did not differ between the subgroups, but CD206$^+$/CD11c$^+$ (double positive; Figure 4F) macrophages were more abundant in the HFF mice. The proportion in the content of M2 and M1 macrophages (i.e., the M2/M1 ratio; Figure 5) decreased between Week 1 and Week 8 in the HFD and tended to decrease in the HFF mice. The M2/M1 ratio tended to be higher in the HFF mice and this difference tended to increase with the duration of the dietary intervention. Both the relatively low number of M1 macrophages in the HFF mice at Week 8, and the relatively high number of double positive macrophages in these mice are consistent with the anti-inflammatory effect of the omega-3 PUFA supplementation [20,46].

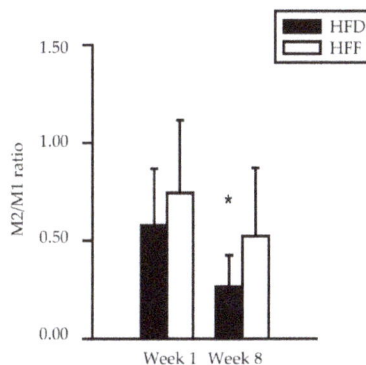

Figure 5. Ratio between M2 and M1 macrophages in eWAT of mice fed HFD or HFF diet for 1 week or 8 weeks as determined by flow cytometry. Data from Figure 4C,E were re-plotted. * Significant difference compared to Week 1 within the diets.

Thus, both qPCR and flow cytometry analysis revealed the lower pro-inflammatory profile of immune cells within eWAT in the HFF compared to the HFD mice at Week 8. However, neither the total number of macrophages nor the numbers of other cells in the leukocyte population, could explain the lower number of eWAT cells in the HFF mice at Week 8 (see the DNA content in Table 1).

2.4. Limited Increase in Adipose Lineage and Endothelial Cells Numbers in eWAT of Mice Fed High-Fat Diet in Response to Omega-3 PUFA

Changes in the immune cells number could not explain the abolishment of eWAT hyperplastic growth by omega-3 PUFA (although the changes in the composition of the immune cells could be important for this mechanism, see Discussion). Therefore, the CD45$^-$ cells contained in the SVF, i.e., the adipose lineage and endothelial cells [45], were characterized (Figure 6A–D; for illustrative flow cytometry plots and the gating strategy, see Figure 6E). In the HFD mice, the number of these cells (recalculated per the whole eWAT depot) was similar in the HFD and HFF mice at Week 1, while in the HFD mice, it increased ~2.7-fold between Week 1 and Week 8. The corresponding increase in the HFF mice was only ~1.2-fold, resulting in a ~2.2-fold lower number of CD45$^-$ cells in the eWAT of the HFF compared to the HFD mice at Week 8 (Figure 6A). The proliferation of CD45$^-$ cells (Figure 6A, striped columns; Supplementary Figure S3A) was similar in both dietary groups at Week 1, and it increased ~8.8-fold (HFD) and ~5.1-fold (HFF) between Week 1 and Week 8. Thus, at Week 8, the fraction of the proliferating cells in the total CD45$^-$ cell population was higher in the HFF than in the HFD mice (Figure 6A; Supplementary Figure S3A).

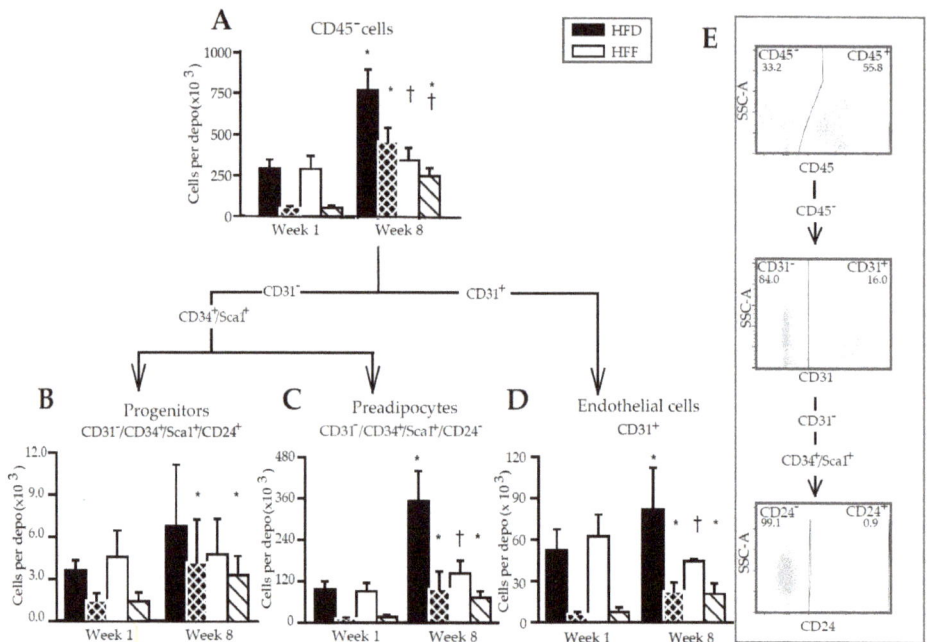

Figure 6. Flow cytometry analysis of non-immune cell subsets in SVF isolated from eWAT. The numbers of cells are calculated per depot. Arrows indicate the gating strategy used. Cells were first gated on size and singularity for further analysis. Single cells were gated on the lack of CD45 expression to identify non-lymfoid cells (**A**). CD45$^-$ cells were then gated on CD31 expression to identify endothelial cells (**D**). CD31$^-$ cells were further subdivided based on the expression of Sca1, CD34 and CD24 into progenitors (CD34$^+$/Sca1$^+$/CD24$^+$; **B**) and preadipocytes (CD34$^+$/Sca1$^+$/CD24$^-$; **C**). Striped columns (black with white stripes, HFD; white with black stripes, HFF) show the amount of proliferating cells per depot, which were detected using antibodies specific for the Ki67 proliferation marker. Illustrative flow cytometry plots and gating strategy are also shown (**E**). Data are means ± SD; n = 5–6. * Significant difference compared to Week 1 for mice fed the same diet; † significant difference between the diets for the same period of dietary intervention.

Further analysis of the CD45$^-$ cell population using the CD31, CD34, Sca1, and CD24 markers enabled the adipose progenitor cells (Figure 6B), preadipocytes (Figure 6C) and endothelial cells (Figure 6D) to be characterized. The eWAT quantity of progenitors was similar in all the groups, irrespective of the duration of high-fat feeding or the omega-3 PUFA supplementation, while the proliferation of these cells increased ~2.8-fold (HFD) and ~2.3-fold (HFF) between Week 1 and Week 8 (Figure 6B; Supplementary Figure S3B).

The eWAT number of preadipocytes did not differ between the HFD and HFF mice at Week 1, and increased much more in the HFD (~3.7- fold) compared with the HFF (~1.6-fold) mice between Week 1 and Week 8, resulting in ~2.5-fold lower number of preadipocytes in the HFF mice compared to the HFD mice at Week 8 (Figure 6C). This was in agreement with the expression of several markers of adipogenesis and mainly of preadipocyte factor 1 (*Pref1*, a marker of preadipocytes and inhibitor of adipocyte differentiation [47]), which was relatively low in both the eWAT and SVF of the HFF mice at Week 8, but was similar in adipocytes isolated from the eWAT of both dietary groups (Supplementary Table S5). Also, the expression of the genes for peroxisome proliferator-activated receptor γ (*Pparg;* a late adipogenic marker; [9]) and platelet-derived growth factor receptor β (*Pdgfrb;* expressed mainly in adipocyte progenitor cells [48]) was relatively low in the SVF isolated from the eWAT of the HFF mice at Week 8 (Supplementary Table S5). The proliferation of preadipocytes was increased in response to high-fat feeding, resulting in a ~7.7-fold (HFD) and ~4.2-fold (HFF) elevation between Week 1 and Week 8 (Figure 6C; Supplementary Figure S3C).

The number of eWAT endothelial cells was similar in all groups, except for Week 8, when the number of these cells was ~1.8-fold lower in the HFF than the HFD mice (Figure 6D). The proliferation of endothelial cells was increased in response to high-fat feeding, i.e., exhibiting a ~3.7-fold (HFD) and ~2.7-fold (HFF) increase between Week 1 and Week 8 (Figure 6D; Supplementary Figure S3D).

Collectively (see also Supplementary Figure S4), the above results documented that counteracting the HFD-driven increase in eWAT cell number by omega-3 PUFA supplementation did not reflect a change in the number of leukocytes. On the contrary, the abolishment of eWAT hyperplasia reflected selective changes in the development of the adipose lineage and endothelial cells, especially in terms of abolishing the increase in the number of preadipocytes and the decrease in the number of endothelial cells. The number of proliferating cells in all the identified classes of CD45$^-$ cells did not differ between the dietary groups (Figure 6A–D); however, when expressed as a percentage, the proportion of proliferating cells was higher in the HFF than the HFD mice at Week 8 (Supplementary Figure S3).

3. Discussion

This study was focused on the mechanism by which omega-3 PUFA limit the accumulation of WAT in mice fed an obesogenic high-fat diet. We confirmed the previous results documenting that both hypertrophy and hyperplasia of eWAT were partially counteracted by the omega-3 PUFA supplementation of the diet (reviewed in [26,32]). The principal new finding was that while the hyperplastic growth of the tissue resulted from the increased number of leukocytes, as well as the adipose lineage and endothelial cells, the amelioration of eWAT hyperplasia by omega-3 PUFA was reflected in the reduced numbers of preadipocytes and adipocytes as well as endothelial cells, but not the immune cells.

Our results support the view that the activity of the immune cells in WAT and tissue metabolism are closely connected ([31]). They suggest that both (i) increased levels of EPA and DHA, and (ii) changing pattern of formation of lipid mediators and cytokines/adipokines in WAT, in response to the omega-3 PUFA supplementation, could trigger the counteraction of the diet-induced hypertrophy and hyperplasia of the tissue. Specifically the time-dependent induction of the anti-inflammatory 5-HEPE and 17,18-diHETE, in the face of the decreased content of pro-inflammatory HETEs (5-HETE, 8-HETE, 12-HETE and 15-HETE), was probably involved (for the biochemical pathways of the formation of these lipid mediators, see reviews [25,26]). Accordingly, a reduced expression of the genes for pro-inflammatory enzyme (*Nos2*) and cytokines (*Tnfa*, *Tgfb* and *Il1b*) was also observed (for more information about these markers, see [29,30]).

Macrophages, adipocytes, as well as other cells contained in WAT represent the source of the above signalling molecules. However, precise identification of the cells involved is not known and was outside the scope of this study. The observed changes in the abundance of the four subtypes of WAT macrophages in response to the omega-3 PUFA supplementation, observed at Week 8, were in general agreement with the involvement of these cells in the change in WAT inflammatory status and the secretion of lipid mediators and adipokines. Thus, the content of the pro-inflammatory M1 macrophages decreased. The double-positive (mixed M1/M2) macrophage content was higher in the HFF than in the HFD mice, in accordance with the possible involvement of these cells in the resolution of WAT inflammation [46] as well as relatively high activity of lipid catabolism in these cells [49], which is linked with the anti-inflammatory macrophage phenotype (reviewed in [25]). A decrease in the content of double-negative macrophages in response to the omega-3 PUFA supplementation was also observed. However, the role of these cells in inflammatory status remains poorly defined. In accordance with the previous study [50], MGCs were detected in the HFF mice at Week 8. MGCs are formed by the fusion of M2 or double-positive macrophages [41], with the participation of scavenger receptor CD36 [51]. These cells have an enhanced reactive oxygen species generating capacity [41] and are engaged in tissue remodeling and repair [42]. Therefore, MGCs probably contributed to tissue remodeling in response to omega-3 PUFA.

Regarding the limitation of the high-fat-diet-induced WAT hypertrophy by the omega-3 PUFA, it should be stressed that this effect was independent of food consumption [33,52]. On the other hand, the induction of fatty acid oxidation in response to omega-3 PUFA was observed in the liver [53], intestine [54], muscle [55,56], and possibly also in brown fat and other tissues (reviewed by us in [25,26,32,35]). In particular, modulation of the cross talk between WAT and liver metabolism could play an important role in the counteraction of eWAT hypertrophy [25,57]. The above metabolic effects of omega-3 PUFA are mediated by (i) these PUFA themselves, (ii) their bioactive metabolites—lipid mediators, or (iii) suppression of tissue levels of endocannabinoids; all these potential mechanisms operate also in WAT (reviewed in [25,26,35]). Multiple receptors and intracellular signalling pathways involved in the modification of WAT immunometabolism by omega-3 PUFA and related lipid mediators (see above) have been identified (reviewed in [26,32]; see Figure 1 of ref. [25]).

Regarding the limitation of the high-fat diet-induced WAT hyperplasia by the omega-3 PUFA, it should be stressed that especially in rodents, WAT exerts a high potential for hyperplastic growth (see [8,13,16–18]). Therefore, the mouse model is instrumental to characterize this omega-3 PUFA effect. This WAT hyperplastic remodeling can be very quick [8,16], as it includes the proliferation of immune cells [13,34,58,59] as well as adipocyte progenitor cells and their differentiation into preadipocytes [8,16,17,60,61]. As for the eWAT immune cells studied here, the strong elevation in the leukocytes (including macrophages) content in response to high-fat feeding was documented using both flow cytometry and immunostaining of the CLS-contained macrophages. Both approaches revealed a trend for a lower macrophage content in the HFF than in the HFD mice at Week 8, but the differences were not significant. These results were consistent with some of the previous studies in mice from our laboratory [33,62] and by others [50]. They are also in agreement with some human studies [63,64], showing no effect of omega-3 PUFA on WAT macrophage content [33,62]. On the other hand, the reduction of WAT macrophage content by omega-3 PUFA was also observed before, both in dietary obese mice [33,34,65,66] and human subjects with insulin resistance [67]. Due to the many variables involved, the reasons for this discrepancy remain unknown.

As for the adipose lineage cells contained in the CD45$^-$ population [45] studied here (except for the mature adipocytes), the expected increase in the number of these cells in response to high-fat feeding was observed (flow cytometry data). Supplementation of the diet with omega-3 PUFA completely eliminated the induction of the CD45$^-$ cells population. The effect on the CD45$^-$ cells population especially reflected the compromised increase in the number of preadipocytes. The immune cells were not involved in the reduction of eWAT cells number by omega-3 PUFA. However, these cells could interact with the adipose lineage cells and contribute to this limitation. For instance, M2 macrophages inhibit the proliferation of adipogenic precursors through the CD206/TGFb signalling pathway [68]. Also 9- and 13-HODE (see Figure 2) are involved in the communication of macrophages with preadipocytes [69].

Furthermore, also a reduction in the endothelial cells content in eWAT in response to the omega-3 PUFA supplementation was observed at Week 8, despite the number of endothelial cells was not affected by the HFD feeding. It has been published that angiogenesis was regulated by PUFA at least in part through the action of the prostanoids (suppressed by prostaglandin E3 and augmented by prostaglandin E2; [70]). Therefore, in the reduction of endothelial cells number, the observed decrease in prostaglandin E2 levels could be involved. Moreover, 12/15 LOX is associated with monocyte-endothelial interaction [71]; indeed lower levels of 12-HETE in the HFF as compared to HFD mice were found (see Supplementary Table S1).

The limitation of this study is the lack of quantitative information regarding the adipocytes abundance in eWAT, however, DNA content measurement in the collagenase-liberated adipocytes from eWAT suggested that mature adipocytes contributed to both (i) the increase in eWAT cell number induced by a high-fat diet, and (ii) the amelioration of this process by omega-3 PUFA supplementation.

Since the proportion of proliferating non-immune cells (including the progenitors and preadipocytes) as well as endothelial cells in the whole population of these cells was higher at Week 8 in the HFF than in the HFD mice, while the eWAT content of these cells was lower in the HFF mice, it is to be inferred that the omega-3 PUFA supplementation likely resulted in increased removal/turnover of the above cell types in the eWAT of the obese mice. Indeed, previous studies described the induction of the apoptosis of preadipocytes/adipocytes by omega-3 PUFA, both in vivo in the WAT of mice [72] and *in vitro* in adipocytes differentiating in cell culture [73,74]. In addition, omega-3 PUFA-derived lipid mediators were shown to be involved in the regulation of apoptosis, e.g., with the products of 5- and 12-LOX (5-HETE and 12-HETE) exerting an inhibitory effect *in vitro* [72,75]. This is in agreement with our lipidomic data at Week 8, showing that: (i) 5-HETE and 12-HETE belonged to the most discriminating analytes between the HFD and HFF mice; and (ii) the levels of both HETEs were relatively low in the HFF mice (see Supplementary Table S1).

In this study, we focused on eWAT, the typical WAT depot forming the majority of abdominal fat in dietary obese mice [33,35,62,76]. However, our previous study documented that the hyperplastic growth of subcutaneous WAT in the mice was also compromised by the omega-3 PUFA supplementation, although a relatively high dose of omega-3 PUFA was required [36]. These results suggested that omega-3 PUFA could reduce the hyperplastic growth of all WAT depots. Fat-depot-specific differences in sensitivity to omega-3 PUFA may exist. That the effect is highly pronounced in WAT in the abdomen may be of practical importance. It has been known for a long time that the accumulation of visceral fat, which characterizes upper body obesity, correlates with metabolic syndrome [77].

This study helps to better understand the mechanism behind the prevention of obesity development by omega-3 PUFA, which is frequently observed in animal models (see our previous studies [33,34,36,52,78], and studies by others; reviewed in [25]) but is of only marginal significance in humans (reviewed in [25]). There may be multiple reasons for this discrepancy, including the dose of omega-3 [35], the effect of the composition of the bulk of dietary lipids [62], possible inter-species differences in intracellular signalling and the formation of lipid mediators involved in the effects of omega-3 PUFA, and others. Whether the reversal of obesity in response to omega-3 PUFA in mice [30,66,76] also reflects in part the reduction of tissue cell number remains to be established.

In conclusion, our results provide evidence for the involvement of omega-3 PUFA in the remodelling of WAT in mice fed a high-fat diet. Changes in macrophages polarization, reflected by their morphology and metabolism, but not the number of immune cells *per se*, contributed to the remodelling process. Prevention of the diet-induced hyperplasia of WAT by omega-3 PUFA could be explained by a limited increase in the number of adipose lineage cells, as well as by the decrease in the number of endothelial cells. To the best of our knowledge, to date the prevention of diet-induced hyperplasia of WAT by omega-3 PUFA is only documented by this and two previous studies from our laboratory [36,37]. Our results support the notion [7,37] that adiposity is closely linked to the control of fat cell turnover and that there could be mechanisms that control fat cell proliferation independently of energy balance.

4. Materials and Methods

4.1. Animals

Male mice (C57BL/6N, Charles River, Germany) were fed the STD diet (3.4% wt/wt as lipids; extruded ssniff R/M-H from Ssniff Spezialdiaten GmbH, Soest, Germany) from the moment they were brought to the institute´s animal house at the age of 6 weeks and maintained on a 12-h light/dark cycle (light from 6:00 a.m.) at 22 °C. At 13 weeks of age, mice were randomly divided into three groups that were subjected to various dietary interventions (i) the STD diet, (ii) a corn oil-based high-fat diet (HFD diet; ~35% wt/wt as lipids; or (iii) an HFD-based diet, in which 15% (wt/wt) of dietary lipids (corn oil) was replaced with the EPA + DHA triglyceride concentrate Epax 1050 TG (HFF diet; Epax 1050 TG contained ~14% EPA and ~46% DHA, wt/wt; EPAX AS, Aalesund, Norway) to achieve a total EPA + DHA concentration of ~30 g/kg diet. The numbers of animals are specified in each caption. For the macronutrient and fatty acid composition of the diets, see ESM Tables 1 and 2 of [34] (the HFD and HFF diets are identical with the cHF and cHF + F diets, respectively). The omega-6/omega-3 ratio based on the fatty acid composition of the diets is 26.5 for HFD and 3.5 for HFF, respectively (see [34]). Both high-fat diets were prepared at the Institute of Physiology in Prague (Prague, Czech Republic) as described previously (see ESM Table 1 of [34]). These diets have already been used in several studies [33–37,43,54,55,62,76].

Two dietary intervention experiments (see above) were performed lasting either 1 or 8 weeks. Animals were killed under ether anesthesia in a random-fed state (between 8:00 and 10:00 a.m.). Body weight and food consumption were recorded daily during Week 1, and then weekly during the later stages of the differential dietary treatment. eWAT was collected and either flash frozen and stored in liquid nitrogen or processed for ex vivo biochemical analyses. All animal procedures were conducted in accordance with all appropriate regulatory standards under protocol 81/2016 (approval date: 2016-10-18) approved by Animal Care and Use Committee of the Czech Academy of Sciences and followed the guidelines for the use and care of laboratory animals of the Institute of Physiology.

4.2. RNA Isolation and Gene Expression Analysis

Total RNA was isolated from eWAT (~100 mg) using TRI Reagent (Sigma-Aldrich, Prague, Czech Republic, see [33]). qPCR and a LightCycler480 (Roche, Prague, Czech Republic) were used to determine the mRNA levels of various transcripts. Data were normalized to the geometrical mean of two reference genes hypoxanthine guanine phosphoribosyl transferase (*Hprt*) and eukaryotic translation elongation factor 1 alpha 1 *(EF1a)* for the analysis using whole eWAT samples and *EF1α* and 18S ribosomal RNA (*Rn18s*) for the analysis using SVF and adipocyte fractions; see Supplementary Table S6 for PCR primer sequences.

4.3. Flow Cytometry

eWAT was enzymatically digested in Krebs-Ringer Bicarbonate Buffer (KRB; pH = 7.4) containing 0.1% collagenase type (Sigma-Aldrich, Munich, Germany) and 4% BSA for 30 min at 37 °C. Released cells were spun down (500× g, 10 min, 4 °C) to separate SVF cells from floating adipocytes. SVF cells were resuspended in KRB containing 10 mM EDTA and 4% BSA, and passed through a 42 μm filter. Red blood cells were lysed using the Lysis Buffer (eBioscience, San Diego, CA, USA). Cells were incubated in Fc block solution for the prevention of non-specific binding (AntiMouse CD16/CD32; eBioScience, San Diego, CA, USA) for 10 min on ice and stained with the indicated antibodies against extracellular markers for 30 min at 4 °C (see Supplementary Tables S3 and S4 for the antibodies). Before intracellular staining, the cells were fixed and permeabilized (Intracellular Fix and Perm Set, eBioScience, San Diego, CA, USA), and then stained with Ki67 antibody for 30 min at 4 °C. After washing, the stained cells were analyzed using a BD LSR II flow cytometer (BD Biosciences, San Jose, CA, USA). Data were analyzed using FlowJo 10.2 software (Tree Star, Ashland, OR, USA).

4.4. Analysis of Lipid Mediators

Lipid mediators were purified from eWAT samples (~100 mg), flash-frozen and stored in liquid nitrogen after dissection, using solid phase extraction procedure as before [35]. Analysis was performed using a UPLC-MS/MS platform (Ultimate 3000 RSLC, Dionex/Thermo and QTRAP 5500, AB SCIEX, Framingham, MA, USA) equipped with a C18 column 150 cm × 2.1 cm, 1.9 μm with a precolumn. Analytes were ionized in negative ion mode and detected with a multiple reaction monitoring method as before [24,35].

4.5. DNA Measurement

DNA was estimated fluorometrically using Hoechst 3328 in tissue and adipocytes samples digested with proteinase K as before [79].

4.6. Histological and Immunohistochemical Analysis of eWAT

These analyses were performed similarly as described previously [28]. Formalin-fixed paraffin-embedded sections (5 μm) were stained using hematoxylin–eosin for the morphometry of adipocytes, or processed by immunohistochemistry or immunofluorescence. The morphometry data are based on approximately 800 cells taken randomly from two to three different eWAT sections per animal. The presence of macrophages in CLS was detected using anti-Mac2 antibodies. The abundance of dying adipocytes marked by CLS in eWAT sections was expressed as % of all adipocytes. In immunofluorescence analyses, perilipin 1-negative adipocytes, surrounded by macrophages (F4/80+ cells) that formed CLS, were considered to represent dying adipocytes. Within the CLS, proliferating (Ki67 stained) nuclei were identified and their relative (% of all 4′,6-diamidine-2′-phenylindole dihydrochloride (DAPI) positive nuclei) content was quantified. All analyses were performed using the imaging software NIS-Elements AR3.0 (Laboratory Imaging, Prague, Czech Republic). For the primary and secondary antibodies specification, see Supplementary Table S7.

4.7. Statistical Analysis

All values are presented as means ± SD. Comparisons were judged to be significant at $p < 0.05$. Data were analyzed by analysis of variance (one-way or two-way ANOVA). SigmaStat 3.5 software (Systat Software, San Jose, CA, USA) was used for statistical evaluation. Logarithmic, square-root or reciprocal transformations were used to stabilize variance or normality of samples when necessary. PCA, a multivariate statistical analysis, was used for the lipidomic data evaluation. Analysis was performed using the statistical software SIMCA-P+12 (Umetrics AB, Malmo, Sweden).

Supplementary Materials: The following are available online at http://www.mdpi.com/1660-3397/16/12/515/s1, Supplementary Table S1: Effects of the omega-3 PUFA supplementation on lipid mediators evaluated in eWAT extracts; Supplementary Table S2: Effect of the omega-3 PUFA supplementation on relative mRNA levels of the genes for enzymes involved in metabolism of polyunsaturated fatty acids; Supplementary Table S3: Antibodies used for flow cytometry; Supplementary Table S4: Specific panels of markers used to identify different cell populations; Supplementary Table S5: Effect of the omega-3 PUFA supplementation on relative mRNA levels of the genes for enzymes involved in adipogenesis; Supplementary Table S6: Sequences of primers; Supplementary Table S7: Antibodies used for immunohistochemistry; Supplementary Figure S1: Morphology and immunohistochemistry of eWAT at Week 1; Supplementary Figure S2 Percentage of proliferating leukocytes and macrophages in SVF of eWAT of mice fed HFD or HFF diet for 1 or 8 weeks determined using flow cytometry; Supplementary Figure S3 Percentage of proliferating CD45- cells, progenitors, preadipocytes and endothelial cells in SVF of eWAT of mice fed HFD or HFF diet for 1 or 8 weeks determined using flow cytometry; Supplementary Figure S4 Flow cytometry analysis of cells subsets in SVF isolated from eWAT.

Author Contributions: Conceptualization, K.A., K.B., O.H., M.R. and J.K.; Methodology, O.H., K.A., K.B., P.J., M.B. and O.K.; Investigation, K.A., O.H., K.B., P.J., M.B. and O.K.; Writing-Original Draft Preparation, K.A., K.B., O.H., M.R. and J.K.; Funding Acquisition, J.K.

Funding: This research was funded by the Czech Science Foundation (16-05151S) and MEYS (LM2015062 Czech-BioImaging).

Acknowledgments: We wish to thank (i) Nathalie Boulet for the help with flow cytometry, and (ii) EPAX AS, Aalesund, Norway for the Epax 1050 TG concentrate.

Conflicts of Interest: The authors declare no conflict of interest.

References

1. Schwartz, M.W.; Seeley, R.J.; Zeltser, L.M.; Drewnowski, A.; Ravussin, E.; Redman, L.M.; Leibel, R.L. Obesity Pathogenesis: An Endocrine Society Scientific Statement. *Endoc. Rev.* **2017**. [CrossRef] [PubMed]
2. Cannon, B.; Nedergaard, J. Brown adipose tissue: Function and physiological significance. *Physiol. Rev.* **2004**, *84*, 277–359. [CrossRef] [PubMed]
3. Kopecky, J. Adipose Tissue and Fat Cell Biology. In *Lipids and Skin Health*; Pappas, A., Ed.; Springer Science: New York, NY, USA, 2015; pp. 201–224.
4. Lee, M.J.; Wu, Y.; Fried, S.K. Adipose tissue heterogeneity: Implication of depot differences in adipose tissue for obesity complications. *Mol. Asp. Med.* **2013**, *34*, 1–11. [CrossRef] [PubMed]

5. Virtue, S.; Vidal-Puig, A. Adipose tissue expandability, lipotoxicity and the Metabolic Syndrome—An allostatic perspective. *Biochim. Biophys. Acta* **2010**, *1801*, 338–349. [CrossRef] [PubMed]

6. Kissebah, A.H.; Krakower, G.R. Regional adiposity and morbidity. *Physiol. Rev.* **1994**, *74*, 761–811. [CrossRef] [PubMed]

7. Spalding, K.L.; Arner, E.; Westermark, P.O.; Bernard, S.; Buchholz, B.A.; Bergmann, O.; Blomqvist, L.; Hoffstedt, J.; Naslund, E.; Britton, T.; et al. Dynamics of fat cell turnover in humans. *Nature* **2008**, *453*, 783–787. [CrossRef] [PubMed]

8. Wang, Q.A.; Tao, C.; Gupta, R.K.; Scherer, P.E. Tracking adipogenesis during white adipose tissue development, expansion and regeneration. *Nat. Med.* **2013**, *19*, 1338–1344. [CrossRef] [PubMed]

9. Berry, R.; Rodeheffer, M.S. Characterization of the adipocyte cellular lineage in vivo. *Nat. Cell Biol.* **2013**, *15*, 302–308. [CrossRef] [PubMed]

10. Nishimura, S.; Manabe, I.; Nagasaki, M.; Hosoya, Y.; Yamashita, H.; Fujita, H.; Ohsugi, M.; Tobe, K.; Kadowaki, T.; Nagai, R.; et al. Adipogenesis in obesity requires close interplay between differentiating adipocytes, stromal cells, and blood vessels. *Diabetes* **2007**, *56*, 1517–1526. [CrossRef] [PubMed]

11. Tran, K.V.; Gealekman, O.; Frontini, A.; Zingaretti, M.C.; Morroni, M.; Giordano, A.; Smorlesi, A.; Perugini, J.; De Matteis, R.; Sbarbati, A.; et al. The vascular endothelium of the adipose tissue gives rise to both white and brown fat cells. *Cell Metab.* **2012**, *15*, 222–229. [CrossRef] [PubMed]

12. Arner, P.; Bernard, S.; Salehpour, M.; Possnert, G.; Liebl, J.; Steier, P.; Buchholz, B.A.; Eriksson, M.; Arner, E.; Hauner, H.; et al. Dynamics of human adipose lipid turnover in health and metabolic disease. *Nature* **2011**, *478*, 110–113. [CrossRef] [PubMed]

13. van Beek, L.; van Klinken, J.B.; Pronk, A.C.; van Dam, A.D.; Dirven, E.; Rensen, P.C.; Koning, F.; Willems van Dijk, K.; van Harmelen, V. The limited storage capacity of gonadal adipose tissue directs the development of metabolic disorders in male C57Bl/6J mice. *Diabetologia* **2015**, *58*, 1601–1609. [CrossRef] [PubMed]

14. Walden, T.B.; Hansen, I.R.; Timmons, J.A.; Cannon, B.; Nedergaard, J. Recruited vs. nonrecruited molecular signatures of brown, "brite," and white adipose tissues. *Am. J. Physiol.-Endocrinol. Metab.* **2012**, *302*, E19–E31. [CrossRef] [PubMed]

15. Chusyd, D.E.; Wang, D.; Huffman, D.M.; Nagy, T.R. Relationships between Rodent White Adipose Fat Pads and Human White Adipose Fat Depots. *Front. Nutr.* **2016**, *3*, 10. [CrossRef] [PubMed]

16. Jeffery, E.; Church, C.D.; Holtrup, B.; Colman, L.; Rodeheffer, M.S. Rapid depot-specific activation of adipocyte precursor cells at the onset of obesity. *Nat. Cell Biol.* **2015**, *17*, 376–385. [CrossRef] [PubMed]

17. Joe, A.W.; Yi, L.; Even, Y.; Vogl, A.W.; Rossi, F.M. Depot-specific differences in adipogenic progenitor abundance and proliferative response to high-fat diet. *Stem Cells* **2009**, *27*, 2563–2570. [CrossRef] [PubMed]

18. Wang, X.; Cheng, M.; Zhao, M.; Ge, A.; Guo, F.; Zhang, M.; Yang, Y.; Liu, L.; Yang, N. Differential effects of high-fat-diet rich in lard oil or soybean oil on osteopontin expression and inflammation of adipose tissue in diet-induced obese rats. *Eur. J. Nutr.* **2013**, *52*, 1181–1189. [CrossRef] [PubMed]

19. Schipper, H.S.; Prakken, B.; Kalkhoven, E.; Boes, M. Adipose tissue-resident immune cells: Key players in immunometabolism. *Trends Endocrinol. Metab.* **2012**, *23*, 407–415. [CrossRef] [PubMed]

20. Lumeng, C.N.; Deyoung, S.M.; Bodzin, J.L.; Saltiel, A.R. Increased inflammatory properties of adipose tissue macrophages recruited during diet-induced obesity. *Diabetes* **2007**, *56*, 16–23. [CrossRef] [PubMed]

21. Pirzgalska, R.M.; Seixas, E.; Seidman, J.S.; Link, V.M.; Sanchez, N.M.; Mahu, I.; Mendes, R.; Gres, V.; Kubasova, N.; Morris, I.; et al. Sympathetic neuron-associated macrophages contribute to obesity by importing and metabolizing norepinephrine. *Nat. Med.* **2017**, *23*, 1309–1318. [CrossRef] [PubMed]

22. Freemerman, A.J.; Johnson, A.R.; Sacks, G.N.; Milner, J.J.; Kirk, E.L.; Troester, M.A.; Macintyre, A.N.; Goraksha-Hicks, P.; Rathmell, J.C.; Makowski, L. Metabolic reprogramming of macrophages: Glucose transporter 1 (GLUT1)-mediated glucose metabolism drives a proinflammatory phenotype. *J. Biol. Chem.* **2014**, *289*, 7884–7896. [CrossRef] [PubMed]

23. Koliwad, S.K.; Streeper, R.S.; Monetti, M.; Cornelissen, I.; Chan, L.; Terayama, K.; Naylor, S.; Rao, M.; Hubbard, B.; Farese, R.V., Jr. DGAT1-dependent triacylglycerol storage by macrophages protects mice from diet-induced insulin resistance and inflammation. *J. Clin. Investig.* **2010**, *120*, 756–767. [CrossRef] [PubMed]

24. Rombaldova, M.; Janovska, P.; Kopecky, J.; Kuda, O. Omega-3 fatty acids promote fatty acid utilization and production of pro-resolving lipid mediators in alternatively activated adipose tissue macrophages. *Biochem. Biophys. Res. Commun.* **2017**, *490*, 1080–1085. [CrossRef] [PubMed]

25. Kuda, O.; Rossmeisl, M.; Kopecky, J. Omega-3 fatty acids and adipose tissue biology. *Mol. Aspects Med.* **2018**, 1–14. [CrossRef] [PubMed]

26. Masoodi, M.; Kuda, O.; Rossmeisl, M.; Flachs, P.; Kopecky, J. Lipid signaling in adipose tissue: Connecting inflammation & metabolism. *Biochim. Biophys. Acta* **2015**, *1851*, 503–518. [CrossRef] [PubMed]

27. Tang, W.; Zeve, D.; Suh, J.M.; Bosnakovski, D.; Kyba, M.; Hammer, R.E.; Tallquist, M.D.; Graff, J.M. White fat progenitor cells reside in the adipose vasculature. *Science* **2008**, *322*, 583–586. [CrossRef] [PubMed]

28. Lee, Y.H.; Petkova, A.P.; Granneman, J.G. Identification of an adipogenic niche for adipose tissue remodeling and restoration. *Cell Metab.* **2013**, *18*, 355–367. [CrossRef] [PubMed]

29. Lee, Y.H.; Thacker, R.I.; Hall, B.E.; Kong, R.; Granneman, J.G. Exploring the activated adipogenic niche: Interactions of macrophages and adipocyte progenitors. *Cell Cycle* **2014**, *13*, 184–190. [CrossRef] [PubMed]

30. Jilkova, Z.M.; Hensler, M.; Medrikova, D.; Janovska, P.; Horakova, O.; Rossmeisl, M.; Flachs, P.; Sell, H.; Eckel, J.; Kopecky, J. Adipose tissue-related proteins locally associated with resolution of inflammation in obese mice. *Int. J. Obes. (Lond.)* **2014**, *38*, 216–223. [CrossRef] [PubMed]

31. Man, K.; Kutyavin, V.I.; Chawla, A. Tissue Immunometabolism: Development, Physiology, and Pathobiology. *Cell Metab.* **2017**, *25*, 11–26. [CrossRef] [PubMed]

32. Flachs, P.; Rossmeisl, M.; Kuda, O.; Kopecky, J. Stimulation of mitochondrial oxidative capacity in white fat independent of UCP1: A key to lean phenotype. *Biochim. Biophys. Acta* **2013**, *1831*, 986–1003. [CrossRef] [PubMed]

33. Flachs, P.; Ruhl, R.; Hensler, M.; Janovska, P.; Zouhar, P.; Kus, V.; Macek, J.Z.; Papp, E.; Kuda, O.; Svobodova, M.; et al. Synergistic induction of lipid catabolism and anti-inflammatory lipids in white fat of dietary obese mice in response to calorie restriction and n-3 fatty acids. *Diabetologia* **2011**, *54*, 2626–2638. [CrossRef] [PubMed]

34. Kuda, O.; Jelenik, T.; Jilkova, Z.; Flachs, P.; Rossmeisl, M.; Hensler, M.; Kazdova, L.; Ogston, N.; Baranowski, M.; Gorski, J.; et al. *n*-3 fatty acids and rosiglitazone improve insulin sensitivity through additive stimulatory effects on muscle glycogen synthesis in mice fed a high-fat diet. *Diabetologia* **2009**, *52*, 941–951. [CrossRef] [PubMed]

35. Rossmeisl, M.; Pavlisova, J.; Janovska, P.; Kuda, O.; Bardova, K.; Hansikova, J.; Svobodova, M.; Oseeva, M.; Veleba, J.; Kopecky, J., Jr.; et al. Differential modulation of white adipose tissue endocannabinoid levels by n-3 fatty acids in obese mice and type 2 diabetic patients. *Biochim. Biophys. Acta* **2018**, *1863*, 712–725. [CrossRef] [PubMed]

36. Ruzickova, J.; Rossmeisl, M.; Prazak, T.; Flachs, P.; Sponarova, J.; Vecka, M.; Tvrzicka, E.; Bryhn, M.; Kopecky, J. Omega-3 PUFA of marine origin limit diet-induced obesity in mice by reducing cellularity of adipose tissue. *Lipids* **2004**, *39*, 1177–1185. [CrossRef] [PubMed]

37. Hensler, M.; Bardova, K.; Jilkova, Z.M.; Wahli, W.; Meztger, D.; Chambon, P.; Kopecky, J.; Flachs, P. The inhibition of fat cell proliferation by n-3 fatty acids in dietary obese mice. *Lipids Health Dis.* **2011**, *10*, 128. [CrossRef] [PubMed]

38. Cinti, S.; Mitchell, G.; Barbatelli, G.; Murano, I.; Ceresi, E.; Faloia, E.; Wang, S.; Fortier, M.; Greenberg, A.S.; Obin, M.S. Adipocyte death defines macrophage localization and function in adipose tissue of obese mice and humans. *J. Lipid Res.* **2005**, *46*, 2347–2355. [CrossRef] [PubMed]

39. Haase, J.; Weyer, U.; Immig, K.; Kloting, N.; Bluher, M.; Eilers, J.; Bechmann, I.; Gericke, M. Local proliferation of macrophages in adipose tissue during obesity-induced inflammation. *Diabetologia* **2014**, *57*, 562–571. [CrossRef] [PubMed]

40. Sobecki, M.; Mrouj, K.; Camasses, A.; Parisis, N.; Nicolas, E.; Lleres, D.; Gerbe, F.; Prieto, S.; Krasinska, L.; David, A.; et al. The cell proliferation antigen Ki-67 organises heterochromatin. *Elife* **2016**, *5*, e13722. [CrossRef] [PubMed]

41. Quinn, M.T.; Schepetkin, I.A. Role of NADPH oxidase in formation and function of multinucleated giant cells. *J. Innate Immun.* **2009**, *1*, 509–526. [CrossRef] [PubMed]

42. Hernandez-Pando, R.; Bornstein, Q.L.; Aguilar Leon, D.; Orozco, E.H.; Madrigal, V.K.; Martinez Cordero, E. Inflammatory cytokine production by immunological and foreign body multinucleated giant cells. *Immunology* **2000**, *100*, 352–358. [CrossRef] [PubMed]

43. Kuda, O.; Rombaldova, M.; Janovska, P.; Flachs, P.; Kopecky, J. Cell type-specific modulation of lipid mediator's formation in murine adipose tissue by omega-3 fatty acids. *Biochem. Biophys. Res. Commun.* **2016**, *469*, 731–736. [CrossRef] [PubMed]

44. Buczynski, M.W.; Dumlao, D.S.; Dennis, E.A. Thematic Review Series: Proteomics. An integrated omics analysis of eicosanoid biology. *J. Lipid Res.* **2009**, *50*, 1015–1038. [CrossRef] [PubMed]

45. Baer, P.C. Adipose-derived mesenchymal stromal/stem cells: An update on their phenotype in vivo and in vitro. *World J. Stem Cells* **2014**, *6*, 256–265. [CrossRef] [PubMed]

46. Bystrom, J.; Evans, I.; Newson, J.; Stables, M.; Toor, I.; van Rooijen, N.; Crawford, M.; Colville-Nash, P.; Farrow, S.; Gilroy, D.W. Resolution-phase macrophages possess a unique inflammatory phenotype that is controlled by cAMP. *Blood* **2008**, *112*, 4117–4127. [CrossRef] [PubMed]

47. Wang, Y.; Kim, K.A.; Kim, J.H.; Sul, H.S. Pref-1, a preadipocyte secreted factor that inhibits adipogenesis. *J. Nutr.* **2006**, *136*, 2953–2956. [CrossRef] [PubMed]

48. Gao, Z.; Daquinag, A.C.; Su, F.; Snyder, B.; Kolonin, M.G. PDGFRalpha/PDGFRbeta signaling balance modulates progenitor cell differentiation into white and beige adipocytes. *Development* **2018**, *145*. [CrossRef] [PubMed]

49. Huang, S.C.; Everts, B.; Ivanova, Y.; O'Sullivan, D.; Nascimento, M.; Smith, A.M.; Beatty, W.; Love-Gregory, L.; Lam, W.Y.; O'Neill, C.M.; et al. Cell-intrinsic lysosomal lipolysis is essential for alternative activation of macrophages. *Nat. Immunol.* **2014**, *15*, 846–855. [CrossRef] [PubMed]

50. Bjursell, M.; Xu, X.; Admyre, T.; Bottcher, G.; Lundin, S.; Nilsson, R.; Stone, V.M.; Morgan, N.G.; Lam, Y.Y.; Storlien, L.H.; et al. The beneficial effects of n-3 polyunsaturated fatty acids on diet induced obesity and impaired glucose control do not require Gpr120. *PLoS ONE* **2014**, *9*, e114942. [CrossRef] [PubMed]

51. Winer, S.; Chan, Y.; Paltser, G.; Truong, D.; Tsui, H.; Bahrami, J.; Dorfman, R.; Wang, Y.; Zielenski, J.; Mastronardi, F.; et al. Normalization of obesity-associated insulin resistance through immunotherapy. *Nat. Med.* **2009**, *15*, 921–929. [CrossRef] [PubMed]

52. Flachs, P.; Horakova, O.; Brauner, P.; Rossmeisl, M.; Pecina, P.; Franssen-van Hal, N.L.; Ruzickova, J.; Sponarova, J.; Drahota, Z.; Vlcek, C.; et al. Polyunsaturated fatty acids of marine origin upregulate mitochondrial biogenesis and induce beta-oxidation in white fat. *Diabetologia* **2005**, *48*, 2365–2375. [CrossRef] [PubMed]

53. Mandard, S.; Muller, M.; Kersten, S. Peroxisome proliferator-activated receptor alpha target genes. *Cell. Mol. Life Sci.* **2004**, *61*, 393–416. [CrossRef] [PubMed]

54. van Schothorst, E.M.; Flachs, P.; Franssen-van Hal, N.L.; Kuda, O.; Bunschoten, A.; Molthoff, J.; Vink, C.; Hooiveld, G.J.; Kopecky, J.; Keijer, J. Induction of lipid oxidation by polyunsaturated fatty acids of marine origin in small intestine of mice fed a high-fat diet. *BMC Genom.* **2009**, *10*, 110. [CrossRef] [PubMed]

55. Horakova, O.; Medrikova, D.; van Schothorst, E.M.; Bunschoten, A.; Flachs, P.; Kus, V.; Kuda, O.; Bardova, K.; Janovska, P.; Hensler, M.; et al. Preservation of metabolic flexibility in skeletal muscle by a combined use of n-3 PUFA and rosiglitazone in dietary obese mice. *PLoS ONE* **2012**, *7*, e43764. [CrossRef] [PubMed]

56. Hessvik, N.P.; Bakke, S.S.; Fredriksson, K.; Boekschoten, M.V.; Fjorkenstad, A.; Koster, G.; Hesselink, M.K.; Kersten, S.; Kase, E.T.; Rustan, A.C.; et al. Metabolic switching of human myotubes is improved by *n*-3 fatty acids. *J. Lipid Res.* **2010**, *51*, 2090–2104. [CrossRef] [PubMed]

57. Flachs, P.; Adamcova, K.; Zouhar, P.; Marques, C.; Janovska, P.; Viegas, I.; Jones, J.G.; Bardova, K.; Svobodova, M.; Hansikova, J.; et al. Induction of lipogenesis in white fat during cold exposure in mice: Link to lean phenotype. *Int. J. Obes. (Lond.)* **2017**, *41*, 372–380. [CrossRef] [PubMed]

58. Fujisaka, S.; Usui, I.; Bukhari, A.; Ikutani, M.; Oya, T.; Kanatani, Y.; Tsuneyama, K.; Nagai, Y.; Takatsu, K.; Urakaze, M.; et al. Regulatory mechanisms for adipose tissue M1 and M2 macrophages in diet-induced obese mice. *Diabetes* **2009**, *58*, 2574–2582. [CrossRef] [PubMed]

59. Lumeng, C.N.; Delproposto, J.B.; Westcott, D.J.; Saltiel, A.R. Phenotypic switching of adipose tissue macrophages with obesity is generated by spatiotemporal differences in macrophage subtypes. *Diabetes* **2008**, *57*, 3239–3246. [CrossRef] [PubMed]

60. Sun, K.; Kusminski, C.M.; Scherer, P.E. Adipose tissue remodeling and obesity. *J. Clin. Investig.* **2011**, *121*, 2094–2101. [CrossRef] [PubMed]

61. Kras, K.M.; Hausman, D.B.; Hausman, G.J.; Martin, R.J. Adipocyte development is dependent upon stem cell recruitment and proliferation of preadipocytes. *Obes. Res.* **1999**, *7*, 491–497. [CrossRef] [PubMed]

62. Pavlisova, J.; Bardova, K.; Stankova, B.; Tvrzicka, E.; Kopecky, J.; Rossmeisl, M. Corn oil versus lard: Metabolic effects of omega-3 fatty acids in mice fed obesogenic diets with different fatty acid composition. *Biochimie* **2016**, *124*, 150–162. [CrossRef] [PubMed]

63. Hames, K.C.; Morgan-Bathke, M.; Harteneck, D.A.; Zhou, L.; Port, J.D.; Lanza, I.R.; Jensen, M.D. Very-long-chain omega-3 fatty acid supplements and adipose tissue functions: A randomized controlled trial. *Am. J. Clin. Nutr.* **2017**. [CrossRef] [PubMed]

64. Holt, P.R.; Aleman, J.O.; Walker, J.M.; Jiang, C.S.; Liang, Y.; de Rosa, J.C.; Giri, D.D.; Iyengar, N.M.; Milne, G.L.; Hudis, C.A.; et al. Docosahexaenoic Acid Supplementation is Not Anti-Inflammatory in Adipose Tissue of Healthy Obese Postmenopausal Women. *Int. J. Nutr.* **2017**, *1*, 31–49. [CrossRef] [PubMed]

65. Claria, J.; Lopez-Vicario, C.; Rius, B.; Titos, E. Pro-resolving actions of SPM in adipose tissue biology. *Mol. Asp. Med.* **2017**, *58*, 83–92. [CrossRef] [PubMed]

66. Rossmeisl, M.; Jilkova, Z.M.; Kuda, O.; Jelenik, T.; Medrikova, D.; Stankova, B.; Kristinsson, B.; Haraldsson, G.G.; Svensen, H.; Stoknes, I.; et al. Metabolic effects of n-3 PUFA as phospholipids are superior to triglycerides in mice fed a high-fat diet: Possible role of endocannabinoids. *PLoS ONE* **2012**, *7*, e38834. [CrossRef] [PubMed]

67. Spencer, M.; Finlin, B.S.; Unal, R.; Zhu, B.; Morris, A.J.; Shipp, L.R.; Lee, J.; Walton, R.G.; Adu, A.; Erfani, R.; et al. Omega-3 fatty acids reduce adipose tissue macrophages in human subjects with insulin resistance. *Diabetes* **2013**, *62*, 1709–1717. [CrossRef] [PubMed]

68. Nawaz, A.; Aminuddin, A.; Kado, T.; Takikawa, A.; Yamamoto, S.; Tsuneyama, K.; Igarashi, Y.; Ikutani, M.; Nishida, Y.; Nagai, Y.; et al. CD206(+) M2-like macrophages regulate systemic glucose metabolism by inhibiting proliferation of adipocyte progenitors. *Nat. Commun.* **2017**, *8*, 286. [CrossRef] [PubMed]

69. Kwon, H.J.; Kim, S.N.; Kim, Y.A.; Lee, Y.H. The contribution of arachidonate 15-lipoxygenase in tissue macrophages to adipose tissue remodeling. *Cell Death Dis.* **2016**, *7*, e2285. [CrossRef] [PubMed]

70. Szymczak, M.; Murray, M.; Petrovic, N. Modulation of angiogenesis by omega-3 polyunsaturated fatty acids is mediated by cyclooxygenases. *Blood* **2008**, *111*, 3514–3521. [CrossRef] [PubMed]

71. Wen, Y.; Gu, J.; Vandenhoff, G.E.; Liu, X.; Nadler, J.L. Role of 12/15-lipoxygenase in the expression of MCP-1 in mouse macrophages. *Am. J. Physiol. Heart Circ. Physiol.* **2008**, *294*, H1933–H1938. [CrossRef] [PubMed]

72. Todorcevic, M.; Hodson, L. The Effect of Marine Derived n-3 Fatty Acids on Adipose Tissue Metabolism and Function. *J. Clin. Med.* **2015**, *5*. [CrossRef] [PubMed]

73. Kim, H.K.; Della-Fera, M.; Lin, J.; Baile, C.A. Docosahexaenoic acid inhibits adipocyte differentiation and induces apoptosis in 3T3-L1 preadipocytes. *J. Nutr.* **2006**, *136*, 2965–2969. [CrossRef] [PubMed]

74. Hanada, H.; Morikawa, K.; Hirota, K.; Nonaka, M.; Umehara, Y. Induction of apoptosis and lipogenesis in human preadipocyte cell line by n-3 PUFAs. *Cell Biol. Int.* **2011**, *35*, 51–59. [CrossRef] [PubMed]

75. Yin, H.; Zhou, Y.; Zhu, M.; Hou, S.; Li, Z.; Zhong, H.; Lu, J.; Meng, T.; Wang, J.; Xia, L.; et al. Role of mitochondria in programmed cell death mediated by arachidonic acid-derived eicosanoids. *Mitochondrion* **2013**, *13*, 209–224. [CrossRef] [PubMed]

76. Kus, V.; Flachs, P.; Kuda, O.; Bardova, K.; Janovska, P.; Svobodova, M.; Jilkova, Z.M.; Rossmeisl, M.; Wang-Sattler, R.; Yu, Z.; et al. Unmasking Differential Effects of Rosiglitazone and Pioglitazone in the Combination Treatment with n-3 Fatty Acids in Mice Fed a High-Fat Diet. *PLoS ONE* **2011**, *6*, e27126. [CrossRef] [PubMed]

77. Despres, J.P.; Lemieux, I. Abdominal obesity and metabolic syndrome. *Nature* **2006**, *444*, 881–887. [CrossRef] [PubMed]

78. Kopecky, J.; Rossmeisl, M.; Flachs, P.; Kuda, O.; Brauner, P.; Jilkova, Z.; Stankova, B.; Tvrzicka, E.; Bryhn, M. n-3 PUFA: Bioavailability and modulation of adipose tissue function. *Proc. Nutr. Soc.* **2009**, *68*, 361–369. [CrossRef] [PubMed]

79. Stefl, B.; Janovska, A.; Hodny, Z.; Rossmeisl, M.; Horakova, M.; Syrovy, I.; Bemova, J.; Bendlova, B.; Kopecky, J. Brown fat is essential for cold-induced thermogenesis but not for obesity resistance in aP2-Ucp mice. *Am. J. Physiol.* **1998**, *274*, E527–E533. [CrossRef] [PubMed]

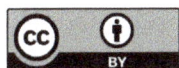

marine drugs

MDPI

Article

Inhibition of Adipogenesis by Diphlorethohydroxycarmalol (DPHC) through AMPK Activation in Adipocytes

Min-Cheol Kang [1,2,†], Yuling Ding [3,†], Hyun-Soo Kim [1], You-Jin Jeon [1] and Seung-Hong Lee [3,*]

[1] Department of Marine Life Sciences, Jeju National University, Jeju 63243, Korea;
    networksun@naver.com (M.-C.K.); gustn783@naver.com (H.-S.K.); youjinj@jejunu.ac.kr (Y.-J.J.)
[2] Korea Food Research Institute, 245 Nongsaengmyeong-Ro Iseo-Myeon, Wanju-Gun,
    Jeollabuk-Do 55365, Korea
[3] Department of Pharmaceutical Engineering, Soonchunhyang University, Asan 31538, Korea;
    dingyuling@naver.com
*   Correspondence: seunghong0815@gmail.com; Tel.: +82-10-4775-3344
†   These authors contributed equally to this study.

Received: 3 December 2018; Accepted: 7 January 2019; Published: 10 January 2019

Abstract: The purpose of this study was to investigate the antiobesity effect and the mechanism of action of diphlorethohydroxycarmalol (DPHC) isolated from *Ishige okamurae* in 3T3-L1 cells. The antiobesity effects were examined by evaluating intracellular fat accumulation in Oil Red O-stained adipocytes. Based on the results, DPHC dose-dependently inhibited the lipid accumulation in 3T3-L1 adipocytes. DPHC significantly inhibited adipocyte-specific proteins such as SREBP-1c, PPARγ, C/EBP α, and adiponectin, as well as adipogenic enzymes, including perilipin, FAS, FABP4, and leptin in adipocytes. These results indicated that DPHC primarily acts by regulating adipogenic-specific proteins through inhibiting fat accumulation and fatty acid synthesis in adipocytes. DPHC treatment significantly increased both AMPK and ACC phosphorylation in adipocytes. These results indicate that DPHC inhibits the fat accumulation by activating AMPK and ACC in 3T3-L1 cells. Taken together, these results suggest that DPHC can be used as a potential therapeutic agent against obesity.

Keywords: adipogenesis; antiobesity; adipocytes; diphlorethohydroxycarmalol (DPHC)

---

1. Introduction

Chronic obesity is one of the most detrimental health issues and a major social problem in the 21st century. In 2017, nearly two billion individuals were reported to be overweight, of which 671 million were obese [1,2]. Excessive food intake and lack of exercise are the most common causes of obesity. Obesity is a metabolic disease characterized by an excessive accumulation of body fat and further associated with complications such as type 2 diabetes, hypertension, hyperlipidemia, and increased risk of cancer and cardiovascular disease [3,4]. Several studies have reported the relationship between obesity and lipid accumulation by evaluating the differentiation of adipocytes. Synthetic antiobesity drugs such as orlistat (Xenical) and sibutramine (Reductil) have widely been used for the treatment of obesity. However, they are associated with side effects including thirst, insomnia, constipation, tension headaches, and steatorrhea [5]. Therapeutic application of natural substances is safer and less toxic than the use of synthetic drugs. Thus, many of the recent investigations have focused on the development of antiobesity agents from natural substances [6,7]. Adipocyte-specific proteins play a crucial role in adipocyte differentiation and lipid accumulation. These include enhancer binding proteins (C/EBP), sterol regulatory element-binding protein 1c (SREBP-1c), peroxisome proliferator activated receptor-γ (PPARγ), adiponectin, perilipin, fatty acid synthase (FAS), fatty acid binding protein (FABP4), and leptin [8]. Adenosine monophosphate-activated protein kinase (AMPK) is a heterotrimeric enzyme, an important mediator involved in regulating energy balance in the human body [9,10]. Many reports show that natural substances could inhibit fat accumulation by suppressing the expression of adipogenic-specific proteins during adipocyte differentiation. Some examples include dioxinodehydroeckol isolated from *Ecklonia cava*, indole derivatives isolated from *Sargassum thunbergii*, ethanol extracts of *Aster yomena*, and *Pinus koraiensis* leaves [11–14].

Ishige okamurae is a brown seaweed widespread in South Korea throughout Japan to China. The ethanolic extract of *I. okamurae* has shown antioxidant, antidiabetes, antihypertension, and antiobesity effects [15–17]. Recent evidence reported that diphlorethohydroxycarmalol (DPHC) isolated from *I. okamurae* could efficiently induce apoptosis via downregulating Bcl-2 while activating Bax caspase-3 and caspase-9 in adipocyte cells [18]. Ihn et al. reported that DPHC suppresses osteoclast differentiation by downregulating the NF-kB signaling pathway [19]. However, none have studied the inhibitory effects of DPHC upon fat accumulation in 3T3-L1 cells and its molecular mechanism. The present study aimed at investigating the effects of DPHC on adipogenesis in adipocytes.

2. Results

2.1. DPHC Inhibited 3T3-L1 Adipocyte Differentiation and Triglyceride Composition

The MTT assay is widely used in evaluating cell viability and toxicity. The effect of DPHC on 3T3-L1 cell viability was measured by the MTT assay in this study. As shown in Figure 1, these data indicate that DPHC does not affect the viability of 3T3-L1 adipocytes at 12.5, 25, 50, and 100 μM concentrations. The Oil Red O staining assay was used to measure the adipocyte differentiation and lipid accumulation in 3T3-L1 adipocytes. These results indicated that DPHC inhibited the lipid accumulation in 3T3-L1 adipocytes in a dose-dependent manner. These results suggest that DPHC possesses potent antiadipogenic effects due to the inhibition of adipocyte differentiation and adipogenesis.

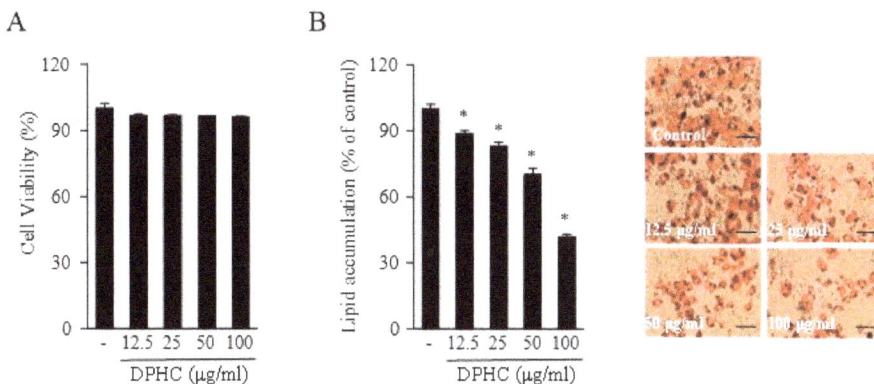

Figure 1. The effect of diphlorethohydroxycarmalol (DPHC) on the cell viability of 3T3-L1 preadipocytes treated for 48 h (**A**). DPHC inhibits intracellular lipid accumulation in 3T3-L1 adipocytes. Lipid accumulation was determined by Oil Red O staining (**B**). Scale bars for B is 50 μm. Data are expressed as the mean of three independent experiments, and the error bars represent the mean ± SE. Significant differences from the control group were identified at * $p < 0.05$.

2.2. Effects of DPHC on the Expression of Adipogenic-Specific Protein Levels during the Differentiation of 3T3-L1 Cells

The expression levels of key adipogenic-specific proteins were investigated to elucidate the molecular mechanisms underlying the inhibitory effect of DPHC on 3T3-L1 adipocyte differentiation. The investigated proteins include CCAAT/enhancer-binding protein-α (C/EBPα), sterol regulatory element binding protein-1c (SREBP-1c), peroxisome proliferator-activated receptor-γ (PPARγ), and adiponectin. As shown in Figure 2, DPHC treatment significantly decreased the levels of the adipogenic-specific proteins C/EBPα, SREBP-1c, PPARγ, and adiponectin in adipocytes. Moreover, it is well known that adipogenic-specific proteins could synergistically activate the downstream promoters of adipocyte-specific proteins, including perilipin, fatty acid synthase (FAS), fatty acid binding protein (FABP4), and leptin, that play a critical role in modulating fatty acid synthesis. We measured the inhibitory effect of DPHC on fatty acid synthesis-related proteins in adipocyte cells. These results show that DPHC could significantly inhibit fatty acid synthesis by downregulating adipogenic-specific proteins, including perilipin, FAS, FABP4, and leptin. Resistin, an adipocyte-derived cytokine, may contribute to the development of obesity. This study showed that DPHC treatment decreased the expression of resistin in the adipocytes. Collectively, DPHC acts by regulating adipogenic-specific proteins through the inhibition of fat accumulation and fatty acid synthesis in adipocyte cells.

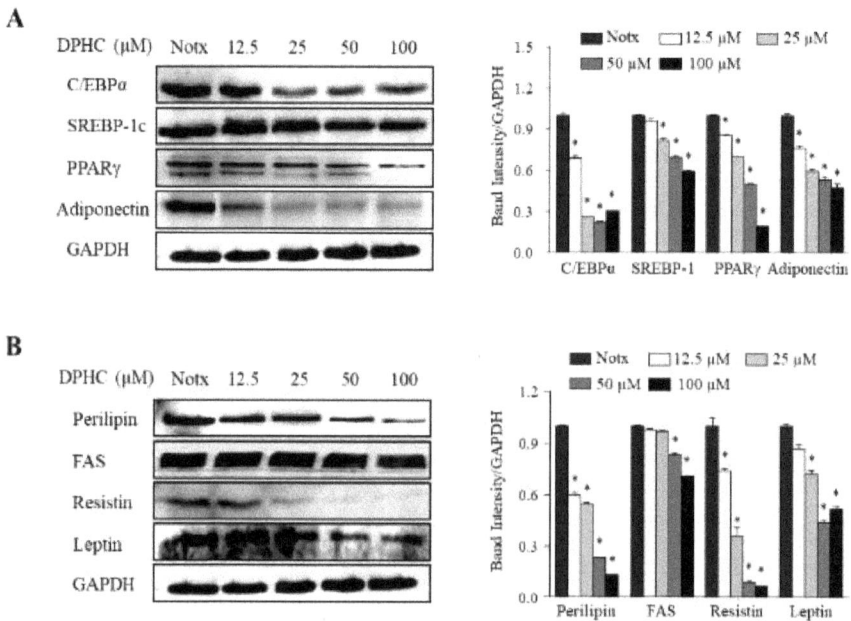

Figure 2. The effect of DPHC treatment on adipogenic-specific protein levels in 3T3-L1 adipocytes. The 3T3-L1 preadipocytes were incubated in a differentiation medium with or without the indicated concentrations of DPHC for eight days (from day 0 to day 8). The expression of sterol regulatory element-binding protein 1c (SREBP-1c), peroxisome proliferator-activated receptor-γ (PPARγ), CCAAT/enhancer-binding protein α (C/EBPα), and adiponectin were assessed by Western blotting (**A**). The expression of perilipin, fatty acid synthase (FAS), fatty acid binding protein (FABP4), and leptin were assessed by Western blotting (**B**). Immunoblot figures are representative of three independent experiments, and each value is expressed as the mean $\pm$ SE of three determinations. Significant differences from the control group were identified at * $p < 0.05$.

2.3. Effects of DPHC on the Activation of AMPK and ACC in 3T3-L1 Adipocytes

The 5′ adenosine monophosphate-activated protein kinase (AMPK) is a major regulator of whole-body energy homeostasis, which gets activated by lower intracellular ATP levels. Recent reports suggest that AMPK plays an important role in the metabolism of energy, glucose, and ATP production [20]. We investigated the effect of DPHC on the phosphorylation of AMPK and acetyl-CoA carboxylase (ACC) in adipocytes. As shown in Figure 3, DPHC treatment significantly increased both AMPK and ACC phosphorylation in 3T3-L1 adipocytes. These results indicate that DPHC could inhibit fat accumulation by activating AMPK and ACC in 3T3-L1 cells.

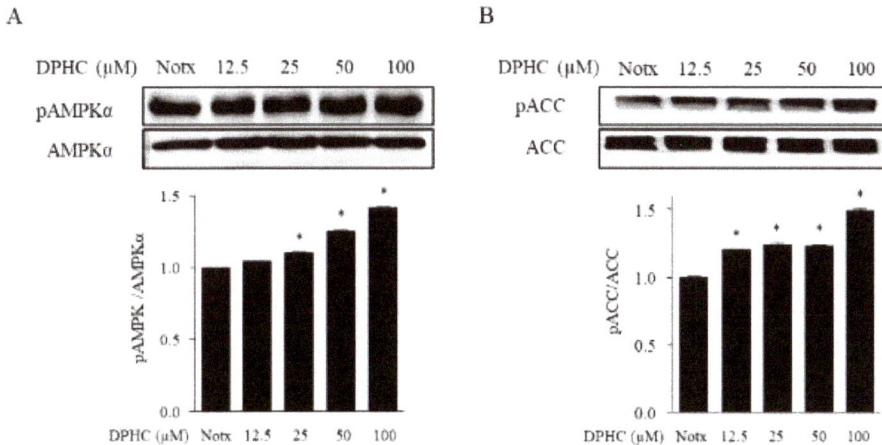

Figure 3. DPHC suppresses the activation of p-AMPKα and p-ACC in 3T3-L1 preadipocytes. 3T3-L1 preadipocytes were maintained in Dulbecco's Modified Eagle Medium (DMEM) with or without different concentrations of DPHC for eight days (from day 0 to day 8) until their differentiation into adipocytes. Immunoblot figures are representative of three independent experiments, and each value is expressed as the mean ± SE of three determinations. Significant differences from the control group were identified at * $p < 0.05$.

3. Discussion

Fat accumulation in adipose tissues is a complex process involving a number of different metabolic and signaling pathways. Adipocytes play a vital role in the regulation of energy intake, energy expenditure, and lipid and carbohydrate metabolism [21]. Excessive fat accumulation in adipocytes increases various risk factors including inflammation, hypertension, and heart diseases. Many recent studies have focused on developing antiobesity agents from natural substances, which could inhibit fat accumulation in adipocytes [22,23]. However, few reports are available on the antiobesity effects of polyphenol compounds from seaweeds. In the present study, investigations were done to evaluate the antiobesity effects of DPHC and its mode of action in adipocytes. Fat accumulation is regarded as a regulatory process, whereas a number of adipocyte-specific proteins are involved in the mediation of lipid synthesis, lipolysis, and glucose uptake in adipocytes. These adipocyte-specific proteins get induced during the differentiation of preadipocytes into adipocytes and play an essential role during adipogenesis. The differentiation of 3T3-L1 preadipocytes into adipocytes is mainly controlled by the family of adipogenic-specific factors, including C/EBPα, SREBP-1c, PPARγ, perilipin, FAS, FABP4, and leptin [24,25]. Thus, reducing the expression of adipogenic-specific factors may be an effective strategy for inhibiting fat accumulation in adipocytes. Several recent studies have focused on the potential of polyphenols such as dieckol, epigallocatechin-3-gallate, and resveratrol upon the inhibition of fat accumulation in differentiating 3T3-L1 cells via measuring the decreased expression levels of adipogenic-specific factors [26–30]. Our results indicate that DPHC treatment plays a critical role in inhibiting fat accumulation via decreasing the expression levels of adipogenesis-associated proteins in 3T3-L1 cells. Activation of AMPK increases glucose transport and fatty acid oxidation in adipocytes. Promising strategies for treating obesity include the reduction of fat accumulation through inhibiting adipogenesis-specific proteins and activating the AMPK pathway. A number of researchers have reported that AMPK is a member of the metabolite-sensing kinase family of proteins and plays a central role in regulating glucose and lipid metabolism. It has previously been reported that activated AMPK inhibits lipogenesis and adipocyte differentiation. Furthermore, ACC is a multi-subunit enzyme that regulates enzymes involved in malonyl-CoA production, fatty acid synthesis, and fatty acid oxidation in adipocytes [31,32].

We found that DPHC treatment could significantly increase both AMPK and ACC phosphorylation in adipocyte cells. These results indicated that DPHC inhibits the fat accumulation by activating AMPK and ACC in adipocytes.

4. Materials and Methods

4.1. Materials

The brown alga *I. okamurae* was collected from the coast of Jeju Island, Korea. All collected samples were washed with tap water to remove salt, sand, and epiphytes attached to the surface, followed by careful rinsing with fresh water and were then maintained in a refrigerator at −20 °C. Next, the frozen samples were lyophilized and homogenized with a grinder before the extraction.

Dulbecco's modified Eagle's medium (DMEM), fetal bovine serum (FBS), bovine serum (BS), phosphate-buffered saline (pH 7.4; PBS), and penicillin–streptomycin (PS) were purchased from Gibco BRL (Grand Island, NY, USA). All chemicals and reagents used were of analytical grade and obtained from commercial sources. 3-Isobutyl-1-methylxanthine (IBMX), dexamethasone, insulin, and 3-(4,5-dimethylthiazol-2-yl)-2,5-diphenyl tetrazolium bromide (MTT) were purchased from Sigma Chemical Co. (St. Louis, MO, USA). Antibodies to CCAAT/enhancer-binding protein-α (C/EBPα; #2295; Cell Signaling), fatty acid binding protein (FABP4; F2120; Cell Signaling), and adenosine monophosphate-activated protein kinase (AMPK; #2535; Cell Signaling) were purchased from Cell Signaling Technology (Bedford, MA, USA). Antibodies to sterol regulatory element binding protein-1c (SREBP-1c; sc-13551; Santa Cruz), peroxisome proliferator-activated receptor-γ (PPARγ; sc-7273; Santa Cruz), adiponectin, perilipin, fatty acid synthase (FAS; sc-715; Santa Cruz), and leptin were obtained from Santa Cruz Biotechnology (Santa Cruz, CA, USA).

4.2. Extraction and Isolation

Dried *I. okamurae* powder was extracted three times with 80% methanol and filtered. The filtrate was rotary-evaporated at 40 °C to obtain the methanol extract, which was suspended in distilled water and partitioned using chloroform. The chloroform fraction was fractionated by silica column chromatography with stepwise elution by a chloroform–methanol mixture (30:1→1:1) to separate the active fractions in the chloroform extract. The active fraction was subjected to further purification using a Sephadex LH-20 column with 100% methanol. The selected active fraction was further purified by reversed-phase high-performance liquid chromatography (HPLC) using a Waters HPLC system (Alliance 2690; Waters Corp., Milford, MA, USA) equipped with a Waters 996 photodiode array detector and C18 column (J'sphere ODS-H80, 250 × 4.6 mm, 4 μm; YMC Co., Kyoto, Japan) by stepwise elution with a methanol–water gradient (UV absorbance detection wavelength, 296 nm; flow rate, 1 mL/min). The eluate was finally purified by high-performance liquid chromatography (HPLC), and the structure of DPHC was determined (Figure 4). The DPHC contents of the 80% methanol extract from *I. okamurae* ranged from ~2 to 3%. The compound was dissolved in dimethyl sulfoxide (DMSO) and employed in experiments in which the final concentration of DMSO in the culture medium was adjusted to <0.01%.

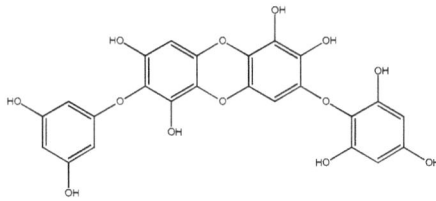

Figure 4. Chemical structure of diphlorethohydroxycarmalol (DPHC).

4.3. Cell Culture

3T3-L1 preadipocytes obtained from the American Type Culture Collection (Rockville, MD, USA) were cultured in DMEM containing 1% PS and 10% bovine calf serum (Gibco BRL) at 37 °C under a 5% CO_2 atmosphere. To induce differentiation, 2-day post-confluent preadipocytes (designated as day 0) culture media was replaced with MDI differentiation medium (DMEM containing 1% PS, 10% FBS, 0.5 mM IBMX, 0.25 μM dexamethasone, and 5 μg/mL insulin) for 2 days. The cells were then maintained for another 2 days in DMEM containing 1% PS, 10% FBS, and 5 μg/mL insulin. Thereafter, the cells were maintained in post-differentiation medium (DMEM containing 1% PS and 10% FBS), with the replacement of the medium every 2 days. To examine the effects of test samples on the differentiation of preadipocytes to adipocytes, the cells were cultured with MDI medium in the presence of test samples. Differentiation was measured by the expression of adipogenic markers and the appearance of lipid droplets and was completed on day 8.

4.4. Cell Viability Assay

Cytotoxicity of DPHC against 3T3-L1 cells was assessed via a colorimetric MTT assay. 3T3-L1 preadipocytes plated on 24-well plates were treated with DPHC at 37 °C for 48 h. MTT stock solution (100 μL; 2 mg/mL in PBS) was then added to each well to a total reaction volume of 600 μL. After 4 h of incubation, the plates were centrifuged ($800\times g$, 5 min) and the supernatant was aspirated. The formazan crystals in each well were dissolved in 300 μL of DMSO, and the absorbance was measured with an ELISA plate reader at 540 nm.

4.5. Determination of Lipid Accumulation by Oil Red O Staining

To induce adipogenesis, 3T3-L1 preadipocytes were seeded in 6-well plates and maintained for two days after reaching confluence. The media was then exchanged with differentiation medium (DMEM containing 10% FBS, 0.5 mM IBMX, 0.25 μM Dex, and 10 μg/mL insulin) and cells were treated with test samples. After two days, the differentiation medium was replaced with adipocyte growth medium (DMEM supplemented with 10% FBS and 5 μg/mL insulin), which was refreshed every two days. After adipocyte differentiation, the cells were stained with Oil Red O for measure lipid content. Briefly, cells were washed with PBS, fixed with 10% buffered formalin and stained with Oil Red O solution (0.5 g in 100 ml isopropanol) for 60 min. After removing the staining solution, the dye retained in the cells was eluted into isopropanol and the optical density was measured at 520 nm. Images were collected on an EVOS microscope (ThermoFisher Scientific, Waltham, MA, USA).

4.6. Western Blot Analysis

Cells were lysed in lysis buffer (20 mM Tris, 5 mM EDTA, 10 mM $Na_4P_2O_7$, 100 mM NaF, 2 mM Na_3VO_4, 1% NP-40, 10 mg/mL aprotinin, 10 mg/mL leupeptin, and 1 mM PMSF) for 1 h and then centrifuged at 12,000 rpm for 15 min at 0 °C. The protein concentrations were determined by using a BCA^{TM} protein assay kit. The lysate containing 40 μg of protein was subjected to electrophoresis on sodium dodecyl sulfate (SDS)–polyacrylamide gels, and the gels were transferred onto nitrocellulose membranes. The membranes were blocked in 5% nonfat dry milk in TBST (25 mM

Tris–HCl, 137 mM NaCl, 2.65 mM KCl, 0.05% Tween 20; pH 7.4) for 1 h. The primary antibodies were used at a 1:1000 dilution. Membranes were incubated with the primary antibodies at 4 °C overnight. Then, the membranes were washed with TBST and incubated with the secondary antibodies (at 1:3000 dilutions). Signals were developed using an Enhanced chemiluminescence (ECL) Western blotting detection kit and exposed to X-ray films.

4.7. Statistical Analysis

Data were analyzed using the Statistical Package for the Social Sciences (SPSS) for Windows (Version 8). Values were expressed as means ± standard error (SE). A *p*-value of less than 0.05 was considered significant.

5. Conclusions

In conclusion, our data demonstrated that DPHC suppressed adipocyte differentiation and fat accumulation by inhibiting adipogenesis-specific proteins in adipocytes. Taken together, these results suggest that DPHC can be a useful candidate and a potential therapeutic agent for treating obesity.

Author Contributions: M.-C.K. and S.-H.L. conceived and designed the experiments; M.-C.K. and Y.D. performed the experiments; M.-C.K. and Y.D. analyzed the data; H.-S.K. contributed reagents/materials/analysis tools; M.-C.K., S.-H.L. and Y.-J.J. wrote the paper.

Funding: This work was supported by the Soonchunhyang University Research Fund (No. 20180406). This research was also supported by the Basic Science Research Program through the National Research Foundation of Korea (NRF) funded by the Ministry of Science, ICT & Future Planning (2018R1C1B6004780).

Conflicts of Interest: The authors declare that they have no conflict of interest.

References

1. Puhl, R.M.; Heuer, C.A. Obesity Stigma: Important Considerations for Public Health. *Am. J. Public Health Res.* **2010**, *100*, 1019–1028. [CrossRef]
2. Tremmel, M.; Gerdtham, U.G.; Nilsson, P.M.; Saha, S. Economic Burden of Obesity: A Systematic Literature Review. *Int. J. Environ. Res. Public Health* **2017**, *14*, 435. [CrossRef]
3. Wilborn, C.; Beckham, J.; Campbell, B.; Harvey, T.; Galbreath, M.; Bounty, P.L.; Nassar, E.; Wismann, J.; Kreider, R. Obesity: Prevalence, Theories, Medical Consequences, Management, and Research Directions. *J. Int. Soc. Sports Nutr.* **2005**, *2*, 4–31. [CrossRef] [PubMed]
4. Moneteiro, R.; Azebedo, I. Chronic Inflammation in Obesity and the Metabolic Syndrome. *Mediat. Inflamm.* **2010**, *2010*, 289645. [CrossRef]
5. Yun, J.W. Possible anti-obesity therapeutics from nature—A review. *Phytochemistry* **2010**, *71*, 14–15. [CrossRef] [PubMed]
6. Mohamed, G.A.; Ibrahim, S.R.M.; Elkhayat, E.S.; Dine, R.S.E. Natural anti-obesity agents. *Bull. Fac. Pharm. Cairo Univ.* **2014**, *52*, 269–284. [CrossRef]
7. Kang, M.C.; Kang, N.; Ko, S.C.; Kim, Y.B.; Jeon, Y.J. Anti-obesity effects of seaweeds of Jeju Island on the differentiation of 3T3-L1 preadipocytes and obese mice fed a high-fat diet. *Food Chem. Toxicol.* **2016**, *90*, 36–44. [CrossRef]
8. Payne, V.A.; Au, W.S.; Lowe, C.E.; Rahman, S.M.; Friedman, J.E.; Rahilly, S.O.; Rochford, J.J. C/EBP transcription factors regulate SREBP1c gene expression during adipogenesis. *Biochem. J.* **2009**, *425*, 215–224. [CrossRef] [PubMed]
9. Gruzman, A.; Babai, G.; Sasson, S. Adenosine Monophosphate-Activated Protein Kinase (AMPK) as a New Target for Antidiabetic Drugs: A Review on Metabolic, Pharmacological and Chemical Considerations. *Rev. Diabet. Stud.* **2009**, *6*, 13–36. [CrossRef]
10. Gaidhu, M.P.; Ceddia, R.B. Remodeling glucose and lipid metabolism throughAMPK activation: Relevance for treating obesityand Type 2 diabetes. *Clin. Lipidol.* **2009**, *4*, 465–477. [CrossRef]
11. Kim, S.K.; Kong, C.S. Anti-adipogenic effect of dioxinodehydroeckol via AMPK activation in 3T3-L1 adipocytes. *Chem. Biol. Interact.* **2010**, *186*, 24–29. [CrossRef]

12. Kang, M.C.; Ding, Y.; Kim, E.A.; Choi, Y.K.; Araujo, T.D.; Heo, S.J.; Lee, S.H. Indole Derivatives Isolated from Brown Alga Sargassum thunbergii Inhibit Adipogenesis through AMPK Activation in 3T3-L1 Preadipocytes. *Mar. Drugs* **2017**, *15*, 119. [CrossRef]

13. Han, M.H.; Jeong, J.S.; Jeong, J.W.; Choi, S.H.; Kim, S.O.; Hong, S.H.; Park, C.; Kim, B.W.; Choi, Y.H. Ethanol extracts of Aster yomena (Kitam.) Honda inhibit adipogenesis through the activation of the AMPK signaling pathway in 3T3-L1 preadipocytes. *Drug Discov. Ther.* **2017**, *11*, 281–287. [PubMed]

14. Lee, M.S.; Cho, S.M.; Lee, M.H.; Lee, E.O.; Kim, S.H.; Lee, H.J. Ethanol extract of Pinus koraiensis leaves containing lambertianic acid exerts anti-obesity and hypolipidemic effects by activating adenosine monophosphate-activated protein kinase (AMPK). *BMC Complement. Altern. Med.* **2016**, *16*, 51. [CrossRef] [PubMed]

15. Kang, M.C.; Lee, S.H.; Lee, W.W.; Kang, N.; Kim, E.A.; Kim, S.Y.; Lee, D.H.; Kim, D.; Jeon, Y.J. Protective effect of fucoxanthin isolated from Ishige okamurae against high-glucose induced oxidative stress in human umbilical vein endothelial cells and zebrafish model. *J. Funct. Foods* **2014**, *11*, 304–312. [CrossRef]

16. Ko, E.Y.; Yoon, W.J.; Lee, H.W.; Heo, S.J.; Ko, Y.H.; Fernando, I.P.S.; Cho, K.; Lee, C.H.; Hur, S.P.; Cho, S.H.; et al. Anti-inflammatory effect of supercritical extract and its constituents from Ishige okamurae. *EXCLI J.* **2016**, *15*, 434–445. [PubMed]

17. Zou, Y.; Qian, Z.J.; Li, Y.; Kim, M.M.; Lee, S.H.; Kim, S.K. Antioxidant effects of phlorotannins isolated from *Ishige okamurae* in free radical mediated oxidative systems. *J. Agric. Food Chem.* **2008**, *56*, 7001–7009. [CrossRef] [PubMed]

18. Park, M.H.; Jeon, Y.J.; Kim, H.J.; Han, J.S. Effect of Diphlorethohydroxycarmalol Isolated from *Ishige okamurae* on Apoptosis in 3 t3-L1 Preadipocytes. *Phytother. Res.* **2012**, *27*, 931–936. [CrossRef] [PubMed]

19. Ihn, H.J.; Kim, J.A.; Cho, H.S.; Shin, H.I.; Kim, G.Y.; Choi, Y.H.; Jeon, Y.J.; Park, E.K. Diphlorethohydroxycarmalol from Ishige okamurae Suppresses Osteoclast Differentiation by Downregulating the NF-κb Signaling Pathway. *Int. J. Mol. Sci.* **2017**, *18*, 2635. [CrossRef]

20. Aguilar, F.M.; Pavillard, L.E.; Giampieri, F.; Bullon, P.; Cordero, M.D. Adenosine Monophosphate (AMP)-Activated Protein Kinase: A New Target for Nutraceutical Compounds. *Int. J. Mol. Sci.* **2017**, *18*, 288. [CrossRef] [PubMed]

21. Rosen, E.D.; Spiegelman, B.M. Adipocytes as regulators of energy balance and glucose homeostasis. *Nature* **2006**, *444*, 847–853. [CrossRef] [PubMed]

22. Prieto-Hontoria, P.L.; Perez-Matute, P.P.; Femandez-Galilea, M.; Bustos, M.; Martinez, J.A.; Moreno-Aliaga, M. Role of obesity-associated dysfunctional adipose tissue in cancer: A molecular nutrition approach. *Biochim. Biophys. Acta* **2011**, *1807*, 664–678. [CrossRef] [PubMed]

23. Sun, N.N.; Wu, T.Y.; Chau, C.F. Natural Dietary and Herbal Products in Anti-Obesity Treatment. *Molecules* **2016**, *21*, 1351. [CrossRef] [PubMed]

24. Coelho, M.; Oliveira, T.; Femandes, R. Biochemistry of adipose tissue: An endocrine organ. *Arch. Med. Sci.* **2013**, *9*, 191–200. [CrossRef] [PubMed]

25. Tung, Y.C.; Hsieh, P.H.; Pan, M.H.; Ho, C.T. Cellular models for the evaluation of the antiobesity effect of selected phytochemicals from food and herbs. *J. Food Drug Anal.* **2017**, *25*, 100–110. [CrossRef] [PubMed]

26. Choi, H.S.; Jeon, H.J.; Lee, O.H.; Lee, B.Y. Dieckol, a major phlorotannin in Ecklonia cava, suppresses lipid accumulation in the adipocytes of high-fat diet-fed zebrafish and mice: Inhibition of early adipogenesis via cell-cycle arrest and AMPKα activation. *Mol. Nutr. Food Res.* **2015**, *59*, 1458–1471. [CrossRef] [PubMed]

27. Chan, C.Y.; Wei, L.; Castro-Munozledo, F.; Koo, W.L. (−)-Epigallocatechin-3-gallate blocks 3T3-L1 adipose conversion by inhibition of cell proliferation and suppression of adipose phenotype expression. *Life Sci.* **2011**, *21*, 779–785. [CrossRef]

28. Chang, C.C.; Lin, K.Y.; Peng, K.Y.; Day, Y.J.; Hung, L.M. Resveratrol exerts anti-obesity effects in high-fat diet obese mice and displays differential dosage effects on cytotoxicity, differentiation, and lipolysis in 3T3-L1 cells. *Endocr. J.* **2016**, *63*, 169–178. [CrossRef]

29. Kim, J.; Yang, G.; Kim, Y.; Kim, J.; Ha, J. AMPK activators: Mechanisms of action and physiological activities. *Exp. Mol. Med.* **2016**, *48*, e224. [CrossRef]

30. Kelly, M.; Ruderman, N.B.; Tomas, E. AMP-activated protein kinase and itsregulation by adiponectin andinterleukin-6. *Scand. J. Food Nutr.* **2006**, *50*, 85–91. [CrossRef]

31. Lago, F.; Gomez, R.; Gomez-Reino, J.J.; Dieguez, C.; Gualillo, O. Adipokines as novel modulators of lipid metabolism. *Cell* **2009**, *2*, 500–510. [CrossRef] [PubMed]
32. Rizzatti, V.; Boschi, F.; Pedrotti, M.; Zoico, E.; Sbarbati, A.; Zamboni, M. Lipid Droplets Characterization in Adipocyte Differentiated 3T3-L1 Cells: Size and Optical Density Distribution. *Eur. J. Histochem.* **2013**, *57*, 159–162. [CrossRef] [PubMed]

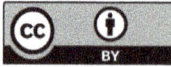

marine drugs

MDPI

Article

Effect of Oral Ingestion of Low-Molecular Collagen Peptides Derived from Skate (*Raja Kenojei*) Skin on Body Fat in Overweight Adults: A Randomized, Double-Blind, Placebo-Controlled Trial

Young Jin Tak [1,2], Yun Jin Kim [1,2], Jeong Gyu Lee [1,2], Yu-Hyun Yi [1,2], Young Hye Cho [3], Geun Hee Kang [4] and Sang Yeoup Lee [3,5,*]

[1]   Department of Family Medicine, Pusan National University School of Medicine, Busandaehak-ro, Mulgeum-eup, Yangsan-si 50612, Korea; 03141998@hanmail.net (Y.J.T.); yujkim@pusan.ac.kr (Y.J.K.); jeklee@pnu.edu (J.G.L.); eeugus@gmail.com (Y.-H.Y.)
[2]   Biomedical Research Institute, Pusan National University Hospital, Busan 602-739, Korea
[3]   Family Medicine Clinic and Research Institute of Convergence of Biomedical Science and Technology, Pusan National University Yangsan Hospital, Yangsan 50612, Korea; younghye82@naver.com
[4]   Yeong San Skate Co., Ltd., Naju 58266, Korea; skate1438@naver.com
[5]   Medical Education Unit, Pusan National University School of Medicine, Yangsan 50612, Korea
*   Correspondence: saylee@pnu.edu; Tel.: +82-10-9134-5959

Received: 2 February 2019; Accepted: 3 March 2019; Published: 7 March 2019

Abstract: Recent animal studies found the potential of a collagen peptide derived from skate skin to have anti-obesity effects through the suppression of fat accumulation and regulation of lipid metabolism. However, no studies have yet been performed in humans. Here, this very first human randomized, placebo-controlled, and double-blinded study was designed to investigate the efficacy and tolerability of skate skin collagen peptides (SCP) for the reduction of body fat in overweight adults. Ninety healthy volunteers (17 men) aged 41.2 ± 10.4 years with a mean body mass index of 25.6 ± 1.9 kg/m^2 were assigned to the intervention group (IG), which received 2000 mg of SCP per day or to the control group (CG) given the placebo for 12 weeks and 81 (90%) participants completed the study. Changes in body fat were evaluated using dual energy X-ray absorptiometry as a primary efficacy endpoint. After 12 weeks of the trial, the percentage of body fat and body fat mass (kg) in IG were found to be significantly better than those of subjects in CG (-1.2% vs. 2.7%, $p = 0.024$ and -1.2 kg vs. 0.3 kg, $p = 0.025$). Application of SCP was well tolerated and no notable adverse effect was reported from both groups. These results suggest the beneficial potential of SCP in the reduction of body fat in overweight adults.

Keywords: Skate skin; *Raja kenojei*; collagen; body fat; obesity

---

1. Introduction

The global burden of cardiovascular diseases (CVD), which is the most common cause of death is increasing rapidly despite tremendous treatment options for diabetes, hypertension and dyslipidemia [1]. It is believed to be mainly attributed to failing to control the growing number of populations who are obese as a sedentary lifestyle and westernized eating habits have become prevalent worldwide [2]. Obesity is the root cause of chronic diseases that have been afflicting about one-third of the total population globally and the crucial factor to solve for prevention of fatal health issues [3]. Although medical experts have been struggling to find out effective treatment options for obese people, there have been only a few medications used to suppress appetite by working on the central neurologic system, which often brings about unexpected side effects such as the urge of suicide, aggravation of depression or other psychological issues [4]. Therefore, it is necessary to discover a material with an anti-adipogenic effect to help lose weight that comes from naturally available sources without any concerns of side effects.

In an attempt to make these possible, numerous products are now being developed and commercialized. Among them is collagen that has been widely used as a material in food, cosmetic, and pharmaceutical industries due to its biological and functional properties [5]. In a recent randomized controlled trial, post-exercise supplementation of a collagen peptide in combination with resistance training was seen to improve body composition and increase muscle strength in 148 elderly sarcopenic men [6]. Especially, collagen peptides derived from sea fish have been recognized as a dietary supplement which is beneficial to blood pressure [7] and glucose control [8], skin moisturizing [9] and improved lipids [10].

Skate is quite a popular food consumed widely in Korea in both a raw and fermented form. From a nutritional perspective, skate is known to contain taurine, which plays a role in the growth and development of cells and is an energy booster, anserine that acts as a buffer for muscles [11]. In addition, it is high in essential fatty acids such as linoleic and linolenic acid, which are beneficial to enhance cognitive functions by reducing a high lipid level [12]. As many healthy nutrients that skate contains are discovered [13,14], its demand has been on the rise in recent years. Accordingly, a great number of by-products such as skin and cartilage remain and go waste in the process of the meat part of the skate. However, the nutritional values of by-products from skate are also reported to be fairly high [15], so these can be a useful resource in the fish-supplements industry [16,17]. Previous information suggests that skate can serve as a good nutrition source for the development of highly functional collagen peptide materials [11].

In very recent study, Woo et al. found the anti-obesity effects of collage peptide derived from skate skin by suppressing fat accumulation and regulation of lipid metabolism in genetic and high-fat diet (HFD)-induced obese animal model [18], presenting that using skate skin might be an effective and safe approach for humans to resolve obesity-related health problems. Although an HFD-induced obese animal is considered to have similar pathophysiology to that of an obese person [19], a well-designed clinical trial is necessary to confirm the effect and safety of skate skin collagen peptide (SCP) in humans. However, the effects of collagen from skate skin on changes in body weight have never been explored in humans. Thus, our study aimed to assess the efficacy and tolerability of SCP for the reduction of excess body fat in overweight adults. We hypothesized that SCP is an effective, safe agent for the treatment of obese people.

2. Results

2.1. General Characteristics of the Study Subjects

Five participants in IG and four in CG withdrew consent for personal reasons that were not considered associated with the trial. The characteristics of these nine participants were similar to ones of the others who completed the study. Compliance was satisfactory with participants taking more than 90% of the supplements given in both IG and CG. Randomization was successful, as the two groups generated were comparable for most variables and no significant differences were observed in the baseline demographic and anthropometric characteristics between the two groups (Table 1). The majority of the participants were women (81.1%) and the mean age of total participants was 41.2 ± 10.4 years. The average BMI of both IG and CG was over 25.6 ± 1.9 kg/m^2, which is more than the cutoff for defining obesity in Korea [20]. Furthermore, no statistically significant intergroup differences were observed for alcohol drinking, smoking, calorie intake and physical activities at baseline. During the whole study period, the double-blind requirement was well maintained.

Table 1. Baseline characteristics of the study subjects.

Variable	Intention to Treat Analysis			Per Protocol Analysis		
	CG (*n* = 45)	IG (*n* = 45)	*p* *	CG (*n* = 41)	IG (*n* = 40)	*p* *
Male (%)	8 (17.8)	9 (20.0)	0.788	8 (19.5)	8 (20.0)	0.956
Age (years)	40.8 ± 11.1	41.7 ± 9.7	0.750	41.1 ± 11.2	41.8 ± 9.9	0.817
BMI (kg/m²)	25.8 ± 1.9	25.5 ± 2.0	0.467	25.8 ± 1.9	25.4 ± 2.0	0.404
Alcohol user (%)	23 (51.1)	18 (40.0)	0.290	20 (48.8)	17 (42.5)	0.570
Smoker (%)	2 (4.4)	1 (2.2)	0.559	2 (4.9)	1 (2.5)	0.573
Calorie intake (kcal/day)	1660 ± 495	1594 ± 357	0.410	1667 ± 515	1601 ± 360	0.427
IPAQ (METs)	1151 (363–1726)	740 (33–2170)	0.813	1158 (396–1658)	903 (33–2655)	0.502

BMI, body mass index; IPAQ, international physical activity questionnaires; SAD, sagittal abdomen distance. Data was presented as mean ± standard deviation or number (%) except for IPAQ with median (interquartile). * By Chi-square test or two sample *t*-test except for IPAQ using Mann-Whitney's U test.

2.2. Changes in Body Composition

There were no significant changes in calorie intake (Δ IG: 133.1 kcal/day, *p* = 0.715 vs. Δ CG: −51.7 kcal/day, *p* = 0.436) and physical activities (Δ IG: −205.6 METs, *p* = 0.166 vs. Δ CG: 129.4 METs, *p* = 0.551) checked at baseline and the 12th week of the trial among the participants, reflecting no additional effect that might have influenced body composition aside from the intervention. After 12 weeks of the trial, CG subjects showed a slight rise in BW by 0.7 kg (*p* = 0.018), and accordingly BMI by 0.3 kg/m² (*p* = 0.015), while IG participants had no significant increase in BW and BMI (Table 2). However, BF in IG after 12 weeks was found to decline (−0.6%, *p* = 0.017) from the baseline with a little decrease of lean body mass. In contrast, there was no change in body composition among CG subjects. In terms of comparison between the groups after 12 weeks, IG subjects turned out to have more body fat loss than the CG ones (−1.2 kg vs. 0.3 kg, *p* = 0.025). This intergroup difference in the percentage of BW change was observed from the sixth week of the trial and lasted until the 12th week (Figure 1).

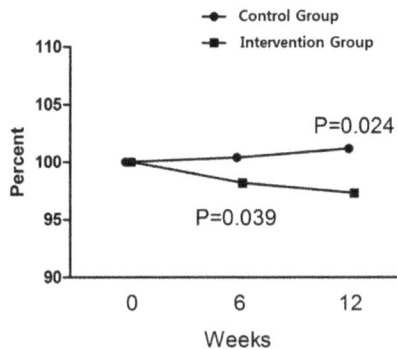

Figure 1. The percentage of changes in body fat during the 12 weeks of the study. *P*-values were derived from Mann-Whitney's U test with the intention to treat analysis (*n* = 90).

2.3. Changes in Laboratory Measurements

In both groups, adiponectin levels rose a bit with a larger increase found in IG although it was not a significant difference between the groups after 12 weeks. When it comes to the lipid profile, no changes were observed except for n aHDL-C decrease in IG.

2.4. Safety

Most of the subjects completed the protocol without adverse symptoms. One subject in IG complained of dyspepsia and decided to withdraw consent for that reason. However, this symptom was not determined to have anything to do with taking SCP. No clinical changes in the levels of liver enzyme, creatinine and glucose were observed in each group. No intergroup differences in these figures were found during the study period (Table 3).

Table 2. Comparison of changes in measurements in the intention to treat (ITT) population.

Variable	Observed Values			Changes from Baseline				
	CG (*n* = 45)	IG (*n* = 45)	*p* *	CG (*n* = 45)	*p* **	IG (*n* = 45)	*p* **	*p* *
Weight (kg)								
Baseline	68.0 ± 8.5	66.6 ± 8.5	0.364 [1]					
At 12 weeks	68.7 ± 8.8	66.8 ± 8.8	0.228 [1]	0.7 ± 1.9	0.018 [4]	0.2 ± 1.3	0.183 [4]	0.155 [2]
SAD (cm)								
Baseline	19.6 ± 2.0	19.3 ± 1.6	0.226 [1]					
At 12 weeks	19.5 ± 2.2	19.2 ± 1.8	0.433 [2]	−0.1 ± 1.1	0.489 [3]	−0.1 ± 1.0	0.701 [4]	0.840 [4]
BMI (kg/m^2)								
Baseline	25.8 ± 1.9	25.5 ± 2.0	0.467 [2]					
At 12 weeks	26.1 ± 2.2	25.6 ± 2.0	0.274 [2]	0.3 ± 0.7	0.015 [3]	0.1 ± 0.5	0.265 [3]	0.153 [1]
Body fat (%)								
Baseline	40.5 ± 4.7	41.2 ± 5.5	0.255 [1]					
At 12 weeks	40.3 ± 4.4	40.6 ± 5.3	0.455 [1]	−0.2 ± 1.4	0.364 [3]	−0.6 ± 1.5	0.017 [4]	0.226 [1]
Fat mass (kg)								
Baseline	27.4 ± 4.0	28.2 ± 7.0	0.744 [1]					
At 12 weeks	27.7 ± 4.0	27.0 ± 4.3	0.458 [2]	0.3 ±1.4	0.154 [3]	−1.2 ± 4.8	0.072 [4]	0.025 [1]
Lean mass (kg)								
Baseline	40.5 ± 7.0	39.8 ± 8.2	0.260 [1]					
At 12 weeks	41.1 ± 7.0	39.8 ± 7.5	0.139 [1]	0.6 ± 1.4	0.154 [3]	−0.1 ± 4.0	0.011 [4]	0.762 [1]
Adiponectin (ug/mL)								
Baseline	3.95 ± 2.0	4.36 ± 2.1	0.314 [1]					
At 12 weeks	4.23 ± 1.8	4.79 ± 2.3	0.456 [1]	0.28 ± 0.7	0.003 [4]	0.43 ± 1.48	0.007 [4]	0.762 [1]
Total Cholesterol (mg/dL)								
Baseline	199.4 ± 28.9	203.0 ± 33.6	0.592 [2]					
At 12 weeks	200.6 ± 32.7	205.8 ± 32.6	0.448 [2]	1.2 ± 24.5	0.753 [3]	2.8 ± 17.9	0.292 [3]	0.288 [1]
Triglyceride (mg/dL)								
Baseline	128.3 ± 114.3	124.2 ± 88.4	0.741 [1]					
At 12 weeks	138.0 ± 85.9	136.8 ± 102.1	0.710 [1]	9.7 ± 95.0	0.009 [4]	12.6 ± 51.2	0.095 [4]	0.301 [1]
HDL-Cholesterol (mg/dL)								
Baseline	55.0 ± 10.5	57.7 ± 13.7	0.290 [2]					
At 12 weeks	54.6 ± 11.2	55.6 ± 12.8	0.490 [1]	−0.4 ± 8.9	0.141 [4]	−2.1 ± 5.9	0.020 [3]	0.665 [1]
LDL-Cholesterol (mg/dL)								
Baseline	118.8 ± 28.1	120.9 ± 26.9	0.711 [2]					
At 12 weeks	119.1 ± 26.8	122.8 ± 27.5	0.529 [2]	0.4 ± 23.8	0.739 [3]	1.8 ± 17.1	0.474 [3]	0.355 [1]

BMI, body mass index; HDL, high density lipoprotein; LDL, low density lipoprotein; SAD, sagittal abdomen distance. Shapiro-Wilk's test was employed for test of normality assumption * *p* values were compared within each group from baseline. ** *p* values were compared between groups. [1] *p* values were derived from Mann-Whitney's U test. [2] *p* values were derived from independent *t* test. [3] *p* values were derived from paired *t* test. [4] *p* values were derived from Wilcoxon's signed rank test.

Table 3. Changes in laboratory results related to safety in the ITT population.

Variable	Control (*n* = 45)			Collagen (*n* = 45)		
	Week 0	Week 12	*p*	Week 0	Week 12	*p*
AST (IU/L)	24.51 ± 7.9	20.93 ± 5.8	0.003	23.84 ± 10.0	24.87 ± 11.8	0.066
ALT (IU/L)	22.31 ± 13.3	20.76 ± 9.5	0.876	24.02 ± 19.7	25.44 ± 20.1	0.932
Cr (mg/dL)	0.69 ± 0.14	0.66 ± 0.1	0.016	0.71 ± 0.1	0.69 ± 0.1	0.812
Glucose (mg/dL)	91.67 ± 11.8	88.6 ± 9.7	0.033	90.07 ± 10.5	89.58 ± 12.6	0.244

AST, aspartate aminotransferase; ALT, alanine aminotransferase; Cr, creatinine. *p* values were compared within each group from baseline.

3. Discussion

To our best knowledge, this study is the first randomized, double-blind, placebo-controlled trial to identify the efficacy, safety, and tolerability of SCP in overweight people. Although the molecular mechanism underlying the anti-obesity effect of fish collagen peptides has now been discovered, the influence of them on body fat in humans had yet to been addressed before our study.

Thus, we aimed to see whether SCP could reduce human body fat as well. Our results showed that oral SCP of 2000 mg daily for 12 weeks decreased a small amount of body fat and was tolerated without reducing calorie intake and increasing physical activities.

The biological underlying mechanism of this current outcome can be found in previous animal studies conducted recently [21,22]. Lee et al. observed in obese mice that the oral administration of fish collagen peptide (FCP) significantly reduced body weight gain induced by HFD without a significant difference in food intake, confirming that FCP has an anti-adipogenic effect in in vitro and in vivo models [21]. Their findings demonstrate that subcritical water-hydrolyzed FCP inhibits lipid accumulation during the differentiation of 3T3-L1 preadipocytes into adipocytes by suppressing the expression of adipogenic master transcription factors such as peroxisome proliferator-activated receptor-γ (PPAR-γ), CCAAT/enhancer binding protein-alpha (C/EBP-α) and adipocyte protein 2 (aP2) genes, which mainly regulate the differentiation and maintenance of adipocytes, leading to a significant decrease in adipocyte size. Moreover, FCP improved the lipid profile showing reduced serum levels of TC, TG, and LDL-C while increased HDL-C. Another study conducted by Astre G et al. confirmed the previous results showing HFD-fed mice supplemented by FCP exhibited a significantly lower weight gain as soon as the 12th week of treatment, whereas no effect was observed in control group mice [22]. Additionally, lower glucose and a decrease of inflammatory cytokines were seen among mice treated with FCD, presenting a potential effect of FCP on insulin sensitivity.

Although Lee et al. [21] and Astre G et al. [22] did not use skate as a source of collagen peptides in their studies, skate skin is also reported as a good source of collagen, consisting of properties of amino acid-rich collagen. The major amino acids of skate skin are arginine, proline, and glutamic acid. Of the total amino acids, approximately 19.8% of arginine and 12% of proline are presented in the skin part [12]. The stability of collagen is proportional to the total amount of collagen and associated with the pyrolidine (proline + hydroxyproline) content [23], thus it can be enhanced by using skate skin. A large amount of skate skin is being disposed of as skate is becoming popular in both the fresh and fermented form owing to the recognition of its high quantity of nutrients and unique flavor in Korea. From an environmental perspective, therefore, it would be a good solution to prevent by-products from being excessively generated.

More recent findings of Woo et al. [18] specifically using collagen peptide derived from skate skin were consistent with the previous research. In this study, a reduced increase in body weight and visceral adipose tissue was observed in the SCD-fed groups compared to the control group. The anti-obesity effects of SCP were attributed to being mediated by regulating transcription factors and enzymes which regulate hepatic lipid metabolism. Histological analysis of the liver revealed that SCP suppressed hepatic lipid accumulation and reduced the lipid droplet size in the adipose tissue. TG-lowering effect of SCP significantly suppressed adipose tissue differentiation in a dose-dependent manner, which was also demonstrated by the histologic results in adipose tissue. Additionally, the researchers observed that the intake of SCP increased the hepatic protein expression of phosphorylated 5' adenosine monophosphate-activated protein kinase (p-AMPK) with elevated adiponectin and reduced leptin levels. As a regulator of energy balance by affecting whole body fuel utilization, AMPK induces fatty acid oxidation and inhibits adipocyte differentiation and the synthesis of hepatic fatty acid, cholesterol [24] emerging as a key target for obesity resolution. It is also involved in the regulation of adiponectin, which can activate p-AMPK [25]. In line with this result, our study showed a slightly larger increase in the adiponectin level in IG than that in CG; although this difference between the groups was not statistically significant. For now, we cannot determine whether this increase in adiponectin shown in the human study is mediated by the same way that SCP works on p-AMPK in an animal model. However, our finding can be clinical evidence that p-AMPK may be a good target with respect to SCP related human experimental study in the future.

In our study, IG saw no statistically significant difference in fat mass (kg). However, there was a significant change in the body fat percentage (%). Methodologically, body fat (%) by DXA indicates the body fat (kg) normalized by total body weight (body fat (%) = body fat (kg)/total body weight (kg)) [26]. Thus, an increase in total body weight causes underestimated body fat (%) and a decrease in body weight comes with overestimated body fat (%) even though actual body fat is the same. Our data shows that the total body weight of CG after 12 weeks was slightly higher than that of IG in which the difference was not statistically significant. This point may be attributable to the non-significance in fat mass (kg) change.

In contrast to those animal studies, the present study failed to find improvements in lipid profile with a slight HDL-C decrease found in IG. The authors cannot infer a convincing explanation for that from the current findings. Presumably, it was probably because HDL-C is known to mainly increase by boosting physical activity [27], which was not conducted in our study. From a clinical point of view, although there was a statistically significant HDL-C reduction in IG, the absolute amount seems not clinically important since both levels of HLD–C before and after SCD administration were still at a desirable level from a CVD prevention perspective. Additionally, lipid metabolism is much more complicated in humans than in animal models and many other factors may have been involved in the process that our study missed including covariates. Furthermore, our primary outcome was a change in body fat. Therefore, the size of the study might not be large enough to identify the effect of SCD on lipids with a study period of 12 weeks. Most importantly, previous animal studies induced weight gain by feeding a high-fat diet in order for mice to reach a hyperlipidemic state before administration of SCD while the majority of our study subjects had normal lipid levels at the baseline and this study did not apply the intervention to the subjects for an improvement in lipid levels.

To fight against obesity and related metabolic disorders, several anti-obesity drugs have been approved by the FDA for the treatment of obesity. However, it is unclear whether these medications actually bring about improved health outcomes including the prevention of CVD and improve the quality of life given that trials of medication-based weight loss interventions showed high study drop-out rates ($\geq$35% in half the included trials) and the differences in these outcomes were small among those on medication compared with placebo [28]. Known adverse effects, financial burden by hefty prices of medications, and failure of the significant outcome of losing weight seem to force obese people to seek alternative treatments with fewer side effects. In this context, many natural products have been tested as potential alternative therapies for obesity and our study was one of them.

Consequently, although the absolute amount was small, body fat loss found in our IG was quite impressive, when considering the fact that the duration of the intervention was relatively short and that the study did not require the participant to engage in any program in order to increase physical activity and cut down on calorie intake so that they could keep their daily routine as they usually had done. Most of the time, subjects who are involved in studies which are designed to demonstrate the efficacy of anti-obesity drugs are provided with dietary advice to decrease calorie intake and are encouraged to participate in moderate physical activity programs at least three times a week, which can be difficult for the subjects to adhere to the trial to the end showing a high drop-out rate and leads to a lower weight loss outcome than expected [29,30]. Additionally, in our study, the reduction in body fat occurred as soon as 6 weeks after taking SCD, showing a significant difference from CG and this gap was sustained until the study ended. On the other hand, recent research has focused on the roles of gastrointestinal peptides in obesity control [31,32]. They are known to be potential regulators of satiety such as cholecystokinin (CCK) and to influence food intake, which is critical when it comes to losing weight [33]. With regards to this point, further study is needed to see if SCD has an impact on gastrointestinal peptides.

The present study has some limitations. We included woman-dominant participants (81%) who are considered relatively better at complying with a study protocol and more conscious about their weight and appearance than men, which may result in a more favorable outcome in weight control intervention. Moreover, since a 24-h dietary recall is affected by day-to-day variation, the one-day investigation may not represent the usual intake of the subjects [34]. The IPAQ also has a substantial measurement error with the tendency to overestimate, although it consists of 27 questions which reflect on the previous seven days' physical activities [35]. These weaknesses of self-report surveys led to the result of a negative caloric balance shown in our subjects. However, the researchers asked the participants not to try to change their eating and physical patterns throughout the trial except for taking SCD so that we could assess the effect of SCD possibly only. In this context, the main purpose of the 24-h dietary recall and IPAQ in our study was to see if there were significant differences of before and after SCD administration in the overall calorie intake or expenditure in the daily routine of the subjects. Consequently, our data showed no changes between the two cited time points as planned. If there were any changes in them, we would have analyzed data adjusting for the amount of calories that the participants consumed and spent. Lastly, the current study was conducted by a single center, which can be limited to generalize the results.

Despite these limitations, our study is considerably valuable owing to several strengths. Firstly, to the best of the authors' knowledge, it is the first clinical study to examine the efficacy and tolerability of SCP on obesity. Moreover, the measurements of body composition were checked by DXA that is more accurate [36] than bioelectrical impedance analysis, which is most commonly used in the clinical study and private clinics due to its lower cost and simplicity to apply [37]. Furthermore, many trials of weight loss interventions have focused on body weight as their primary efficacy endpoint [28]. However, when it comes to resolution of obesity, what is fundamentally important is whether the intervention can effectively reduce body fat, not just body weight. The current study measured the change in body fat by using a reliable quantitative method through DXA.

We confirmed that there was no toxicity or severe adverse effect when SCP was applied to humans. More importantly, only SCD supplement for three months without having to change dietary habits and physical performance decreased more body fat than the placebo significantly (-1.2 kg vs. $+0.3$ kg, $p = 0.025$) and its effect came out as soon as six weeks after it was taken whereas no effect was observed in CG. The study suggests that SCD can help reduce excess body fat and it can be considered a potential alternative treatment for obesity itself and associated disorders. If it is combined with exercise and dietary intervention, the effect of SCD can be greater. However, a replicated study with a larger population is needed so as to reconfirm this favorable effect of SCP on body composition and to elucidate the mechanism responsible for the action of SCP in humans.

4. Materials and Methods

4.1. Study Design and Study Subjects

The present study was designed as a randomized, placebo-controlled, double-blind controlled clinical trial and approved by the Institutional Review Board at Pusan National University Yangsan Hospital (IRB No. 02-2017-012). We carried out the study in accordance with the principles of the Declaration of Helsinki from 26 June 2017 through 5 June 2018. Written informed consents following a fully detailed description of the study protocol were obtained from all participants before enrollment. This trial is registered with ClinicalTrials.gov Identifier: NCT03409705.

Eligible subjects were overweight, or obese, defined according to the guidelines of the Korean Society for the Study of Obesity [20]. One hundred adults aged between 20 and 60 years with any value from 23 to 30 kg/m^2 of body mass index (BMI) were enrolled through recruitment posting at a tertiary hospital in Yangsan. The individuals were excluded if they had any conditions as following; (1) previously taken any medication or supplements that can cause a change in body weight within the past one month including anti-depressants, anti-absorptive agents, appetite suppressors and any other hormonal products, (2) history of engagement in commercial anti-obesity programs within the past three months, (3) being treated for hyperthyroidism or hypothyroidism, (4) alcohol abuser, (5) quit smoking within three months of enrollment, (6) uncontrolled blood pressure, blood glucose, or gastrointestinal symptoms, (7) an aspartate aminotransferase (AST) or alanine aminotransferase (ALT) serum level greater than 80 mg/dL or a creatinine (Cr) level greater than 1.5 mg/dL, (8) pregnant or lactating women or (9) allergic to the ingredient involved. In addition, for safety reasons, candidates diagnosed with cardiovascular diseases or any cancer during the six months prior to study commencement were also excluded. Four participants met the exclusion criteria and ten participants declined to participate.

4.2. Randomization

One hundred adults were recruited for screening and 90 (90%) participants were finally enrolled. After undergoing baseline measurements, they were randomly assigned to either one of the two groups through block randomization methods using randomized numbers and given identification numbers on recruitment: the intervention group (IG) (*n* = 45), which received 2000 mg of SCP per day in the form of capsules, or the control group (*n* = 45) which was given a placebo (Figure 2). Randomization codes were created by an expert in statistics using nQuery Advisor 7.0. Those who were responsible for deciding on study eligibility and conducting the measurements were kept unaware of the results of the randomization throughout the whole study process. All of the participants were asked to visit the center four times in total (visit 1; for screening, visit 2; randomization and start taking supplements, visit 3; 6 weeks after intervention, visit 4; 12 weeks later).

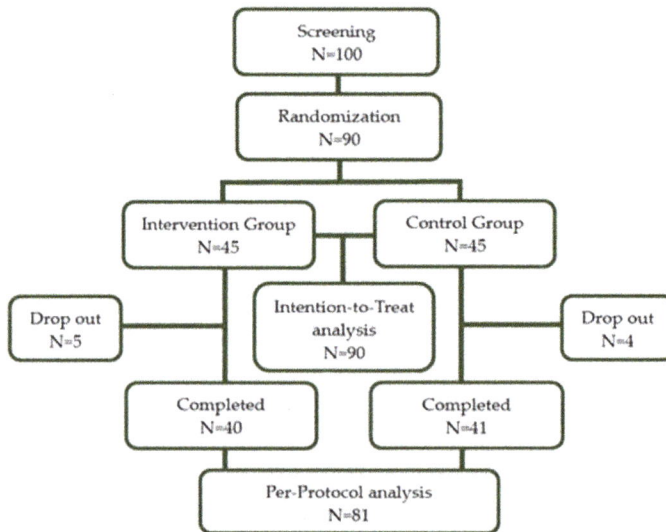

Figure 2. Flow diagram of the study subjects.

4.3. Intervention

The dosage of SCP applied to the subjects had been determined based on the results from previous animal studies where mice fed 300 mg of SCP daily had shown a significant reduction in body fat without any adverse events. Given the dosage of 300 mg applied to mice of which an average body weight was in these studies [18,19], 2000 mg of SCP was considered appropriate to be given to humans with an average body weight of 60 kg according to the guidance for estimating the maximum safe starting dose in initial clinical trials for therapeutics in adult healthy volunteers [38]. Two capsules (500 mg per capsule) of SCP were taken twice a day in the morning and evening by the subjects in IG (total four capsules each day) for 12 weeks. Subjects in CG were given the placebos with the same protocol and duration. Capsules were visually identical and supplied by Serom Co., Ltd. (Jeonnam, South Korea). Compliance was assessed by counting the remaining capsules at every visit and less than 80% of the taken number of capsules was considered to have dropped out from the study. Reports of any adverse event or unpredicted drug reaction were reported throughout the study.

4.4. Evaluation of Dietary Intake and Physical Activities

At baseline and the 12th week of the trial, the study subjects were asked to answer the questionnaire on dietary intake and physical activities that mainly determine the change in body weight so as to check if there was a significant alteration in their daily routine and to take into account the extra possible effect on their body composition. Dietary intake was investigated by the 24-h recall, which is an open-label nutritional survey method for estimating all food products ingested by the study subjects during the previous 24 h, together with dietary information (time, location, types of food, amount, and cooking method) and hereby reflecting the recent calorie intake of individuals [39,40]. Alcohol drinking was defined as consumption of alcohol with an average of seven cups for men and five or more for women, more than two times a week [41] Frequency, intensity and type of physical activities that the participants had done during the previous weeks were reported using the international physical activity questionnaires (IPAQ) [35] and the number of physical activities were represented as the metabolic equivalent of task (METs).

4.5. Measurements

As the primary outcome was changed into body fat mass (kg) and body fat percent of each subject, dual-energy X-ray absorptiometry (DXA) (Lunar Prodigy 8.50, Lunar Radiation Corp., Madison, WI, USA) was implemented twice at baseline and 12th week of the study. The fat mass percentage was calculated as fat mass/(fat mass + lean mass + bone mineral content). Secondary outcome variables were changes in BMI, sagittal abdomen distance (SAD), fat mass (kg) and lean mass (kg) checked by DXA, lipid profile (triglyceride (TG), total cholesterol (TC), high density lipoprotein cholesterol (HDL-C), low density lipoprotein cholesterol (LDL-C)), free fatty acid (FFA), and adiponectin. The participants were asked to maintain a fasting state for at least 4 h before the test. SAD was measured while the participants were lying supine on their back. A caliper with two sliding arms attached parallel to a vertical scale (Holtain-Kahn Abdominal Caliper 50 cm (98.609XL), U.K.) (Holtain-Kahn Abdominal Caliper Extra Long 50 cm (Holtain Model 609 XL), Seritex Inc, 1 Madison St. East Rutherford, NJ, USA) according to the standard method for the use of the caliper [42]. The upper arm of the caliper was lowered without compressing the abdomen and the arm of the caliper was placed at the level of L4–L5 under the participant. The reading on the vertical scale with a normal exhalation was noted in cm. BMI was calculated by dividing weight (kg) by height squared (m^2). To measure blood pressure (BP), a mercury sphygmomanometer was used in the sitting position after a 10-min rest period. Two readings of systolic and diastolic BP were checked at 3-min intervals, and averages were recorded in the analysis. Blood samples were collected at baseline and after 12 weeks of study after a 12-h fast. Fasting blood glucose was reported using a glucose oxidase test method (LX-20, Beckman Coulter, Fullerton, CA, USA). Serum AST, ALT, and Cr were measured using a Toshiba TBA200FR biochemical analyzer (Toshiba Co. Ltd., Tokyo, Japan).

4.6. Statistical Methods

The sample size of the study was calculated based on the research by Min et al. [43]. The estimated sample size was 45 patients per group for an 80% power to detect a difference in the mean investigator assessment score of 0.8, assuming a standard deviation of 1.2472 in the primary outcome variables and an alpha error of 5% with a 10% of drop-off rate. When a result of a test was unavailable, the last recorded data entry was included in the analysis (the last observation carried forward method). Efficacy analysis was conducted on both an intention to treat (ITT) basis on subjects that received at least one dose of SCP or placebo and that underwent at least one assessment post-baseline and per protocol (PP) only including data from subjects that completed the study protocol as planned. The Shapiro-Wilk's test was employed to test the normality assumption. Intergroup comparisons of baseline characteristics and their changes at the 12th week of the trial were done using the two-sample *t*-test for continuous variables (or Mann-Whitney's U test in case of valuables showing non-normal distributions) or the chi-square test for categorical variables (or Fisher's exact test in case of valuables showing non-normal distributions). Intragroup comparisons were conducted using the paired *t*-test for continuous variables (or Mann-Whitney's U test in case of valuables showing non-normal distributions). An analysis of covariance (ANCOVA) was performed to compare intergroup differences in outcomes after adjustment for physical activities and covariates that had shown a statistical significance between the groups at baseline. A *p*-value of less than 0.05 was considered statistically significant. SPSS version 22.0 (SPSS Statistics for Windows Version 22.0, Armonk, NY, IBM Corp) was employed for the analysis.

Author Contributions: Conceptualization, S.Y.L.; Formal analysis, Y.-H.Y.; Investigation, J.G.L.; Methodology, Y.H.C.; Project administration, G.H.K.; Supervision, Y.J.K.; Writing—original draft, Y.J.T.

Funding: This research received no external funding.

Acknowledgments: The authors would like to acknowledge the excellent technical assistance provided by Ye Li Lee, a senior researcher from Integrated Research Institute for Natural Ingredients and Functional Foods at Pusan National University Hospital.

Conflicts of Interest: The authors declare no conflict of interest.

References

1. Aminde, L.N.; Veerman, L. Interventions for the prevention of cardiovascular diseases: A protocol for a systematic review of economic evaluations in low-income and middle-income countries. *BMJ Open* **2016**, *6*, e013668. [CrossRef] [PubMed]
2. GBD 2015 Obesity Collaborators; Afshin, A.; Forouzanfar, M.H.; Reitsma, M.B.; Sur, P.; Estep, K.; Lee, A.; Marczak, L.; Mokdad, A.H.; Moradi-Lakeh, M.; et al. Health Effects of Overweight and Obesity in 195 Countries over 25 Years. *N. Engl. J. Med.* **2017**, *377*, 13–27. [PubMed]
3. Kreidieh, D.; Itani, L.; El Masri, D.; Tannir, H.; Citarella, R.; El Ghoch, M. Association between Sarcopenic Obesity, Type 2 Diabetes, and Hypertension in Overweight and Obese Treatment-Seeking Adult Women. *J. Cardiovasc. Dev. Dis.* **2018**, *5*, 51. [CrossRef] [PubMed]
4. Yao, F.; MacKenzie, R.G. Obesity Drug Update: The Lost Decade? *Pharmaceuticals* **2010**, *3*, 3494–3521. [CrossRef]
5. Hays, N.P.; Kim, H.; Wells, A.M.; Kajkenova, O.; Evans, W.J. Effects of whey and fortified collagen hydrolysate protein supplements on nitrogen balance and body composition in older women. *J. Am. Diet. Assoc.* **2009**, *109*, 1082–1087. [CrossRef] [PubMed]
6. Zdzieblik, D.; Oesser, S.; Baumstark, M.W.; Gollhofer, A.; König, D. Collagen peptide supplementation in combination with resistance training improves body composition and increases muscle strength in elderly sarcopenic men: A randomised controlled trial. *Br. J. Nutr.* **2015**, *114*, 1237–1245. [CrossRef] [PubMed]
7. Fahmi, A.; Morimura, S.; Guo, H.-C.; Shigematsu, T.; Kida, K.; Uemura, Y. Production of angiotensin I converting enzyme inhibitory peptides from sea bream scales. *Process Biochem.* **2004**, *39*, 1195–1200. [CrossRef]
8. Zhu, C.-F.; Li, G.-Z.; Peng, H.-B.; Zhang, F.; Chen, Y.; Li, Y. Treatment with marine collagen peptides modulates glucose and lipid metabolism in Chinese patients with type 2 diabetes mellitus. *Appl. Physiol. Nutr. Metab.* **2010**, *35*, 797–804. [CrossRef] [PubMed]
9. Tanaka, M.; Koyama, Y.-I.; Nomura, Y. Effects of collagen peptide ingestion on UV-B-induced skin damage. *Biosci. Biotechnol. Biochem.* **2009**, *73*, 930–932. [CrossRef] [PubMed]
10. Wang, J.; Xie, Y.; Pei, X.; Yang, R.; Zhang, Z.; Li, Y. The lipid-lowering and antioxidative effects of marine collagen peptides. *Chin. J. Prev. Med.* **2008**, *42*, 226–230.
11. Baek, J.M.; Kang, K.H.; Kim, S.H.; Noh, J.S.; Jeong, K.S. Development of high functional collagen peptide materials using skate skins. *J. Environ. Sci. Int.* **2016**, *25*, 579–588. [CrossRef]
12. Cho, S.H.; Michael, L.; Eun, J.B. Nutritional composition and microflora of the fresh and fermented skate (*Raja Kenojei*) skins. *Int. J. Food Sci. Nutr.* **2004**, *55*, 45–51. [CrossRef] [PubMed]
13. Hu, F.Y.; Chi, C.F.; Wang, B.; Deng, S.G. Two Novel Antioxidant Nonapeptides from Protein Hydrolysate of Skate (Raja porosa) muscle. *Mar. Drugs* **2015**, *13*, 1993–2009. [CrossRef] [PubMed]
14. Pan, X.; Zhao, Y.Q.; Hu, F.Y.; Chi, C.F.; Wang, B. Anticancer Activity of a Hexapeptide from Skate (Raja porosa) Cartilage Protein Hydrolysate in HeLa Cells. *Mar. Drugs* **2016**, *14*, 153. [CrossRef] [PubMed]

15. Song, Y.O.; Kim, M.; Woo, M.; Baek, J.M.; Kang, K.H.; Kim, S.H.; Roh, S.S.; Park, C.H.; Jeong, K.S.; Noh, J.S. Chondroitin Sulfate-Rich Extract of Skate Cartilage Attenuates Lipopolysaccharide-Induced Liver Damage in Mice. *Mar. Drugs* **2017**, *15*, 178. [CrossRef] [PubMed]

16. Takeshi, N.; Nobutaka, S. Isolation of collagen from fish waste material-skin, bone and fins. *Food Chem.* **2000**, *68*, 227–281.

17. Nam, H.K.; Lee, M.K. Studies on the fatty acids and cholesterol level of Raja skate. *J. Korean Oil Chem. Soc.* **1995**, *12*, 55–58.

18. Woo, M.J.; Song, Y.O.; Kang, K.H.; Noh, J.S. Anti-Obesity Effects of Collagen Peptide Derived from Skate (*Raja kenojei*) Skin Through Regulation of Lipid Metabolism. *Mar. Drugs* **2018**, *16*, 306. [CrossRef] [PubMed]

19. Kim, J.H.; Kim, O.-K.; Yoon, H.-G.; Park, J.; You, Y.; Kim, K.; Lee, Y.-H.; Choi, K.-C.; Lee, J.; Jun, W. Anti-obesity effect of extract from fermented Curcuma longa L. through regulation of adipogenesis and lipolysis pathway in high-fat diet-induced obese rats. *Food Nutr. Res.* **2016**, *60*, 30428. [CrossRef] [PubMed]

20. Lee, S.Y.; Park, H.S.; Kim, D.J.; Han, J.H.; Kim, S.M.; Cho, G.J.; Kim, D.Y.; Kwon, H.S.; Kim, S.R.; Lee, C.B.; et al. Appropriate waist circumference cutoff points for central obesity in Korean adults. *Clin. Pract.* **2007**, *75*, 72–80. [CrossRef] [PubMed]

21. Lee, E.J.; Hur, J.W.; Ham, S.A.; Jo, Y.; Lee, S.Y.; Choi, M.J.; Seo, H.G. Fish collagen peptide inhibits the adipogenic differentiation of preadipocytes and ameliorates obesity in high fat diet-fed mice. *Int. J. Biol. Macromol.* **2017**, *104*, 281–286. [CrossRef] [PubMed]

22. Astre, G.; Deleruyelle, S.; Dortignac, A.; Bonnet, C.; Valet, P.; Dray, C. Diet-induced obesity and associated disorders are prevented by natural bioactive type 1 fish collagen peptides (Naticol®) treatment. *J. Physiol. Biochem.* **2018**, *74*, 647–654. [CrossRef] [PubMed]

23. Johnston-Banks, F.A. Gelatine. In *Food Gels*; Harris, P., Ed.; Elsevier Applied Science: London, UK; New York, NY, USA, 1990; pp. 258–259.

24. Lage, R.; Diéguez, C.; Vidal-Puig, A.; López, M. AMPK: A metabolic gauge regulating whole-body energy homeostasis. *Trends Mol. Med.* **2008**, *14*, 539–549. [CrossRef] [PubMed]

25. Da Costa Guerra, J.F.; Maciel, P.S.; de Abreu, I.C.M.E.; Pereira, R.R.; Silva, M.; de Morais Cardoso, L.; Pinheiro-Sant'Ana, H.M.; de Lima, W.G.; Silva, M.E.; Pedrosa, M.L. Dietary açaí attenuates hepatic steatosis via adiponectin-mediated effects on lipid metabolism in high-fat diet mice. *J. Funct. Foods* **2015**, *14*, 192–202. [CrossRef]

26. Toombs, R.J.; Ducher, G.; Shepherd, J.A.; De Souza, M.J. The impact of recent technological advances on the trueness and precision of DXA to assess body composition. *Obesity* **2012**, *20*, 30–39. [CrossRef] [PubMed]

27. Kraus, W.E.; Houmard, J.A.; Duscha, B.D.; Knetzger, K.J.; Wharton, M.B.; McCartney, J.S.; Bales, C.W.; Henes, S.; Samsa, G.P.; Otvos, J.D.; et al. Effects of the amount and intensity of exercise on plasma lipoproteins. *N. Engl. J. Med.* **2002**, *347*, 1483–1492. [CrossRef] [PubMed]

28. LeBlanc, E.L.; Patnode, C.D.; Webber, E.M.; Redmond, N.; Rushkin, M.; O'Connor, E.A. Behavioral and Pharmacotherapy Weight Loss Interventions to Prevent Obesity-Related Morbidity and Mortality in Adults: An Updated Systematic Review for the U.S. Preventive Services Task Force. *JAMA* **2018**, *320*, 1172–1191. [CrossRef] [PubMed]

29. Khera, R.; Murad, M.H.; Chandar, A.K.; Dulai, P.S.; Wang, Z.; Prokop, L.J.; Loomba, R.; Camilleri, M.; Singh, S. Association of Pharmacological Treatments for Obesity with Weight Loss and Adverse Events: A Systematic Review and Meta-analysis. *JAMA* **2016**, *315*, 2424–2434. [CrossRef] [PubMed]

30. Smith, S.R.; Weissman, N.J.; Anderson, C.M.; Sanchez, M.; Chuang, E.; Stubbe, S.; Bays, H.; Shanahan, W.R.; Behavioral Modification and Lorcaserin for Overweight and Obesity Management (BLOOM) Study Group. Multicenter, Placebo-Controlled Trial of Lorcaserin for Weight Management. *N. Engl. J. Med.* **2010**, *363*, 245–256. [CrossRef] [PubMed]

31. Steinert, R.E.; Christine, F.B.; Asarian, L.; Horowitz, M.; Beglinger, C.; Geary, N. Ghrelin, CCK, GLP-1, and PYY(3–36): Secretory Controls and Physiological Roles in Eating and Glycemia in Health, Obesity, and After RYGB. *Physiol. Rev.* **2017**, *97*, 411–463. [CrossRef] [PubMed]

32. Mishra, A.K.; Dubey, V.; Ghosh, A.R. Obesity: An overview of possible role(s) of gut hormones, lipid sensing and gut microbiota. *Metabolism* **2016**, *65*, 48–65. [CrossRef] [PubMed]

33. Bray, G.A.; Tartaglia, L.A. Medicinal strategies in the treatment of obesity. *Nature* **2000**, *404*, 672–677. [CrossRef] [PubMed]

34. Whitton, C.; Ho, J.C.Y.; Tay, Z.; Rebello, S.A.; Lu, Y.; Ong, C.N.; van Dam, R.M. Relative Validity and Reproducibility of a Food Frequency Questionnaire for Assessing Dietary Intakes in a Multi-Ethnic Asian Population Using 24-h Dietary Recalls and Biomarkers. *Nutrients* **2017**, *9*, 1059. [CrossRef] [PubMed]

35. Craig, C.L.; Marshall, A.L.; Sjöström, M.; Bauman, A.E.; Booth, M.L.; Ainsworth, B.E.; Pratt, M.; Ekelund, U.; Yngve, A.; Sallis, J.F.; et al. International Physical Activity Questionnaire: 12-Country Reliability and Validity. *Med. Sci. Sports Exerc.* **2003**, *35*, 1381–1395. [CrossRef] [PubMed]

36. Rothney, M.P.; Brychta, R.J.; Schaefer, E.V.; Chen, K.Y.; Skarulis, M.C. Body composition measured by dual-energy X-ray absorptiometry half-body scans in obese adults. *Obesity* **2009**, *17*, 1281–1286. [CrossRef] [PubMed]

37. Coppini, L.Z.; Waitzberg, D.L.; Campos, A.C. Limitations and validation of bioelectrical impedance analysis in morbidly obese patients. *Curr. Opin. Clin. Nutr. Metab. Care* **2005**, *8*, 329–332. [CrossRef] [PubMed]

38. U.S. Department of Health and Human Services Food and Drug Administration Center for Drug Evaluation and Research (CDER). Guidance for Industry Estimating the Maximum Safe Starting Dose in Initial Clinical Trials for Therapeutics in Adult Healthy Volunteers. July 2005; Pharmacology and Toxicology. APPENDIX B, Analysis of Body Weight Effects on HED Calculations; p. 19. Available online: https://www.fda.gov/downloads/Drugs/Guidances/UCM078932.pdf%23search=%27guidekines+for+industry+sfe+starting%27 (accessed on 7 March 2019).

39. Rural Development Administration, National Institute of Agricultural Sciences. *Food Composition Table*; Rural Development Administration, National Institute of Agricultural Sciences: Wanju, Korea, 2011.

40. Jung, H.J.; Lee, S.E.; Kim, D.; Noh, H.; Song, S.; Kang, M. Development and feasibility of a web-based program 'Diet Evaluation System (DES)' in urban and community nutrition survey in Korea. *Korean J. Health Promot.* **2013**, *13*, 107–115. (In Korean)

41. Bradstock, K.; Forman, M.R.; Binkin, N.J.; Gentry, E.M.; Hogelin, G.C.; Williamson, D.F.; Trowbridge, F.L. Alcohol use and health behavior lifestyles among U.S. women: The behavioral risk factor surveys. *Addict. Behav.* **1988**, *13*, 61–71. [CrossRef]

42. Sampaio, L.R.; Simões, E.J.; Assis, A.M.; Ramos, L.R. Validity and reliability of the sagittal abdominal diameter as a predictor of visceral abdominal fat. *Arq. Bras. Endocrinol. Metabol.* **2007**, *51*, 980–986. [CrossRef] [PubMed]

43. Min, K.S.; Han, D.S.; Kwon, S.O.; Yeo, K.M.; Kim, B.N.; Ly, S. The effect of Sargassum confusum on reduction of body fat in obese women. *J. Nutr. Health* **2014**, *47*, 23–32. [CrossRef]

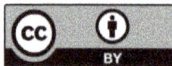

marine drugs

MDPI

Review

Anti-Obesity and Anti-Diabetic Effects of *Ishige okamurae*

Hye-Won Yang, K.H.N. Fernando, Jae-Young Oh, Xining Li, You-Jin Jeon * and BoMi Ryu *

Department of Marine Life Science, Jeju National University, Jeju 63243, Korea; koty221@naver.com (H.-W.Y.); hiruninfdo@gmail.com (K.H.N.F.); ojy0724@naver.com (J.-Y.O.); xiningmarinesci666@naver.com (X.L.)
* Correspondence: youjin2014@gmail.com (Y.-J.Y.); ryu.bomi@gmail.com (B.R.); Tel.: +82-64-754-3475 (B.R.)

Received: 15 March 2019; Accepted: 25 March 2019; Published: 29 March 2019

Abstract: Obesity is associated with several health complications and can lead to the development of metabolic syndrome. Some of its deleterious consequences are related to insulin resistance, which adversely affects blood glucose regulation. At present, there is a growing concern regarding healthy food consumption, owing to awareness about obesity. Seaweeds are well-known for their nutritional benefits. The brown alga *Ishige okamurae* (IO) has been studied as a dietary supplement and exhibits various biological activities in vitro and in vivo. The bioactive compounds isolated from IO extract are known to possess anti-obesity and anti-diabetic properties, elicited via the regulation of lipid metabolism and glucose homeostasis. This review focuses on IO extract and its bioactive compounds that exhibit therapeutic effects through several cellular mechanisms in obesity and diabetes. The information discussed in the present review may provide evidence to develop nutraceuticals from IO.

Keywords: *Ishige okamurae*; marine alga; obesity; diabetes; nutraceuticals

---

1. Introduction

Over the past 50 years, obesity has become a global public health issue that negatively affects quality of life and increases the risk of various illnesses and healthcare costs worldwide [1–3]. Obesity is considered a risk factor for coronary artery diseases, cerebrovascular accidents, type-2 diabetes mellitus, systemic hypertension, various cancers, fatty liver disease, osteoarthritis, and gynecological disorders [4]. An understanding of the molecular basis of obesity-associated diseases is required to approach its prevention. The properties of adipose tissue and adipocytes in obesity have been studied [5], and Higdon and Frei [6] also emphasized that obesity is a chronic oxidative stress condition due to an imbalance among tissue active oxygen, reactive oxygen species (ROS) and antioxidants.

Oxidative stress also plays a key role in the pathogenesis of many other progressive diseases including diabetes, atherosclerosis and cancer [7–9]. In addition, lipid accumulation has been correlated with various markers of systemic oxidative stress [10]. Furukawa et al. [11] reported that oxidative stress mediates the obesity-associated development of metabolic syndrome via two mechanisms: (1) increased oxidative stress due to lipid accumulation leads to dysregulated production of adipocytokines, and (2) selective increase in ROS production due to lipid accumulation leads to elevation in systemic oxidative stress. Oxidative stress can activate a series of stress pathways involving a family of serine/threonine kinases, resulting in a negative effect on insulin signaling [12], and an increase in the production of free radicals or impaired antioxidant defenses. Diabetes is characterized by hyperglycemia and insufficiency in the secretion or action of endogenous insulin [13]. An increase in oxidative stress can lead to hyperglycemia in both type-1 and type-2 diabetes [14,15]. Tan et al. [16] showed that hydrogen peroxide (H_2O_2) stimulated the inhibition of insulin-induced glucose uptake in vitro. In that study, oxidative stress directly causes insulin resistance via overactivation of extracellular signal-related kinase (ERK).

Current available therapies for obesity and diabetes have either limited efficacy or cause side effects. Therefore, many studies have suggested that natural sources can be used as complementary treatments and preventive materials with less toxic and fewer side effects [17]. Marine algae have been identified as rich sources of structurally diverse bioactive compounds including pigments, fucoidans, phycocolloids, and phlorotannis, with nutraceutical and biomedical potential [18,19]. *Ishige okamurae* (IO) is an edible brown seaweed found in temperate coastal areas, such as the Korean peninsula [20]. It is abundant along the coast of Jeju Island and is a potential functional food. In this review, we discuss the anti-obesity and anti-diabetic effects of IO extract and its cellular mechanisms of action. We also suggest its use as a potential nutraceutical source.

2. Anti-Obesity and Anti-Diabetic Properties of IO Extract

Ishige is a genus of brown algae with two species—*Ishige foliacea* and IO. Studies on the extracts of *Ishige*, including *Ishige foliacea* and IO, have reported various in vitro and in vivo activities, such as antioxidant, anti-diabetic, and anti-obesogenic effects [21–23]. Owing to these bioactivities, these extracts have been gaining increased attention in recent years for potential nutraceutical application in metabolic syndrome.

Metabolic syndrome is characterized by an increase in ROS levels, which cannot be counteracted by endogenous antioxidant systems [24]. The increase in ROS levels plays a key role in the development of metabolic diseases, which could lead to changes in glucose uptake, exacerbating diabetes mellitus, obesity, cardiovascular diseases, or cancer [24,25]. The antioxidant properties of *Ishige foliacea* and IO methanol extracts have been investigated in terms of their free-radical which includes 1,1-diphenyl-2-picryl hydrazyl (DPPH); 2,2-azobis(3-ethylbenzothiazoline-6-sulfonate (ABTS) and nitrite scavenging activity [21]. Furthermore, Heo and Jeon [26] reported that IO enzymatically extracted with different carbohydrases and proteases exhibits antioxidative effects. In particular, Ultraflo extract, which is a carbohydrase-based enzymatic extract, can scavenge free radicals, and Kojizyme extract, which is a protease-based extract, can reduce the DNA damage caused by hydrogen peroxide (H_2O_2). Thus, the antioxidant efficacy of IO extracts indicates that it is a potential functional food, which can be used as a supplement for patients with metabolic syndrome.

Diabetes and obesity are common, closely interrelated disorders and are caused by poor metabolic conditions. Obesity, a characteristic feature of metabolic syndrome, involves the accumulation of abnormal or excessive fat that may interfere with the maintenance of an optimal state of health [27]. It is also associated with a systemic increase in oxidative stress, resulting in adipokine imbalance [28]. Previous in vitro and in vivo studies have suggested that oxidative stress can cause obesity through increased proliferation of pre-adipocytes and increased size of differentiated adipocytes [29,30].

Cha and Cheon [31] showed that IO extract can inhibit lipid accumulation induced during adipogenesis of 3T3-L1 preadipocytes. The concerted regulation of gene expression by various adipogenic factors is required for the differentiation of preadipocytes to adipocytes. Furthermore, research on the mechanism underlying preadipocyte mitogenesis and differentiation into adipocytes may help understand the initiation and progression of obesity and its associated diseases. Peroxisome proliferator-activated receptors (PPARγ) has been studied for its involvement in the regulation of nutrient sensing and glucose and lipid metabolism [32]. Expression level of PPARγ is highest in adipose tissue [33] when it regulates the transcriptional cascade involved in adipocyte differentiation [34]. The hormone nuclear receptor PPARγ plays an important role in the regulation of downstream adipogenic genes [33]. Expression levels of PPARγ mRNA were significantly decreased by the IO extract during 10 days of induction [31]. Thus, the antioxidant effect of IO extract can inhibit the accumulation of lipids and modulate PPARγ expression. Although IO extract can decrease the levels of PPARγ, previous studies showed the effect of IO extract against obesity through other adipogenic transcription factors. The IO extract can suppress the increase in lipid droplet size by reducing the expression of adipogenic transcription factors in white adipose tissue (WAT), which is larger in a high-fat diet (HFD)-fed mice than in mice on a normal diet [35,36]. Therefore, IO extract can reduce body weight gain by preventing an increase in WAT mass and ameliorating HFD-induced obesity.

Adipose tissue helps maintain glucose and lipid homeostasis through the secretion of various factors and through neural networks [37–39]. Diabetes in obese people occurs mostly due to insulin resistance and subsequent hyperinsulinemia through adipogenesis and the insulin signaling pathway. In addition, oxidative stress has been linked with disruption of insulin secretion by pancreatic β-cells [40], glucose transport in muscle [8], and adipocytokines [41].

A widely used preclinical model of diabetes is *db/db* mice, characterized by hyperglycemia, hyperinsulinemia, hyperleptinemia, and obesity, similar to type-2 diabetes [42]. C57BL/KsJ-*db/db* mice were fed a standard semi-synthetic diet (AIN-93G) with IO extract (0.5%, w/w; IO extract supplementation), resulting in downregulated fasting blood glucose levels. IO extract supplementation controlled blood glucose levels during the intraperitoneal glucose tolerance test (IPGTT) [22]. Homeostatic model assessment (HOMA) is a method for assessing insulin resistance (IR) and is a useful index of insulin sensitivity [43]. It has been shown that HOMA-IR is lowered following IO extract supplementation [22]. Previous studies have suggested that therapeutic agents may be required to prevent hyperglycemic conditions in patients with early-stage type-2 diabetes. IO extract supplementation significantly lowered glycated hemoglobin (HbA1c) levels [22], which is useful for monitoring glycemic control in diabetic patients [44]. Taken together, IO extract supplementation can control blood glucose levels and improve insulin resistance in *db/db* mice. We suggest that IO extract can be used as an antidiabetic supplement.

3. Composition of IO

Many brown algae species are used as food ingredients and supplements and possess a variety of biological activities. These biological activities are related to the presence of polyphenols, polysaccharides and pigments. Among polyphenols, one of the most common classes of secondary metabolites derived from polymerized phloroglucinol units are phlorotannins [45]. Phlorotannins are tannin derivatives composed of several phloroglucinol units isolated from brown algae [19]. It has been reported that brown algae are richer in phlorotannins than other marine algae. Polyphenols can react with oxidants in one-electron reactions, pairing with the free electron of the oxidant to become chemically inactive. Therefore, polyphenols act as antioxidants that inhibit the formation of free radicals in biological systems [46]. In addition, previous studies have examined various biological activities associated with polyphenols from brown algae, including antioxidant, anti-coagulant, anti-bacterial, anti-inflammatory, and anti-cancer effects [18,47,48]. Thus, phlorotannins isolated from brown seaweeds represent the most widely studied class of secondary metabolites in marine organisms, with potential use in the nutraceutical and functional food industry.

Yoon et al. [49] studied the secondary metabolites of IO extract with antioxidant effects, including phloroglucinol, 6,6′-bieckol, and diphlorethohydroxycarmalol (DPHC). Octaphlorethol A (OPA) was also isolated and purified from IO extract [50]. Recently, a novel polyphenol-compound, ishophloroglucin A (IPA) with α-glucosidase inhibitory activity was isolated from IO extract [51]. Zou et al. [52] evaluated the antioxidant effects of 6,6′-bieckol and DPHC by using the electron spin resonance (ESR) technique. The two phlorotannins displayed potent radical scavenging activities against DPPH as well as hydroxyl, alkyl, and superoxide radicals. Moreover, effective concentration (EC_{50}) values of phlorotannins, defined as the concentration at which the radicals were scavenged by 50%, are summarized in Table 1. Heo and Jeon [53] reported the cytoprotective effect of DPHC in Vero cells against oxidative stress induced by hydrogen peroxide (H_2O_2).

Table 1. EC$_{50}$ values of phlorotannins from *Ishige okamurae*.

	EC$_{50}$ (μM $\pm$ SD)			
	DPPH	Hydroxyl	Alkyl	Superoxide
6,6'-bieckol	9.1 $\pm$ 0.4	23.7 $\pm$ 1.1	17.3 $\pm$ 1.0	15.4 $\pm$ 0.9
Diphlorethohydroxycarmalol (DPHC)	10.5 $\pm$ 0.5	27.1 $\pm$ 0.9	18.8 $\pm$ 1.2	16.7 $\pm$ 0.6
Phloroglucinol	Not determined	408.5 $\pm$ 3.7	103.5 $\pm$ 1.9	124.7 $\pm$ 2.4

Several studies have reported that among the pigments of brown algae, fucoxanthin can reduce oxidative stress and symptoms of metabolic syndrome via its anti-diabetic and anti-obesogenic effects [54–57]. In addition, Kang et al. [58] reported that fucoxanthin isolated from IO can reduce high glucose-induced oxidative stress in human umbilical vein endothelial cells (HUVEC) and in zebrafish models. Taken together, the antioxidative effects of IO may be effective as supplementary treatment of metabolic syndrome, including obesity and diabetes.

3.1. Anti-Obesity Effect of IO

When caloric expenditure is lower than caloric intake, adipocytes play a critical role by storing triacylglycerol and regulating metabolism in obesity. In fat tissue, adipocyte differentiation and lipid accumulation occur through adipocyte-specific proteins including enhancer binding protein (C/EBP), sterol-regulatory element-binding protein 1c (SREBP-1c), peroxisome proliferator activated receptor-γ (PPARγ), adiponectin, perilipin, fatty acid synthase (FAS), fatty acid binding protein (FABP4), and leptin [59]. According to Cha and Cheon [31], IO extract is known to inhibit lipid accumulation, which is induced during adipogenesis from 3T3-L1 preadipocytes. Previous studies have focused on the inhibition of lipid accumulation in 3T3-L1 cells through decreased expression levels of adipogenic-specific factors by polyphenols such as dieckol [60], epigallocatechin-3-gallate [61], and resveratrol [62]. Several studies have found that IO extract inhibited fat accumulation in 3T3-L1 cells through a molecular mechanism involving adipocyte-specific proteins.

DPHC from IO extract has potential antiadipogenic effects elicited via the inhibition of adipocyte differentiation and adipogenesis. Kang et al. [63] reported that levels of the adipogenesis-specific proteins including C/EBPα, SREBP-1c, PPARγ, and adiponectin were decreased to activate molecular mechanisms involved in 3T3-L1 adipocyte differentiation. These transcription factors are highly expressed in adipocytes and are involved in the mediation of lipid synthesis, lipolysis, and glucose uptake in adipocytes. DPHC can disrupt fatty acid synthesis by downregulating adipocyte-specific proteins including perilipin, FAS, FABP4, and leptin. Furthermore, DPHC can activate adenosine monophosphate-activated protein kinase (AMPK) and acetyl-CoA carboxylase (ACC), resulting in the inhibition of lipogenesis, adipocyte differentiation, and fatty acid synthesis in adipocytes. Besides the increase in AMPK and ACC, preadipocyte apoptosis also has an anti-obesity effect. Park et al. [64] reported that DPHC induced apoptosis in 3T3-L1 preadipocytes through the intrinsic pathway by regulating the protein levels of Fas, Bax, Bcl-2, caspase-9, caspase-3, and PARP. Taken together, DPHC can be used as a potential therapeutic agent against obesity.

3.2. Anti-Diabetic Activity of IO

Diabetes, a serious chronic metabolic disease, may develop with obesity and ageing in the general population. In addition, rapidly increasing blood glucose levels are a result of the hydrolysis of starch by pancreatic α-amylase and glucose uptake by intestinal α-glucosidases. These enzymes play a crucial role in the effective regulation of glucose absorption [65]. Therefore, an important strategy for suppressing postprandial hyperglycemia is the inhibition of α-amylase and α-glucosidase activities [66,67]. A previous study with C57BL/KsJ-*db/db* mice showed that IO extract supplementation prevented insulin resistance and regulated blood glucose levels in hyperglycemia [22].

Lee and Jeon [19] focused on developing potential anti-diabetic nutraceutical and functional foods from phlorotannins.

Furthermore, several studies found that IO extract showed anti-diabetic activity by inhibiting α-amylase and α-glucosidases. Phlorotannins isolated from IO extract have excellent anti-diabetic properties. DPHC (IC_{50} = 0.53 ± 0.08 and 0.16 ± 0.01 mM) showed effective inhibitory effects against α-amylase and α-glucosidase compared to acarbose (IC_{50} = 1.10 ± 0.07 and 1.05 ± 0.03 mM), which was used as the positive control [68]. DPHC significantly suppressed the increase in postprandial blood glucose levels in both streptozotocin-induced diabetic and normal mice after the consumption of starch [68]. Moreover, Lee et al. [69] described that DPHC treatment protected high glucose-induced damage in RINm5F pancreatic β-cells. The dysfunction of pancreatic β-cells has a central role in the pathogenesis of type-2 diabetes [70]. Therefore, DPHC can delay the absorption of dietary carbohydrates and improve secretory responsiveness of insulin following stimulation with glucose.

Recently, IPA, a novel polyphenol-compound derived from IO extract showed a solid α-glucosidase inhibitory activity [51]. The study showed the application of IPA in standardizing the inhibition of α-glucosidase activity of IO extract and proposed IPA potential in the application of marine-derived nutraceuticals.

4. Potential Nutraceutical Use of IO

The role of food is to provide enough nutrients to meet metabolic requirements, which is relevant to well-being, good health, and disease management [71]. Recently, consumer awareness of bioactive compounds as functional ingredients has increased, and knowledge about their various health benefits is increasing. Seaweeds are rich sources of structurally diverse bioactive compounds with valuable nutraceutical, pharmaceutical and cosmeceutical potentials [72]. Antioxidant properties of seaweeds enable their use as nutraceuticals and functional food ingredients [73]. A considerable number of bioactive compounds has been isolated from seaweeds and evaluated for their potential as functional food ingredients to assist in the treatment of metabolic diseases such as cancer, hypertension and diabetes [73].

IO is an edible brown seaweed that grows on rocks in the upper and middle intertidal zones in the northwest Pacific Ocean (Korea, Japan, and China), where it forms continuous bands [20]. As shown in Table 2, previous studies have discussed the usefulness of bioactive compounds from IO as functional ingredients [49,58,74]. Additionally, the antioxidant properties of the methanol extract and enzymatic extract from IO were evaluated to develop potential functional food materials against oxidative stress [21,26]. IO extract is rich in secondary metabolites such as phlorotannins, carotenoids, and polysaccharides with various bioactive properties.

Table 2. Bioactivities of functional ingredients from *Ishige okamurae*.

Functional Ingredient	Bioactivities	References
Methanolic extract	Antioxidant, anti-MMP, and anti-diabetic	[21,22,74]
Ethanolic extract	Anti-inflammatory	[75]
Enzymatic extract	Antioxidant	[26]
Fermented extract	Radioprotective and antioxidant	[76]
6,6′-Bieckol	Cholinesterase inhibition	[49]
Diphlorethohydroxycarmalol (DPHC)	Antioxidant, anti-cancer, anti-HIV, anti-obesity, and anti-diabetic	[52,53,64,68,69,77–79]
Fucoxanthin	Antioxidant, anti-inflammatory	[58,80]
Ishigoside	Antioxidant	[20]
Ishophloroglucin A (IPA)	α-glucosidases inhibition	[51]
Phloroglucinol	Cholinesterase inhibition	[49]

6,6′-bieckol is another phlorotannin from IO which possesses in vitro and in vivo neuroprotective effects. 6,6′-bieckol suppresses acetylcholinesterase (AChE) activity with an IC_{50} value of

46.42 ± 1.19 μM [49]. AChE plays a key role in the regulation of several physiological reactions by hydrolyzing the neurotransmitter acetylcholine in the cholinergic synapses [81,82]. In addition, Alzheimer's disease (AD) is related to a deficit in cholinergic functions in the brain [83]. Thus, the application of 6,6′-bieckol as an alternative for AChE inhibitors suggests a therapeutic potential in AD. Fucoxanthin, an accessory pigment in chloroplasts, is a well-known brown seaweed carotenoid with numerous important bioactive properties [84]. It is also one of the major constituents of IO. Kim et al. [80] showed that fucoxanthin from IO reduced the production of nitric oxide (NO) and inflammatory mediators, including inducible nitric oxide synthase (iNOS) and cyclooxygenase-2 (COX-2), and inhibited nuclear factor (NF)-κB activation and mitogen-activated protein kinases (MAPKs; JNK, ERK and p38) signal pathways in LPS-stimulated RAW264.7. In LPS-treated macrophages, pro-inflammatory cytokines and gene expression were upregulated through NF-κB activation and MAPK signaling pathways [85,86]. Cancer is characterized by uncontrolled cell growth and spread [87]. Fucoxanthin has the potential to inhibit the proliferation of melanoma cell lines (B16F10 cells) through cell cycle arrest during the G0/G1 phase and the apoptotic pathway [64]. Fucoxanthin also decreases Bcl-xL expression level, which is a critical regulator of the apoptotic pathway. Moreover, it has been shown that fucoxanthin suppressed in vivo growth of B16F10 melanoma in Balb/c mice. Therefore, researchers have been interested in identifying new anti-cancer drugs from marine sources, which supposedly have fewer adverse side effects unlike synthetic drugs [88].

5. Conclusions

Obesity is associated with lipid accumulation together with oxidative stress, which increases insulin resistance and eventually results in diabetes. In this review, we have discussed the antioxidant properties of IO extract and the mechanisms of action underpinning its anti-obesity and anti-diabetic effects (Figure 1).

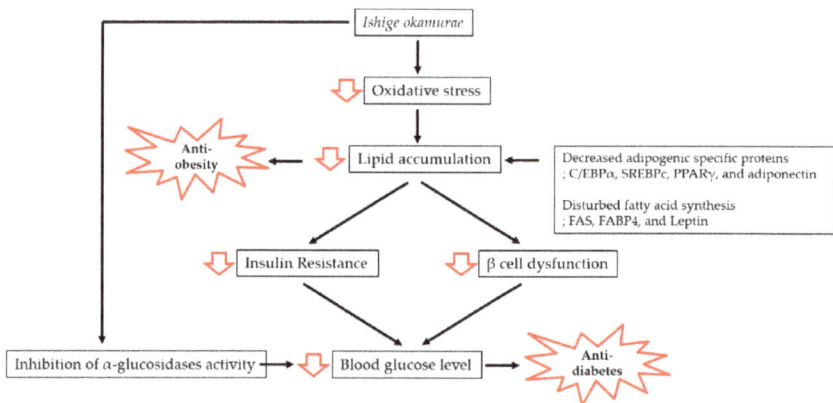

Figure 1. Mechanisms involved in the anti-obesity and anti-diabetic effects of *Ishige okamurae*.

The significant health benefits associated with IO may represent an interesting progress in the search for novel functional applications. IO can also be used as a therapeutic agent and functional food against metabolic syndrome.

Author Contributions: H.-W.Y.: Collection and assembly of data, manuscript writing; K.H.N.F., J.-Y.O., X.L.: Collection and assembly of data and addition of valuable comments; Y.-J.J.: final approval of manuscript; B.R.: Conception and design, data analysis and interpretation, final approval of manuscript. All the authors read and approved the final version of the manuscript.

Funding: This research was a part of the project titled 'Development of functional food products with natural materials derived from marine resources', funded by the Ministry of Oceans and Fisheries, Korea.

Mar. Drugs **2019**, *17*, 202

Conflicts of Interest: The authors declare no conflict of interest

References

1. World Health Organization. World Health Organization Obesity and Overweight Fact Sheet. 2016. Available online: https://www.who.int/news-room/fact-sheets/detail/obesity-and-overweight (accessed on 29 March 2019).

2. Scully, T. Society at large: The increasing prevalence of obesity is a worldwide phenomenon, affecting peoples from diverse cultural and economic backgrounds. *Nature* **2014**, *508*, S50. [CrossRef]

3. Ng, M.; Fleming, T.; Robinson, M.; Thomson, B.; Graetz, N.; Margono, C.; Mullany, E.C.; Biryukov, S.; Abbafati, C.; Abera, S.F. Global, regional, and national prevalence of overweight and obesity in children and adults during 1980–2013: A systematic analysis for the Global Burden of Disease Study 2013. *Lancet* **2014**, *384*, 766–781. [CrossRef]

4. Mozaffarian, D. Dietary and policy priorities for cardiovascular disease, diabetes, and obesity: A comprehensive review. *Circulation* **2016**, *133*, 187–225. [CrossRef]

5. Fernández-Sánchez, A.; Madrigal-Santillán, E.; Bautista, M.; Esquivel-Soto, J.; Morales-González, Á.; Esquivel-Chirino, C.; Durante-Montiel, I.; Sánchez-Rivera, G.; Valadez-Vega, C.; Morales-González, J.A. Inflammation, oxidative stress, and obesity. *Int. J. Mol. Sci.* **2011**, *12*, 3117–3132. [CrossRef]

6. Higdon, J.V.; Frei, B. Obesity and oxidative stress: A direct link to CVD? *Am. Heart Assoc.* **2003**, *23*, 365–367. [CrossRef]

7. Matsuda, M.; Shimomura, I. Increased oxidative stress in obesity: Implications for metabolic syndrome, diabetes, hypertension, dyslipidemia, atherosclerosis, and cancer. *Obes. Res. Clin. Pr.* **2013**, *7*, 330–341. [CrossRef]

8. Maddux, B.A.; See, W.; Lawrence, J.C.; Goldfine, A.L.; Goldfine, I.D.; Evans, J.L. Protection against oxidative stress-induced insulin resistance in rat L6 muscle cells by micromolar concentrations of α-lipoic acid. *Diabetes* **2001**, *50*, 404–410. [CrossRef]

9. Nakazono, K.; Watanabe, N.; Matsuno, K.; Sasaki, J.; Sato, T.; Inoue, M. Does superoxide underlie the pathogenesis of hypertension? *Proc. Natl. Acad. Sci. USA* **1991**, *88*, 10045–10048. [CrossRef]

10. Keaney, J.F., Jr.; Larson, M.G.; Vasan, R.S.; Wilson, P.W.; Lipinska, I.; Corey, D.; Massaro, J.M.; Sutherland, P.; Vita, J.A.; Benjamin, E.J. Obesity and systemic oxidative stress: Clinical correlates of oxidative stress in the Framingham Study. *Arterioscl. Throm. Vasc.* **2003**, *23*, 434–439. [CrossRef] [PubMed]

11. Furukawa, S.; Fujita, T.; Shimabukuro, M.; Iwaki, M.; Yamada, Y.; Nakajima, Y.; Nakayama, O.; Makishima, M.; Matsuda, M.; Shimomura, I. Increased oxidative stress in obesity and its impact on metabolic syndrome. *J. Clin. Investig.* **2017**, *114*, 1752–1761. [CrossRef]

12. Rains, J.L.; Jain, S.K. Oxidative stress, insulin signaling, and diabetes. *Free Radic. Biol. Med.* **2011**, *50*, 567–575. [CrossRef]

13. Maritim, A.; Sanders, A.; Watkins Iii, J. Diabetes, oxidative stress, and antioxidants: A review. *J. Biochem. Mol. Toxicol.* **2003**, *17*, 24–38. [CrossRef]

14. Jain, S.K. Hyperglycemia can cause membrane lipid peroxidation and osmotic fragility in human red blood cells. *J. Biol. Chem.* **1989**, *264*, 21340–21345.

15. Jain, S.K.; Levine, S.N.; Duett, J.; Hollier, B. Elevated lipid peroxidation levels in red blood cells of streptozotocin-treated diabetic rats. *Metabolism* **1990**, *39*, 971–975. [CrossRef]

16. Tan, Y.; Ichikawa, T.; Li, J.; Si, Q.; Yang, H.; Chen, X.; Goldblatt, C.S.; Meyer, C.J.; Li, X.; Cai, L. Diabetic downregulation of Nrf2 activity via ERK contributes to oxidative stress–induced insulin resistance in cardiac cells in vitro and in vivo. *Diabetes* **2011**, *60*, 625–633. [CrossRef]

17. Chang, M.S.; Oh, M.S.; Jung, K.J.; Park, S.; Choi, S.B.; Ko, B.-S.; Park, S.K. Effects of Okchun-San, a herbal formulation, on blood glucose levels and body weight in a model of Type 2 diabetes. *J. Ethnopharmacol.* **2006**, *103*, 491–495. [CrossRef]

18. Heo, S.-J.; Kim, J.-P.; Jung, W.-K.; Lee, N.-H.; Kang, H.-S.; Jun, E.-M.; Park, S.-H.; Kang, S.-M.; Lee, Y.-J.; Park, P.-J. Identification of chemical structure and free radical scavenging activity of diphlorethohydroxycarmalol isolated from a brown alga, Ishige okamurae. *J. Microbiol. Biotechnol.* **2008**, *18*, 676–681.

19. Lee, S.-H.; Jeon, Y.-J. Anti-diabetic effects of brown algae derived phlorotannins, marine polyphenols through diverse mechanisms. *Fitoterapia* **2013**, *86*, 129–136. [CrossRef]
20. Lee, K.M.; Boo, G.H.; Riosmena-Rodriguez, R.; Shin, J.A.; Boo, S.M. Classification of the genus Ishige (ishigeales, phaeophyceae) in the north Pacific Ocean with recognition of Ishige foliacea based on plastid rbcl and mitochondrial cox3 gene sequences 1. *J. Phycol.* **2009**, *45*, 906–913. [CrossRef]
21. Ahn, S.-M.; Hong, Y.-K.; Kwon, G.-S.; Sohn, H.-Y. Evaluation of antioxidant and nitrite scavenging activity of seaweed extracts. *J. Life Sci.* **2011**, *21*, 576–583. [CrossRef]
22. Min, K.-H.; Kim, H.-J.; Jeon, Y.-J.; Han, J.-S. Ishige okamurae ameliorates hyperglycemia and insulin resistance in C57BL/KsJ-db/db mice. *Diabetes Res. Clin. Pr.* **2011**, *93*, 70–76. [CrossRef] [PubMed]
23. Kang, M.-C.; Kang, N.; Ko, S.-C.; Kim, Y.-B.; Jeon, Y.-J. Anti-obesity effects of seaweeds of Jeju Island on the differentiation of 3T3-L1 preadipocytes and obese mice fed a high-fat diet. *Food Chem. Toxicol.* **2016**, *90*, 36–44. [CrossRef] [PubMed]
24. Casuso, R.A.; Huertas, J.R. Antioxidant Supplements in Obesity and Metabolic Syndrome: Angels or Demons. In *Obesity*; Elsevier: Amsterdam, The Netherlands, 2018; pp. 263–275.
25. Acin-Perez, R.; Enriquez, J.A. The function of the respiratory supercomplexes: The plasticity model. *BBA-Bioenergetics* **2014**, *1837*, 444–450. [CrossRef]
26. Heo, S.-J.; Jeon, Y.-J. Radical scavenging capacity and cytoprotective effect of enzymatic digests of Ishige okamurae. *J. Appl. Phycol.* **2008**, *20*, 1087–1095. [CrossRef]
27. Ellulu, M.S.; Patimah, I.; Khaza'ai, H.; Rahmat, A.; Abed, Y. Obesity and inflammation: The linking mechanism and the complications. *Arch. Med. Sci. AMS* **2017**, *13*, 851. [CrossRef]
28. Holguin, F.; Fitzpatrick, A. Obesity, asthma, and oxidative stress. *J. Appl. Physiol.* **2009**, *108*, 754–759. [CrossRef]
29. Lee, H.; Lee, Y.J.; Choi, H.; Ko, E.H.; Kim, J.-W. Reactive oxygen species facilitate adipocyte differentiation by accelerating mitotic clonal expansion. *J. Biol. Chem.* **2009**, *284*, 10601–10609. [CrossRef] [PubMed]
30. Fajas, L. Adipogenesis: A cross-talk between cell proliferation and cell differentiation. *Ann. Med.* **2003**, *35*, 79–85. [CrossRef] [PubMed]
31. Cha, S.-Y.; Cheon, Y.-P. Suppressive Effects of an Ishige okamurae extract on 3T3-L1 Preadipocyte Differentiation. *Dev. Reprod.* **2013**, *17*, 451. [CrossRef] [PubMed]
32. Polvani, S.; Tarocchi, M.; Tempesti, S.; Bencini, L.; Galli, A. Peroxisome proliferator activated receptors at the crossroad of obesity, diabetes, and pancreatic cancer. *World J. Gastroenterol.* **2016**, *22*, 2441. [CrossRef] [PubMed]
33. Tontonoz, P.; Hu, E.; Spiegelman, B.M. Stimulation of adipogenesis in fibroblasts by PPARγ2, a lipid-activated transcription factor. *Cell* **1994**, *79*, 1147–1156. [CrossRef]
34. Rosen, E.D.; Sarraf, P.; Troy, A.E.; Bradwin, G.; Moore, K.; Milstone, D.S.; Spiegelman, B.M.; Mortensen, R.M. PPARγ is required for the differentiation of adipose tissue in vivo and in vitro. *Mol. Cell* **1999**, *4*, 611–617. [CrossRef]
35. Hong, S.J.; Lee, J.-H.; Kim, E.J.; Yang, H.J.; Park, J.-S.; Hong, S.-K. Anti-obesity and anti-diabetic effect of neoagarooligosaccharides on high-fat diet-induced obesity in mice. *Mar. Drugs* **2017**, *15*, 90. [CrossRef]
36. Seo, Y.-J.; Lee, K.; Song, J.-H.; Chei, S.; Lee, B.-Y. Ishige okamurae extract suppresses obesity and hepatic steatosis in high fat diet-induced obese mice. *Nutrients* **2018**, *10*, 1802. [CrossRef]
37. Yamauchi, T.; Kamon, J.; Minokoshi, Y.A.; Ito, Y.; Waki, H.; Uchida, S.; Yamashita, S.; Noda, M.; Kita, S.; Ueki, K. Adiponectin stimulates glucose utilization and fatty-acid oxidation by activating AMP-activated protein kinase. *Nat. Med.* **2002**, *8*, 1288. [CrossRef]
38. Watanabe, M.; Houten, S.M.; Mataki, C.; Christoffolete, M.A.; Kim, B.W.; Sato, H.; Messaddeq, N.; Harney, J.W.; Ezaki, O.; Kodama, T. Bile acids induce energy expenditure by promoting intracellular thyroid hormone activation. *Nature* **2006**, *439*, 484. [CrossRef]
39. Uno, K.; Katagiri, H.; Yamada, T.; Ishigaki, Y.; Ogihara, T.; Imai, J.; Hasegawa, Y.; Gao, J.; Kaneko, K.; Iwasaki, H. Neuronal pathway from the liver modulates energy expenditure and systemic insulin sensitivity. *Science* **2006**, *312*, 1656–1659. [CrossRef]
40. Matsuoka, T.-A.; Kajimoto, Y.; Watada, H.; Kaneto, H.; Kishimoto, M.; Umayahara, Y.; Fujitani, Y.; Kamada, T.; Kawamori, R.; Yamasaki, Y. Glycation-dependent, reactive oxygen species-mediated suppression of the insulin gene promoter activity in HIT cells. *J. Clin. Investig.* **1997**, *99*, 144–150. [CrossRef] [PubMed]

41. Rudich, A.; Tirosh, A.; Potashnik, R.; Hemi, R.; Kanety, H.; Bashan, N. Prolonged oxidative stress impairs insulin-induced GLUT4 translocation in 3T3-L1 adipocytes. *Diabetes* **1998**, *47*, 1562–1569. [CrossRef] [PubMed]

42. Kodama, H.; Fujita, M.; Yamazaki, M.; Yamaguchi, I. The possible role of age-related increase in the plasma glucagon/insulin ratio in the enhanced hepatic gluco neogenesis and hyperglycemia in genetically diabetic (C57BL/KsJ-db/db) mice. *JPN J. Pharmacol.* **1994**, *66*, 281–287. [CrossRef]

43. Haffner, S.M.; Miettinen, H.; Stern, M.P. The homeostasis model in the San Antonio heart study. *Diabetes Care* **1997**, *20*, 1087–1092. [CrossRef]

44. Tahara, Y.; Shima, K. Kinetics of HbA1c, glycated albumin, and fructosamine and analysis of their weight functions against preceding plasma glucose level. *Diabetes Care* **1995**, *18*, 440–447. [CrossRef] [PubMed]

45. Singh, I.P.; Bharate, S.B. Phloroglucinol compounds of natural origin. *Nat. Prod. Rep.* **2006**, *23*, 558–591. [CrossRef]

46. Handique, J.; Baruah, J. Polyphenolic compounds: An overview. *React. Funct. Polym.* **2002**, *52*, 163–188. [CrossRef]

47. Mayer, A.M.; Hamann, M.T. Marine pharmacology in 2001–2002: Marine compounds with anthelmintic, antibacterial, anticoagulant, antidiabetic, antifungal, anti-inflammatory, antimalarial, antiplatelet, antiprotozoal, antituberculosis, and antiviral activities; affecting the cardiovascular, immune and nervous systems and other miscellaneous mechanisms of action. *Comp. Biochem. Physiol. C: Toxicol. Pharmacol.* **2005**, *140*, 265–286.

48. Kong, C.-S.; Kim, J.-A.; Yoon, N.-Y.; Kim, S.-K. Induction of apoptosis by phloroglucinol derivative from Ecklonia cava in MCF-7 human breast cancer cells. *Food Chem. Toxicol.* **2009**, *47*, 1653–1658. [CrossRef] [PubMed]

49. Yoon, N.Y.; Lee, S.-H.; Kim, S.-K. Phlorotannins from Ishige okamurae and their acetyl-and butyrylcholinesterase inhibitory effects. *J. Funct. Foods* **2009**, *1*, 331–335. [CrossRef]

50. Kim, H.-H.; Kim, H.-S.; Ko, J.-Y.; Kim, C.-Y.; Lee, J.-H.; Jeon, Y.-J. A single-step isolation of useful antioxidant compounds from Ishige okamurae by using centrifugal partition chromatography. *Fish Aquat. Sci.* **2016**, *19*, 22. [CrossRef]

51. Ryu, B.; Jiang, Y.; Kim, H.-S.; Hyun, J.-M.; Lim, S.-B.; Li, Y.; Jeon, Y.-J. Ishophloroglucin A, a novel phlorotannin for standardizing the anti-α-glucosidase activity of Ishige okamurae. *Mar. Drugs* **2018**, *16*, 436. [CrossRef]

52. Zou, Y.; Qian, Z.-J.; Li, Y.; Kim, M.-M.; Lee, S.-H.; Kim, S.-K. Antioxidant effects of phlorotannins isolated from Ishige okamurae in free radical mediated oxidative systems. *J. Agric. Food Chem.* **2008**, *56*, 7001–7009. [CrossRef] [PubMed]

53. Heo, S.-J.; Jeon, Y.-J. Evaluation of diphlorethohydroxycarmalol isolated from Ishige okamurae for radical scavenging activity and its protective effect against H2O2-induced cell damage. *Process Biochem.* **2009**, *44*, 412–418. [CrossRef]

54. Kumar, S.; Hosokawa, M.; Miyashita, K. Fucoxanthin: A marine carotenoid exerting anti-cancer effects by affecting multiple mechanisms. *Mar. Drugs* **2013**, *11*, 5130–5147. [CrossRef]

55. Liu, C.-L.; Liang, A.-L.; Hu, M.-L. Protective effects of fucoxanthin against ferric nitrilotriacetate-induced oxidative stress in murine hepatic BNL CL. 2 cells. *Toxicol. In Vitro* **2011**, *25*, 1314–1319. [CrossRef]

56. Maeda, H.; Hosokawa, M.; Sashima, T.; Funayama, K.; Miyashita, K. Fucoxanthin from edible seaweed, Undaria pinnatifida, shows antiobesity effect through UCP1 expression in white adipose tissues. *Biochem. Biophys. Res. Commun.* **2005**, *332*, 392–397. [CrossRef] [PubMed]

57. Maeda, H.; Hosokawa, M.; Sashima, T.; Miyashita, K. Dietary combination of fucoxanthin and fish oil attenuates the weight gain of white adipose tissue and decreases blood glucose in obese/diabetic KK-Ay mice. *J. Agric. Food Chem.* **2007**, *55*, 7701–7706. [CrossRef] [PubMed]

58. Kang, M.-C.; Lee, S.-H.; Lee, W.-W.; Kang, N.; Kim, E.-A.; Kim, S.Y.; Lee, D.H.; Kim, D.; Jeon, Y.-J. Protective effect of fucoxanthin isolated from Ishige okamurae against high-glucose induced oxidative stress in human umbilical vein endothelial cells and zebrafish model. *J. Funct. Foods* **2014**, *11*, 304–312. [CrossRef]

59. Payne, V.A.; Au, W.-S.; Lowe, C.E.; Rahman, S.M.; Friedman, J.E.; O'Rahilly, S.; Rochford, J.J. C/EBP transcription factors regulate SREBP1c gene expression during adipogenesis. *Biochem. J.* **2010**, *425*, 215–224. [CrossRef]

60. Choi, H.S.; Jeon, H.J.; Lee, O.H.; Lee, B.Y. Dieckol, a major phlorotannin in Ecklonia cava, suppresses lipid accumulation in the adipocytes of high-fat diet-fed zebrafish and mice: Inhibition of early adipogenesis via cell-cycle arrest and AMPKα activation. *Mol. Nutr. Food Res.* **2015**, *59*, 1458–1471. [CrossRef]

61. Chan, C.Y.; Wei, L.; Castro-Muñozledo, F.; Koo, W.L. (−)-Epigallocatechin-3-gallate blocks 3T3-L1 adipose conversion by inhibition of cell proliferation and suppression of adipose phenotype expression. *Life Sci.* **2011**, *89*, 779–785. [CrossRef]

62. Chang, C.-C.; Lin, K.-Y.; Peng, K.-Y.; Day, Y.-J.; Hung, L.-M. Resveratrol exerts anti-obesity effects in high-fat diet obese mice and displays differential dosage effects on cytotoxicity, differentiation, and lipolysis in 3T3-L1 cells. *Endocr. J.* **2016**, *63*, 169–178. [CrossRef]

63. Kang, M.-C.; Ding, Y.; Kim, H.-S.; Jeon, Y.-J.; Lee, S.-H. Inhibition of Adipogenesis by Diphlorethohydroxycarmalol (DPHC) through AMPK activation in adipocytes. *Mar. Drugs* **2019**, *17*, 44. [CrossRef] [PubMed]

64. Park, M.H.; Jeon, Y.J.; Kim, H.J.; Han, J.S. Effect of Diphlorethohydroxycarmalol isolated from ishige okamurae on apoptosis in 3 t3-L1 preadipocytes. *Phytother. Res.* **2013**, *27*, 931–936. [CrossRef] [PubMed]

65. Gray, G.M. Carbohydrate digestion and absorption: Role of the small intestine. *N. Engl. J. Med.* **1975**, *292*, 1225–1230. [CrossRef]

66. Dong, H.-Q.; Li, M.; Zhu, F.; Liu, F.-L.; Huang, J.-B. Inhibitory potential of trilobatin from Lithocarpus polystachyus Rehd against α-glucosidase and α-amylase linked to type 2 diabetes. *Food Chem.* **2012**, *130*, 261–266. [CrossRef]

67. Collado-González, J.; Grosso, C.; Valentão, P.; Andrade, P.B.; Ferreres, F.; Durand, T.; Guy, A.; Galano, J.-M.; Torrecillas, A.; Gil-Izquierdo, Á. Inhibition of α-glucosidase and α-amylase by Spanish extra virgin olive oils: The involvement of bioactive compounds other than oleuropein and hydroxytyrosol. *Food Chem.* **2017**, *235*, 298–307. [CrossRef]

68. Heo, S.-J.; Hwang, J.-Y.; Choi, J.-I.; Han, J.-S.; Kim, H.-J.; Jeon, Y.-J. Diphlorethohydroxycarmalol isolated from Ishige okamurae, a brown algae, a potent α-glucosidase and α-amylase inhibitor, alleviates postprandial hyperglycemia in diabetic mice. *Eur. J. Pharmacol.* **2009**, *615*, 252–256. [CrossRef] [PubMed]

69. Lee, S.-H.; Choi, J.-I.; Heo, S.-J.; Park, M.-H.; Park, P.-J.; Jeon, B.-T.; Kim, S.-K.; Han, J.-S.; Jeon, Y.-J. Diphlorethohydroxycarmalol isolated from Pae (Ishige okamurae) protects high glucose-induced damage in RINm5F pancreatic β cells via its antioxidant effects. *Food Sci. Biotechnol.* **2012**, *21*, 239–246. [CrossRef]

70. Stumvoll, M.; Goldstein, B.J.; van Haeften, T.W. Type 2 diabetes: Principles of pathogenesis and therapy. *Lancet* **2005**, *365*, 1333–1346. [CrossRef]

71. Roberfroid, M.B. Concepts and strategy of functional food science: The European perspective. *Am. J. Clin. Nutr.* **2000**, *71*, 1660S–1664S. [CrossRef]

72. Barrow, C.; Shahidi, F. *Marine Nutraceuticals and Functional Foods*; CRC Press: Boca Raton, FL, USA, 2007.

73. Kim, S.-K.; Mendis, E. Bioactive compounds from marine processing byproducts—A review. *Food Res. Int.* **2006**, *39*, 383–393. [CrossRef]

74. Zou, Y.; Li, Y.; Kim, M.-M.; Lee, S.-H.; Kim, S.-K. Ishigoside, a new glyceroglycolipid isolated from the brown alga Ishige okamurae. *Biotechnol. Bioprocess Eng.* **2009**, *14*, 20–26. [CrossRef]

75. Bae, M.J.; Karadeniz, F.; Ahn, B.-N.; Kong, C.-S. Evaluation of effective MMP inhibitors from eight different brown algae in human fibrosarcoma HT1080 cells. *PNF* **2015**, *20*, 153. [CrossRef] [PubMed]

76. Kim, M.M.; Rajapakse, N.; Kim, S.K. Anti-inflammatory effect of Ishige okamurae ethanolic extract via inhibition of NF-κB transcription factor in RAW 264.7 cells. *Phytother. Res.* **2009**, *23*, 628–634. [CrossRef] [PubMed]

77. Lee, W.; Kang, N.; Kim, E.-A.; Yang, H.-W.; Oh, J.-Y.; Fernando, I.P.S.; Kim, K.-N.; Ahn, G.; Jeon, Y.-J. Radioprotective effects of a polysaccharide purified from Lactobacillus plantarum-fermented Ishige okamurae against oxidative stress caused by gamma ray-irradiation in zebrafish in vivo model. *J. Funct. Foods* **2017**, *28*, 83–89. [CrossRef]

78. Heo, S.-J.; Hwang, J.-Y.; Choi, J.-I.; Lee, S.-H.; Park, P.-J.; Kang, D.-H.; Oh, C.; Kim, D.-W.; Han, J.-S.; Jeon, Y.-J. Protective effect of diphlorethohydroxycarmalol isolated from Ishige okamurae against high glucose-induced-oxidative stress in human umbilical vein endothelial cells. *Food Chem. Toxicol.* **2010**, *48*, 1448–1454. [CrossRef]

79. Heo, S.-J.; Cha, S.-H.; Kim, K.-N.; Lee, S.-H.; Ahn, G.; Kang, D.-H.; Oh, C.; Choi, Y.-U.; Affan, A.; Kim, D. Neuroprotective effect of phlorotannin isolated from Ishige okamurae against H 2 O 2-induced oxidative stress in murine hippocampal neuronal cells, HT22. *Appl. Biochem. Biotechnol.* **2012**, *166*, 1520–1532. [CrossRef]

80. Ahn, M.J.; Yoon, K.D.; Kim, C.; Kim, J.; Shin, C.G.; Kim, J. Inhibitory activity on HIV-1 reverse transcriptase and integrase of a carmalol derivative from a brown Alga, Ishige okamurae. *Phytother. Res.* **2006**, *20*, 711–713. [CrossRef]

81. Kim, K.-N.; Heo, S.-J.; Yoon, W.-J.; Kang, S.-M.; Ahn, G.; Yi, T.-H.; Jeon, Y.-J. Fucoxanthin inhibits the inflammatory response by suppressing the activation of NF-κB and MAPKs in lipopolysaccharide-induced RAW 264.7 macrophages. *Eur. J. Pharmacol.* **2010**, *649*, 369–375. [CrossRef] [PubMed]

82. Milatovic, D.; Dettbarn, W.-D. Modification of acetylcholinesterase during adaptation to chronic, subacute paraoxon application in rat. *Toxicol. Appl. Pharmacol.* **1996**, *136*, 20–28. [CrossRef]

83. Schetinger, M.R.; Porto, N.M.; Moretto, M.B.; Morsch, V.M.; da Rocha, J.B.T.; Vieira, V.; Moro, F.; Neis, R.T.; Bittencourt, S.; Bonacorso, H.G. New benzodiazepines alter acetylcholinesterase and ATPDase activities. *Neurochem. Res.* **2000**, *25*, 949–955. [CrossRef]

84. Greig, N.H.; Utsuki, T.; Yu, Q.-S.; Zhu, X.; Holloway, H.W.; Perry, T.; Lee, B.; Ingram, D.K.; Lahiri, D.K. A new therapeutic target in Alzheimer's disease treatment: Attention to butyrylcholinesterase. *Curr. Med. Res. Opin.* **2001**, *17*, 159–165. [CrossRef] [PubMed]

85. Hosokawa, M. Fucoxanthin as a bioactive and nutritionally beneficial marine carotenoid. *Carotenoid Sci.* **2006**, *10*, 15–28.

86. Pahl, H.L. Activators and target genes of Rel/NF-κB transcription factors. *Oncogene* **1999**, *18*, 6853. [CrossRef] [PubMed]

87. Uto, T.; Fujii, M.; Hou, D.-X. 6-(Methylsulfinyl) hexyl isothiocyanate suppresses inducible nitric oxide synthase expression through the inhibition of Janus kinase 2-mediated JNK pathway in lipopolysaccharide-activated murine macrophages. *Biochem. Pharmacol.* **2005**, *70*, 1211–1221. [CrossRef] [PubMed]

88. Balkwill, F.; Coussens, L.M. Cancer: An inflammatory link. *Nature* **2004**, *431*, 405. [CrossRef] [PubMed]

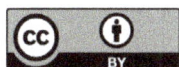

marine drugs

MDPI

Article

Chlorophyll Derivatives from Marine Cyanobacteria with Lipid-Reducing Activities

Sara Freitas [1,2,†], Natália Gonçalves Silva [1,†], Maria Lígia Sousa [1], Tiago Ribeiro [1], Filipa Rosa [1], Pedro N. Leão [1], Vitor Vasconcelos [1,2], Mariana Alves Reis [1] and Ralph Urbatzka [1,2,*]

[1] Interdisciplinary Center of Marine and Environmental Research (CIIMAR/CIMAR), University of Porto, Terminal de Cruzeiros de Leixões, Av. General Norton de Matos s/n, 4450-208 Matosinhos, Portugal; sfreitas@ciimar.up.pt (S.F.); nsilva@ciimar.up.pt (N.G.S.); msousa@ciimar.up.pt (M.L.S.); tribeiro@ciimar.up.pt (T.R.); frosa@ciimar.up.pt (F.R.); pleao@ciimar.up.pt (P.N.L.); vmvascon@fc.up.pt (V.V.); mreis@ciimar.up.pt (M.A.R.)
[2] FCUP, Faculty of Science, Department of Biology, University of Porto, Rua do Campo, Alegre, 4169-007 Porto, Portugal
*   Correspondence: rurbatzka@ciimar.up.pt; Tel.: +351-223-401-818
†   These authors contributed equally to this paper.

Received: 26 March 2019; Accepted: 14 April 2019; Published: 17 April 2019

Abstract: Marine organisms, particularly cyanobacteria, are important resources for the production of bioactive secondary metabolites for the treatment of human diseases. In this study, a bioassay-guided approach was used to discover metabolites with lipid-reducing activity. Two chlorophyll derivatives were successfully isolated, the previously described 13^2-hydroxy-pheophytin a (**1**) and the new compound 13^2-hydroxy-pheofarnesin a (**2**). The structure elucidation of the new compound **2** was established based on one- and two-dimensional (1D and 2D) NMR spectroscopy and mass spectrometry. Compounds **1** and **2** showed significant neutral lipid-reducing activity in the zebrafish Nile red metabolism assay after 48 h of exposure with a half maximal effective concentration (EC_{50}) of 8.9 ± 0.4 µM for **1** and 15.5 ± 1.3 µM for **2**. Both compounds additionally reduced neutral lipid accumulation in 3T3-L1 multicellular spheroids of murine preadipocytes. Molecular profiling of mRNA expression of some target genes was evaluated for the higher potent compound **1**, which indicated altered peroxisome proliferator activated receptor gamma (PPARγ) mRNA expression. Lipolysis was not affected. Different food materials (*Spirulina*, *Chlorella*, spinach, and cabbage) were evaluated for the presence of **1**, and the cyanobacterium *Spirulina*, with GRAS (generally regarded as safe) status for human consumption, contained high amounts of **1**. In summary, known and novel chlorophyll derivatives were discovered from marine cyanobacteria with relevant lipid-reducing activities, which in the future may be developed into nutraceuticals.

Keywords: zebrafish Nile red fat metabolism assay; anti-obesity drugs; chlorophyll derivatives; murine pre-adipocytes; PPARγ

1. Introduction

In recent years, the discovery of natural products was extended to new pharmaceutical targets in addition to the traditional targets explored in the past decades, for example, in the search of new anti-obesogenic compounds [1]. Obesity is a complex metabolic disease characterized by an abnormal fat accumulation in adipocytes which are also important regulators of the whole metabolism and homeostasis [2]. This disease is an increasing epidemic, since a considerable percentage of the world's population is overweight, which is associated with several chronic diseases like diabetes, cardiovascular diseases, and cancer [2,3].

The ineffective pharmacological treatment of current anti-obesity drugs available on the market is due to the limitation of long-term success, potentially dangerous side effects, and high costs [4]. Alternatively, some natural products and derived compounds are being used in the clinic to treat obesity, for example, orlistat, a synthetic derivative of lipostatin isolated from *Streptomyces toxytricini* [5]. Yoshinone A isolated from the marine cyanobacterium *Leptolyngbya* sp., and other marine natural products containing a 7-en-γ-pyrone moiety showed promising anti-obesogenic activity [6].

Although the marine environment is a rich source of new natural products with a high range of applications [7], this environment is still largely underexploited due to inaccessibility and difficulties in retrieving these organisms from their habitat into laboratorial cultures. Cyanobacteria, a group of ancient photoautotrophic microorganisms, are interesting resources for natural product discovery in marine environments [8]. These organisms are known to produce a wide range of bioactive secondary metabolites and most often adapt well to laboratorial culture conditions [9,10]. Our in-house cyanobacterial culture collection (LEGEcc) currently harbors about 500 cyanobacterial strains isolated from the Portuguese coast and other environments that overall represent a largely untapped source for discovery of new secondary metabolites [11]. Some natural compounds were already successfully isolated from this collection, for example, hierridin B [12], bartolosides (A–K) [13,14], and portoamides (A–D) [15], all with cytotoxic activity on cancer cell lines.

Zebrafish (*Danio rerio*) is an attractive model organism for biomedical research. In the study of complex metabolic disorders like obesity, the use of more complex in vivo model systems as small whole animal models can bring significant advantages. For drug discovery, zebrafish assays can be used complementary to rodent assays with easier handling, high predictive validity and cost-efficiency, while compatible with high-throughput screening [16]. Zebrafish possess higher physiological relevance than cellular in vitro models, more interactions between tissues and have genetic homology to mammals, as well as significant similarities in lipid metabolism [16,17]. The original procedure of the zebrafish Nile red fat metabolism assay was published by Jones et al. [18] and analyzed the capacity of compounds to reduce neutral lipids in zebrafish larvae in vivo. The authors concluded that the zebrafish organism model can be used for identifying non-toxic molecules for treating clinical obesity due the conservation of signal transduction pathways that regulate lipid metabolism.

The aim of this study was to uncover new cyanobacterial compounds with lipid-reducing activity using the zebrafish Nile red fat metabolism assay optimized in our laboratory. We report the isolation and structural elucidation of a known and a novel chlorophyll derivative from the marine cyanobacteria *Cyanobium* sp. LEGE 07175 and *Nodosilinea* sp. LEGE 06001, respectively. Their lipid-reducing activity was additionally evaluated in a three-dimensional (3D) cell culture model of murine pre-adipocytes. Initial molecular profiling was performed for the more potent compound **1**. Furthermore, the presence of **1** was evaluated in different photoautotrophic organisms (*Spirulina*, *Chlorella*, spinach, and cabbage), with GRAS (generally regarded as safe) status for human consumption.

2. Results

2.1. Isolation of Compound **1**

Compound **1** was obtained as a green dark amorphous solid from the cyanobacterium *Cyanobium* sp. LEGE 07175. The isolation required several chromatographic steps and was guided by a strong reduction of lipid content observed in the zebrafish Nile red fat metabolism assay. An LC-ESI-LRMS (liquid chromatography-electrospray ionization-low resolution mass spectrometry) analysis revealed a mass consistent with 13^2-hydroxy-pheophytin a (data not shown), through comparison with spectroscopic data reported on the literature [19,20]. An HR-ESI-MS analysis was performed and showed a monoisotopic *m/z* 887.5697 value for $[M + H]^+$ consistent with the molecular formula of $C_{55}H_{74}N_4O_6$ of 13^2-hydroxy-pheophytin a (Figure 1). One- and two-dimensional (1D and 2D) NMR experiments and HR-ESI-MS/MS analysis also corroborated this assignment, revealing the typical resonances and correlations of this chlorophyll derivative [19,20].

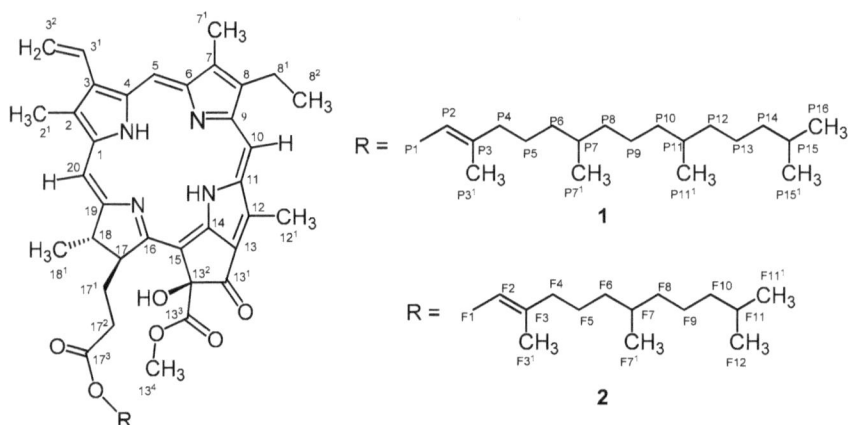

Figure 1. Planar structure of compounds **1** and **2**.

2.2. Isolation and Sctructure Elucidation of Compound 2

The zebrafish Nile red fat metabolism assay-guided fractionation of the CH_2Cl_2/MeOH (dichloromethane/methanol) extract of the cyanobacterium *Nodosilinea* sp. LEGE 06001 yielded compound **2** as a brownish green amorphous solid. The molecular formula was determined as $C_{50}H_{64}N_4O_6$ on the basis of HR-ESI-MS data, *m/z* 817.4522 [M + H]$^+$, which demanded 15 degrees of unsaturation. The ^{1}H and ^{13}C NMR data for compound **2** showed similarities to what was observed for **1**, indicating that **2** could be a chlorophyll derivative. Comparison of the HR-ESI-MS/MS data between **1** and **2** suggested that compound **2** bears a farnesyl moiety instead of a phytyl group. The difference between the mass of the pseudomolecular ion at *m/z* 817.4522 [M + H]$^+$ and the fragment at *m/z* 609.2697 [M + 2H − farnesyl]$^+$ (Δ *m/z* 208.1825) is consistent with the presence of a farnesyl substituent as opposed to phytyl (Δ *m/z* 279.36; *m/z* 909.55 [M + Na]$^+$ and *m/z* 607.20 [M − phytol]$^+$) [18]. Therefore, compound **2** was named 13^2-hydroxy-pheofarnesin a.

The ^{1}H NMR spectrum of **2** (Table 1) showed all the typical resonances of the porphyrin ring: three singlets and an aromatic methyl multiplet (δ_H 1.59 m, 3.28 s, 3.44 s, 3.90 s), one methyl triplet (δ_H 1.72) and two diastereotopic benzylic proton signals (δ_H 3.64, 3.77) corresponding to an aromatic ethyl substituent, three olefinic singlets (δ_H 8.71, 9.56, 9.77), a methyl singlet (δ_H 3.76) corresponding to a methoxy group, and a vinyl moiety (δ_H 6.19, 6.35, 8.03) with the characteristic exomethylene coupling pattern (*J* = 18.7 and *J* = 11.4 Hz). The attached farnesyl moiety was recognized by a large number of overlapping proton signals of aliphatic methylene and methyl functions. Indicative proton resonances were the oxymethylene resonances (δ_H 4.44, 4.5 at F1), the vinylic resonances for H-F2 (δ_H 5.14), and H$_3$-F3^1 (δ_H 1.61), as well as those for the geminal dimethyl at F11^1 and F12 (δ_H 0.85 d).

Table 1. ^{1}H and ^{13}C (600 MHz) data (δ, ppm) of compound **2** at 600 MHz in CDCl$_3$ (deuterated chloroform).

Position	δ_H (*J* in Hz)	δ_C	Position	δ_H (*J* in Hz)	δ_C
1		141.3	15		102.0/100.4 [2]
2		131.5	16		166.3
2 [1]	3.44 s	11.5	17	4.07 dd (7.4)	53.1
3		133.4	17 [1]	2.56 dd (7.7)	30.7
				1.83 dd (9.1)	
3 [1]	8.03 dd (11.5, 17.8)	128.3	17 [2]	2.46 m	31.7
				2.17 m	
3 [2]	6.35 d (18.7)	122.1	17 [3]		173.4
	6.19 d (11.4)				
4		135.9	18	4.46 m (7.8)	49.7
5	9.56 s	99.1	18 [1]	1.59 m	21.7
6		155.7	19		171
7		136.6	20	8.71 s	93.3
7 [1]	3.28 s	10.8	F1	4.5 m 4.44 m (6.8)	60.8
8		145.6	F2	5.14 t (6.5)	117.1
8 [1]	3.77 m	19.0	F3		
	3.64 m				
8 [2]	1.72 t (7.7)	17.0	F3 [1]	1.61 s	15.8
9		149.9	F4	1.89 m (7.7)	39.9
10	9.77 s	103.4	F5	1.29 m (7.4)	22-24 [1]
11		128.8	F6	1.01 m	36.6
12		131.5	F7	1.33 m	32.1
12 [1]	3.90 s	11.9	F7 [1]	0.8 m	19.2
13		133.2	F8	2.35 t (7.5)	32.6
13 [1]		1	F9	1.65 m (7.3)	24.3
13 [2]-OH	6.11 s	110.4/102.0 [2]	F10	1.11 m	38.9
13 [3]		170.8	F11	1.51 m	27.4
13 [4]-OCH$_3$	3.76 s	53.4	F11 [1]	0.85 m (6.6)	22.1
14		140.2	F12	0.85 m (6.6)	22.1

[1] ^{13}C spectra signal not detected or very-low-intensity signal. [2] Assignment undetermined due lack of specific correlations.

The ^{13}C NMR and 2D NMR data (COSY, HSQC, and HMBC) for **2** allowed the assignment of all carbons on the porphyrin ring and the location of the functional groups, with the exception of the carboxyl group at C-13^1 (Figure 2 and Figure S10, Supplementary Materials). The connection between the four pyrrole rings was established by the long-range HMBC correlations (Figure 2) of the olefinic protons H-5 to C-4 (ring A), H-10 to C-8 (ring B), C-11, and C-12 (ring C), and H-20 with C-18 (ring D), C-1, and C-2 (ring A). The presence of the methoxycarbonyl group was deduced from the long-range HMBC correlation of the singlet protons of a methyl group resonating at δ_H 3.76 H$_3$-13^4 to a carbonyl carbon (δ_C 170.8 C-13^3). This assignment was corroborated by comparison with reported data for similar moieties [19,21,22]. A singlet at δ_H 6.11 without an HSQC correlation, but with HMBC correlations to C-13^2, C-13^3, and C-15 suggested the presence of a hydroxy group in ring E. Its position at C-13^2 was deduced by the significant low field shifts of carbons at 13^2 and 15 (δ_C 100.4 and 102, respectively). Moreover, the HMBC data allowed the connection of the farnesyl moiety to the porphyrin system by a long correlation of the methylene group H$_2$-F1 (δ_H 4.44/4.5) with the carboxyl group at C-17^3. The assignments from F1 to F12 were confirmed through ^{1}H-^{1}H TOCSY and ^{1}H-^{1}H COSY experiments (Figure 2 and Figure S12, Supplementary Materials).

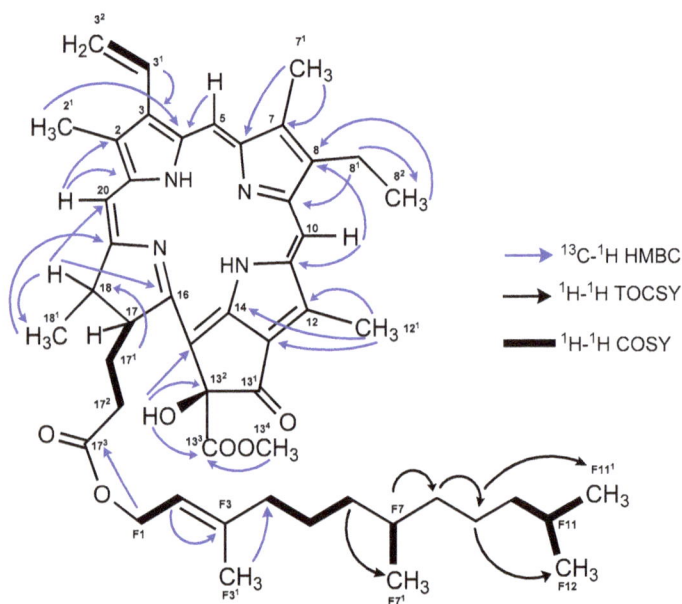

Figure 2. Key ^{13}C-^{1}H HMBC, ^{1}H-^{1}H COSY, and ^{1}H-^{1}H TOCSY correlations for **2**.

The relative stereochemistry of **2** was confirmed by ROESY experiments and comparison with literature data. Strong ROESY interactions between H-17/H_2-17^2 and H_2-17^2/H_3-18^1 indicated that these protons lay on the same side of the molecule plane (Figure S13, Supplementary Materials). Moreover, the alpha (α) orientation of these protons results from the natural biosynthesis of chlorophylls, in which occurs a stereo-specific reduction of the C-17/C-18 bond of ring D [23]. The stereochemistry of the hydroxy group at C-13^2 varies naturally to an alpha or beta position ($\delta_{OH\beta}$ 5.47 to 5.53 in CDCl$_3$ [19,24]; $\delta_{OH\alpha}$ 5.35 in CDCl$_3$ [24]). A correlation of the stereochemistry at C-13^2 was studied in several pheophytin derivatives comparing the shielding level of the H-17 [25]. It was established that, when the hydroxy group was located on the same side of the molecular plane as H-17 (H-17α and OHα-13^2), the proton was distinctly deshielded, displaying chemical shifts between δ_H 4.54 and 4.69. By contrast, when the hydroxy group had β orientation and the H-17 had α orientation, there was a lack of significant deshielding, and the chemical shift was between δ_H 4.13 and 4.29. Thus, despite any strong ROESY signal being observed for this chiral center, the stereochemistry was determined as S (OHβ-13^2) in accordance with these findings. Therefore, the structure of compound **2** was identified as 13^2(S)-hydroxy-pheofarnesin a.

2.3. Lipid-Reducing Activity of 1 and 2, but not of Chlorophyll a and b

To characterize the lipid-reducing activity of the two isolated chlorophyll derivatives, the zebrafish Nile red fat metabolism assay was used. Exposure of the zebrafish larvae to compounds **1** and **2** resulted in significant neutral lipid-reducing activity in this assay after 48 h (Figure 3A). A significant decrease in Nile red staining was observed for compound **1** at 10, 5, and 2.5 µg/mL, and for compound **2** at 10 and 5 µg/mL (Figure 3B), with half maximal effective concentration (EC$_{50}$) values of 8.9 ± 0.4 µM (7.5 ± 0.3 µg/mL) for **1** and 15.5 ± 1.3 µM (12.7 ± 1.3 µg/mL) for **2**. Toxicity and malformations were evaluated on zebrafish larvae exposed to these two compounds considering general toxicity (death after 24 h or 48 h) and malformations of larval morphological features. No such adverse effects were observed for both compounds. REV (resveratrol) was used as a positive control at a final concentration of 50 µM and significantly reduced the Nile red lipid staining in all bioassays. The solvent control,

0.1% DMSO (dimethyl sulfoxide), did not cause any observable toxicity or malformations toward the zebrafish larvae. Chlorophylls a and b were tested for lipid-reducing activity in this same assay, but neither reduced the fluorescence intensity of Nile red in any of the tested concentrations (156 ng/mL to 10 µg/mL) as shown in Figure 3B.

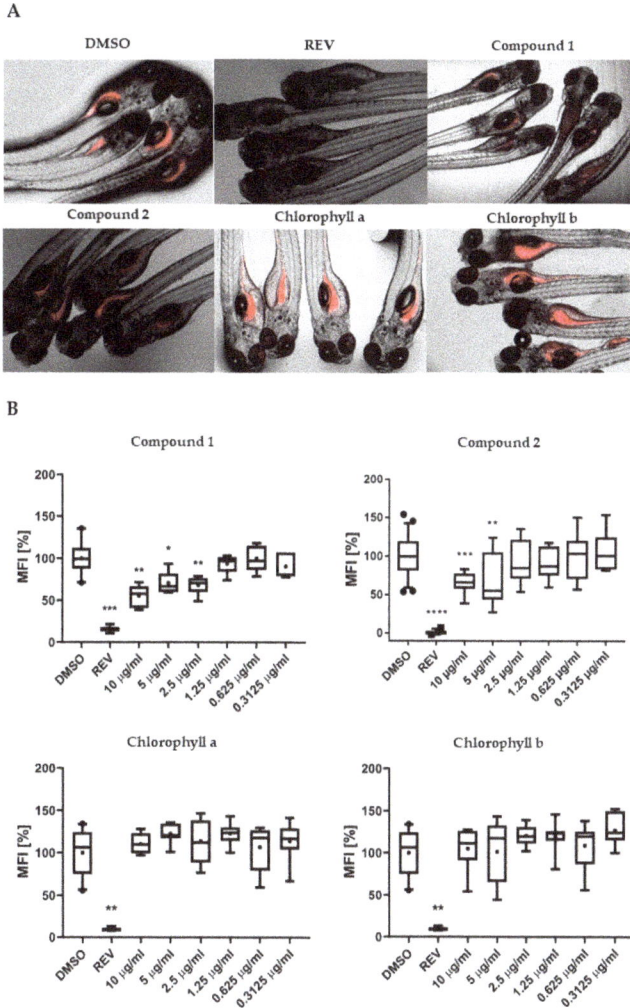

Figure 3. (**A**) Representation of the zebrafish Nile red fat metabolism assay. Strong fluorescence signal is present in zebrafish larvae from the solvent control around the yolk sac and stomach/intestine. Compounds **1** and **2** decreased the Nile red staining, in contrast to chlorophyll a and b. (**B**) Quantification of lipid-reducing activity in the zebrafish Nile red fat metabolism assay after exposure over 48 h. Solvent control was 0.1% dimethyl sulfoxide (DMSO) and positive control was 50 µM resveratrol (REV). Values are expressed as mean fluorescence intensity (MFI) relative to the DMSO group and are derived from six to eight individual larvae per treatment group. The data are represented as box-whisker plots from the fifth to 95th percentiles. Asterisks highlight significant altered fluorescence intensities that indicate changes of neutral lipid level (**** $p < 0.0001$; *** $p < 0.001$; ** $p < 0.01$; * $p < 0.05$).

2.4. Confirmation of Lipid-Reducing Activity in Differentiated 3T3-L1 Spheroids, and Analysis of Lipolysis

The lipid-reducing activity of **1** and **2** was evaluated in 3T3-L1 spheroids, obtained after a seven-day differentiation period (Figure S16). A significant reduction of lipid accumulation was observed following 48 h of exposure to **1** at 7.5, 15, and 30 µg/mL, and to **2** at 30 µg/mL (Figure 4A). The concentrations were chosen based on the EC_{50} values of compound **1** and **2** in the zebrafish fat metabolism assay. The uptake of this lipids was blocked without affecting cell differentiation, since the impairment of lipid accumulation did not occur in spheroids at the beginning of adipogenesis. No significant reduction of viability of spheroids was observed for exposure to **1** and **2** at 7.5 to 30 µg/mL. Lipases hydrolyze triglycerides into glycerol and free fatty acids making the latter available for cell incorporation [26]. By analysis of the free glycerol content, we observed that compounds **1** and **2** did not induce lipolysis on spheroids of differentiated adipocytes.

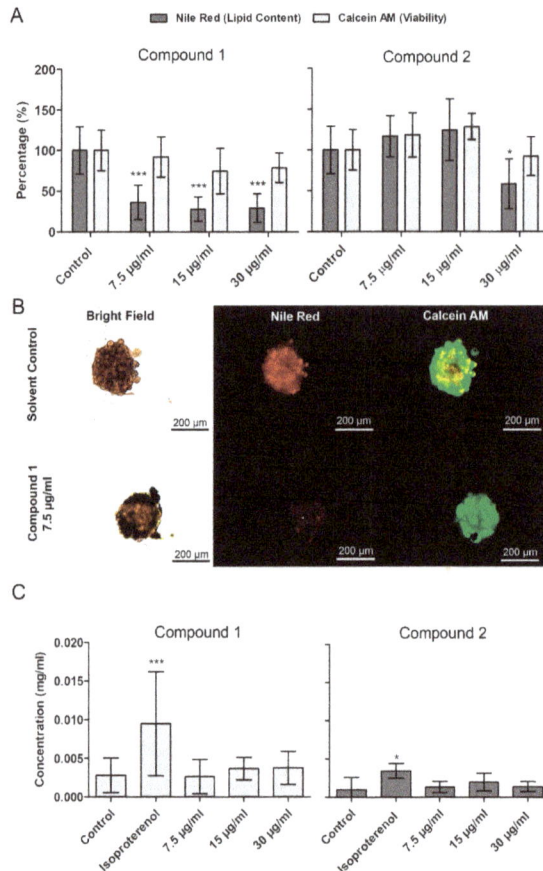

Figure 4. Quantification of lipid content (Nile red) and viability (calcein AM) in differentiated 3T3-L1 spheroids after exposure to **1** and **2** over 48 h. (**A**) Results of quantification of fluorescence by CellProfiler software (mean ± SD). (**B**) Representative images from fluorescence microscopy. Statistical differences to the solvent control were analyzed by one-way ANOVA, followed by a Dunnett's multiple comparison post-test (*** $p < 0.001$, ** $p < 0.01$, * $p < 0.05$). (**C**) Quantification of free glycerol on the medium where 3T3-L1 organoids were exposed to **1** and **2** over 48 h. Data represent means ± SD. No significant alterations on free glycerol content in the medium were observed. Kolmogorov–Smirnov test was used to test normality of the data, followed by a Dunnett's multiple comparison post-test (*** $p < 0.001$, ** $p < 0.01$, * $p < 0.05$).

2.5. qPCR Indicates PPARγ for **1**

In order to study the effects of **1** in lipid metabolism at the transcriptional level, the messenger RNA (mRNA) expression of *fasn*, *mtp*, *pparγ*, and *sirt1* was analyzed in pools of zebrafish larvae, which were exposed to **1** at the EC_{50} concentration for 48h. *Pparγ* mRNA was increased two-fold in response to exposure, while the other genes did not show any significant alteration of their mRNA expression level (Figure 5).

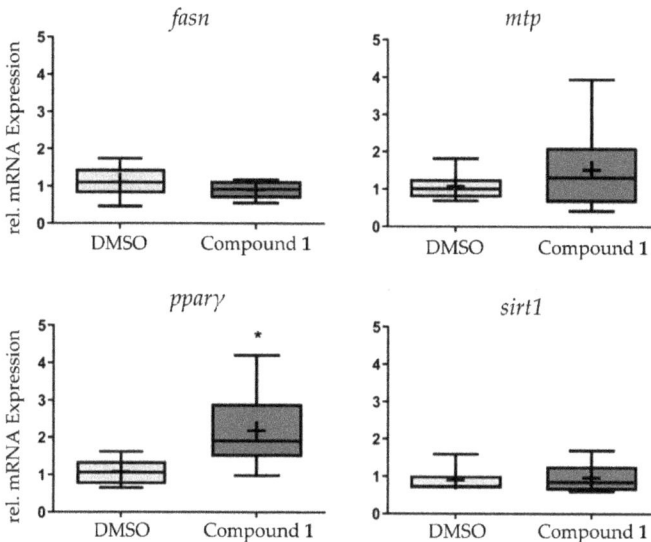

Figure 5. Analysis of messenger RNA (mRNA) expression of *fasn*, *mtp*, *pparγ*, and *sirt1* after exposure to **1** at the half maximal effective concentration (EC_{50}) for 48 h. Data are presented as box-whisker plots (5–95%) from *n* = 8 replicates, consisting of each replicate from a pool of 10 zebrafish larvae. Significant differences are presented as asterisks, * $p < 0.05$.

2.6. Quantification in Different Source Material of **1**

To understand whether metabolite **1** could be found in biomass suitable for human consumption, the presence of the compound was analyzed by LC-ESI-MS in methanolic extyracts derived from various algae- and plant-based materials. When compared to the strain producing **1**, i.e., *Cyanobium* sp. LEGE 07175 (100%), *Spirulina* sp. biomass contained a slightly higher amount of **1** (120.4%), while lower values were observed for *Chlorella vulgaris* (18.0%), spinach (14.7%), and cabbage (33.0%), as shown in Figure 6.

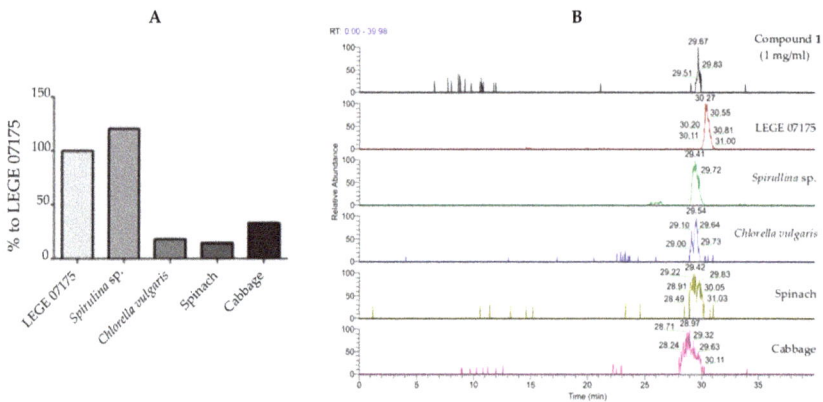

Figure 6. Comparative quantification of **1** in different materials. (**A**) Quantification data are shown as percentage relative to the producing strain of **1**. Samples were prepared at 1 mg/mL in MeOH (100%). (**B**) LC-ESI-MS analysis of the selected samples showing the presence of **1** in all selected materials, compared to the standard (compound **1**) retention time. The peaks selected for analysis had a mass range of *m/z* 887.5593–887.5793 and the following retention times: Compound 1, 29.67 min; LEGE 07175, 30.27 min; *Spirulina* sp., 29.41 min; *Chlorella vulgaris*, 29.54 min; spinach, 29.42 min; and cabbage, 28.97 min.

3. Discussion

Chlorophylls are among the most abundant biological molecules on earth, essential for photosynthesis and ubiquitous in photoautotrophic organisms including cyanobacteria. Chlorophylls are porphyrins, which comprise closed and completely conjugated rings, also referred to as tetrapyrroles. The structure of chlorophyll a, the most widely distributed chlorophyll in nature, features a chelated magnesium atom in the center of tetrapyrrole macrocycle, a characteristic isocyclic fifth ring (ring E) conjoined with ring C, a vinyl group at carbon-3, a ketone at carbon-13^1, a carbomethoxy group at carbon-13^2, and a propionic acid moiety at carbon-17 esterified with phytol [27–30]. Numerous structural alterations occur naturally for chlorophyll a, for example, the formation of magnesium-free pheophorbides and pheophytins, as well as metallo-chlorophyll derivatives. Pheophytin a and pheophorbide a possess some biological properties beneficial for human health including antioxidant properties [31], anti-inflammatory activity [31,32], anti-mutagenic activity [33], cytotoxic effects on cancer cells [34], antiviral activity against hepatitis C virus [35], antimicrobial activity [36], and induction of neuro-differentiation [37]. Regarding metabolic diseases, pheophytin a and pheophorbide a isolated from *Laminaria japonica* inhibited the formation of AGE (advanced glycation end-products) (half maximal inhibitory concentration (IC_{50}) 228.71 µM and 49.43 µM, respectively) and of aldose reductase activity (IC_{50} >100 µM and 12.31 µM, respectively) [38]. Reduction of lipid content in differentiated murine 3T3-L1 preadipocytes was shown for a pheophytin (a and b)-rich extract of a plant at 100 µg/mL [39].

However, for the herein presented chlorophyll derivative **1**, only a few bioactivities are known. For example, 13^2(S)-hydroxy-pheophytin a (compound **1**) was shown to have some cytotoxicity (9.9–24.8 µM) on different cancer cells [40]. An anti-proliferative effect on LNCaP cells (prostate cancer) was shown for **1** with an IC_{50} of 20 µM [41]. A methanolic extract from a red alga containing **1** as a minor component amongst seven other compounds (major peaks were unidentified compounds) showed anti-inflammatory activity in vitro at 10 µg/mL [42]. Here, we observed for the first time the lipid-reducing activity of **1** and of the novel compound **2** in the zebrafish Nile red fat metabolism assay. Both effectively reduced the fluorescent staining of neutral lipids with EC_{50} concentrations of 8.9 and 15.5 µM, respectively. Interestingly, neither chlorophyll a nor chlorophyll b showed any activity in that same assay, which highlights the importance of the structural differences found in compounds 1 and 2 for the observed lipid-reducing activity. The zebrafish Nile red fat metabolism assay belongs to the category of small whole animal assays, which have a higher physiological relevance compared to the traditionally used cell assays. Zebrafish larvae were shown to react with known lipid modulator drugs in a similar manner as humans [18]. The zebrafish Nile red fat metabolism assay was already successfully used to identify structurally modified polyphenolic compounds with lipid-reducing activity with EC_{50} values of 0.07–1.67 µM [43], as well as anthraquinone compounds from a marine fungus with EC_{50} values of 0.17–0.95 µM [44]. In comparison to such studies, chlorophyll derivatives 1 and 2 showed lower potency (micromolar range). However, chlorophyll molecules are ubiquitous to photoautotrophic organisms, and may be easy to purify from sources with GRAS status (generally regarded as safe) for human consumption. Here, we quantified the more potent compound 1 by LC–MS/MS in various sources (*Spirulina*, *Chlorella*, cabbage, and spinach) in comparison to our cyanobacterial strain. Compound 1 is produced in a higher quantity in *Spirulina*, but is also present in lower quantity in cabbage, spinach, or *Chlorella*. This result is in line with a study that showed that, amongst chlorophylls, the hydroxy-pheophytins are present in low quantity in different microalgae species [45].

The differentiation of murine 3T3-L1 preadipocytes is one of the most used bioassays to identify compounds that interfere with adipogenesis or that act on differentiated adipocytes. In a comparative study utilizing 3T3-L1 adipocytes, zebrafish staining of neutral lipids and the diet-induced obese mice, an effect of chrysophanic acid was detected consistently in all three model systems [46]. Here, we intended to confirm the lipid-reducing activity of 1 and 2 observed for zebrafish larvae in another model system and selected 3T3-L1 preadipocytes. Since 3D cell culture systems present a physiologically relevant alternative to monolayer cell culture, we analyzed the possibility to grow multicellular spheroids (MCS) with 3T3-L1 cells and to induce their differentiation. A similar approach was chosen for immortalized preadipocytes, as well as primary cells from the stromal vascular fractions isolated from adipose tissue from human and mice [47]. Previously, spheroids of 3T3-L1 cells were formed by surface coatings of ELP-PEI (elastin-like polypeptide conjugated to polyethyleneimine), and such spheroids showed higher TG (triglycerides) content and uptake of FA (fatty acids) compared to monolayer cells [48]. The lipid-reducing activity of 1 and 2 was confirmed in MCS from 3T3-L1, as well as the higher potency of 1 that was chosen for the following analyses regarding its molecular mode of action. Toxicity and malformations were evaluated in the same zebrafish whole small animal assay, and, for both 1 and 2, no general toxicity or malformations were observed. Accordingly, exposure of MCS of differentiated 3T3-L1 did not show any significant viability reduction for both compounds.

In order to get initial insights into the mechanism of action of 1, lipolysis was analyzed in the MCS of differentiated 3T3-L1 cells, but such activity was not confirmed. The qPCR analysis of some target genes in zebrafish showed a two-fold induction of *ppary* in response to 1. Peroxisome proliferator activated receptors are involved in the regulation of lipid and carbohydrate metabolism, and PPARγ plays a key role in adipocyte differentiation, lipid storage, and lipogenesis [49]. The yolk cells in zebrafish were shown to process lipids during development, and the exposure of zebrafish with a PPARγ antagonist changed the composition of the lipid profile of 5DPF larvae with increasing/decreasing effects on different lipid species, mainly phospholipids [50]. Studies in mice and clinical trials of PPARγ agonists as thiazolidinediones showed that PPARγ had a role on the distribution of body fat [51]. As a response to TZD (thiazolidinedione) treatment, the metabolically more harmful adipose tissue (the visceral adipose tissue) decreased, while subcutaneous adipose tissue increased, which in part explained the beneficial effects of TZD. Hypothetically, the observed *ppary* induction in zebrafish in response to 1 may be responsible, to some degree, for the regulation of lipid distribution or alteration of lipid profiles, but our data are not conclusive in this regard. Future studies are needed to identify the mechanism of action of 1.

Recent studies indicated the existence of absorption and metabolization of oxidized chlorophyll derivatives in both in vitro and in vivo models, establishing a good indication for the future success of compound **1** as a nutraceutical. On the one hand, Chen and Roca demonstrated that oxidized derivatives have a preferential absorption in Caco-2 human intestinal cells (heterogeneous human epithelial colorectal adenocarcinoma cells) over phytylated and other chlorophylls [52]. On the other hand, Vieira et al. highlighted that derivatives with phytyl chains are available for absorption from dietary sources and accumulate to be further metabolized in mice liver [53].

4. Materials and Methods

4.1. General Experimental Procedures

One- and two-dimensional (1D and 2D) NMR spectra were acquired with a 400-MHz Bruker Avance III (Bruker, Karlsruhe, Germany) for samples in DMSO-d_6 and with a 600-MHz Bruker Avance III HD frequency for samples in CDCl$_3$ and DMSO-d_6 (deuterated dimethyl sulfoxide). Both chemical shifts (^{1}H and ^{13}C) are expressed in δ (ppm), referenced to the solvent used, and the proton coupling constants *J* are given in hertz (Hz). Spectra were assigned using appropriate COSY, HSQC, HMBC, TOCSY, and ROESY sequences.

LC-ESI-HRMS analysis was performed on an UltiMate 3000 HPLC (Thermo Fisher Scientific, Waltham, MA, USA) using an ACE Ultracore 2.5 SuperC18 (ACE, United Kingdom), 75 × 2.1 mm inner diameter (id) and the column oven was set to 40 °C. The samples were eluted at 0.35 mL/min over a gradient of 99.5% solvent A (95% H$_2$O, 5% MeOH, 0.1% *v/v* HCOOH) to reach 10% solvent B (95% isopropanol, 5% MeOH, 0.1% *v/v* HCOOH) for 0.5 min, followed by an increase to 60% solvent B for 8 min and by another increase to 90% for 1 min, maintaining those isocratic conditions for over 6 min and returning to the initial conditions for over 1.5 min, before equilibrating for a final 2 min. Analyses were done on a Q Exactive Focus Hybrid Quadrupole Orbitrap Mass Spectrometer (Thermo Fisher Scientific) in the negative and positive ion mode (switching) and controlled by Xcalibur 4.1. The capillary voltage of the heated electrospray ionization (HESI) was set to 3.8 kV. The capillary temperature was 300 °C. The sheath gas and auxiliary gas flow rates were at 35 and 10 (arbitrary units as provided by the software settings).

LC-ESI-HRMS/MS analysis was performed using the same equipment and conditions mentioned previously but with the following gradient: 99.5% solvent A to reach 10% solvent B for 0.5 min, followed by an increase to 60% solvent B for 8 min and by another increase to 90% for 1 min, maintaining those isocratic conditions for over 9 min and returning to the initial conditions for 2 min, before equilibrating for a final 2 min. The UV absorbance of the eluate was monitored at 254 nm, 410 nm, and 665 nm and a full MS scan at the resolution of 70,000 FWHM (full width at half maximum; range of 150–2000 *m/z*), and data-dependent MS2 (ddMS2, Discovery mode) at the resolution of 17,500 FWHM (isolation window used was 3.0 amu and normalized collision energy was 35).

Reverse-phase HPLC data were obtained with a Waters Alliance e2695 instrument coupled with a PDA (photodiode array) detector (Mildford, MA, USA) for compound **2** and a Waters 1525 binary pump, coupled to a Waters 2487 detector (monitored wavelengths: 230 and 254 nm) for compound **1**. The software Empower 2 was used for data interpretation.

Precoated silica gel plates (Merck, KGaA, 60 F-254, 0.5 mm) were used for preparative TLC with visualization under UV light (λ 254 nm).

The phase contrast and red fluorescence images of zebrafish bioassays were obtained with a Leica DM6000B microscope.

4.2. Cyanobacterial Growth, Extraction and Fractionation

Initial screening assays led to the selection of two cyanobacterial strains, *Cyanobium* sp. LEGE 07175 and *Nodosilinea* sp. LEGE 06001 isolated from the Portuguese coast [11] and maintained in the LEGEcc in CIIMAR, Matosinhos, Portugal. Strains were cultured in Z8 medium supplemented with marine tropical salt (25 g/L), at 25 °C, with a photoperiod of 14 h/10 h light and dark, respectively, and at a light intensity of 10–30 μmol photons·m^{-2}·s^{-1}. *Cyanobium* sp. LEGE 07175 cultures were grown in 20-L flasks with constant aeration and, at the exponential phase, cells were harvested through centrifugation, before being frozen and freeze-dried. For the *Nodosilinea* sp. LEGE 06001 strain, available freeze-dried biomass was used, which followed the same growth conditions. The biomass of LEGE 07175 (13 g) and LEGE 06001 (56.5 g) was extracted by repeated percolation with a warm mixture of CH_2Cl_2/MeOH (2:1, *v/v*), yielding a crude extract of 1.9 g and 8.74 g, respectively. Both crude extracts were fractionated by normal-phase (Si gel 60, 0.015–0.040 mm, Merck KGaA, Darmstadt, Germany) VLC (vacuum liquid chromatography) with an increasing polarity grade, from 90% *n*-hex to 100% EtOAc and 100% MeOH [12], giving a total of nine fractions each.

4.3. Compound 1 Isolation and Structure Elucidation

VLC fractions E and F (3:2 and 4:1 EtOAc/*n*-Hex, *v/v*; ethyl acetate/hexane) showed a lipid-reducing activity with the zebrafish assay; thus, they were pooled and further sub-fractionated by gravity column chromatography using Si gel 60 (0.040–0.063 mm, Merck KGaA, Darmstadt, Germany) as a stationary phase and a gradient of increasing polarity from 1:3 EtOAc/*n*-hex (*v/v*) to MeOH producing 12 fractions. The sub-fractions E4 to E6, eluted in 1:3 to 2:3 EtOAc/*n*-hex (*v/v*) demonstrated the previous bioactivity, so they were joined. Then, a SPE (solid-phase extraction) separation was performed, using an Si 5g cartridge (Strata SI-1, Phenomenex) and a gradient of 3:2 EtOAc/*n*-hex (*v/v*) to MeOH, yielding 14 fractions. Sub-fractions E4E and E4F eluted in 3:2 EtOAc/*n*-hex (*v/v*) demonstrated bioactivity and, thus, were submitted to HPLC using a Synergi 4u Fusion (250 × 10 mm 80 Å RP, Phenomenex, Torrance, California, USA) column and using a linear gradient from 7:3 MeCN (aq; acetonitrile) to MeCN for 30 min, before being maintained for 30 min at MeCN (3 mL/min flow). Compound **1** was isolated as the major component at 60 min RT (real-time), yielding 17 mg of pure compound. It was then subjected to LRMS analysis, with a chromatographic column Luna-C18 (250 mm × 4.6 mm, 5 μm, 100 Å, Phenomenex). Samples were eluted at 0.8 mL/min with a gradient starting with 80% H_2O/MeCN and passing to 100% MeCN in 20 min before maintaining in isocratic conditions for 10 min and returning to the initial conditions for 3 min, followed by 5 min of stabilizing. The monoisotopic mass value 887.33 *m/z* appeared to be the major compound. Through a search of this mass, a hit was found, corresponding to 13^2-hydroxy-pheophytin a. Then, 1D and 2D NMR analysis, together with HR-ESI-MS and MS/MS analysis, was performed to confirm the hit (Figures S1–S7, Supplementary Materials).

13^2-hydroxy-pheophytin a (1): green dark powder, HR-ESI-MS *m/z* 887.5697 [M + H]$^+$, *m/z* 909.5493 [M + Na]$^+$, $C_{55}H_{74}N_4O_6$. HR-ESI-MS/MS *m/z* 869.5542 [M − OH]$^+$, *m/z* 609.2696 [M − phytol]$^+$, *m/z* 591.2602 [M − OH − phytol]$^+$. **^{13}C NMR** (101 MHz, DMSO-d_6) δ 192.53 (C-13^1), 172.88 (C-17^3), 172.46 (C-13^3), 168.67 (C-19), 160.59 (C-14), 156.19 (C-16), 153.93 (C-1), 151.07 (C-6), 147.35 (C-3), 147.29 (C-11), 146.71 (C-13), 145.42 (C-9), 143.79 (C-8), 141.79 (C-P3), 138.47 (C-4), 135.18 (C-2), 133.78 (C-7), 130.34 (C-3^1), 128.08 (C-12), 120.01 (C-3^2), 118.05 (C-P2), 109.61 (C-15), 106.97 (C-10), 99.65 (C-5), 93.24 (C-20), 89.88 (C-13^2), 60.40 (C-P1), 52.19 (C-13^4), 48.81 (C-17), 48.66 (C-18), 36.65-23.65 (C-P4-P14), 29.93 (C-17^1), 29.90 (C-17^2), 22.76 (C-18^1), 22.54 (C-P15^1), 22.45 (C-P16), 19.58 (C-P7^1), 19.50 (C-P11^1), 18.88 (C-8^1), 17.72 (C-8^2), 15.84 (C-P3^1), 12.53 (C-12^1), 12.25 (C-2^1), 10.87 (C-7^1) ppm.

^{1}H NMR (400 MHz, DMSO-d_6) δ 9.70 (1H, *s*, H-10), 9.35 (1H, *s*, H-5), 8.53 (1H, *s*, H-20), 8.14 (1H, *dd*, *J* = 17.7, 11.5 Hz, H-3^1), 7.24 (1H, *s*, H-13^2-OH), 6.23 (1H, *dd*, *J* = 17.8, 1.8 Hz, H-3^2E), 6.02 (1H, *dd*, *J* = 11.6, 1.7 Hz, H-3^2Z), 5.06 (1H, *m*, H-P2), 4.53 (1H, *m*, H-17), 4.47 (1H, *m*, H-18), 4.37 (2H, *d*, *J* = 7.1 Hz, H-P1), 3.79 (2H, *q*, *J* = 7.6 Hz, H-8^1), 3.61 (3H, *s*, H-12^1), 3.50 (3H, *s*, H-13^4), 3.30 (3H, *s*, H-2^1), 3.27 (1H, *s*, H-7^1), 2.68–1.75 (H-P4-P14), 2.3–1.8 (H-17^1-H-17^2), 1.68 (3H, *t*, *J* = 7.6 Hz, H-8^2), 1.55 (3H, *d*, *J* = 7.2 Hz, H-18^1), 0.82 (6H, *d*, *J* = 6.6 Hz, H-P15^1, H-P16), 0.77 (3H, *d*, *J* = 6.6 Hz, H-P7^1), 0.72 (3H, *d*, *J* = 6.6 Hz, H-P11^1) ppm.

4.4. Compound 2 Isolation and Structure Elucidation

Fraction E (35.27 mg), resulting from the VLC separation and eluted with *n*-hex/EtOAc (2:3, *v/v*), had the most interesting activity in the zebrafish bioassay, and was, thus, further fractionated over prepacked normal-phase SPE SiO2 cartridges (55 µm, 70 Å, 2 g, Phenomenex) using CH$_2$Cl$_2$/MeOH (from 1:0 to 0:1, *v/v*), resulting in seven sub-fractions (E1 to E7). Subsequently, sub-fraction E4 eluted with a mixture of CH$_2$Cl$_2$/MeOH (1:0 and 99:1, *v/v*) had the desirable bioactivity level. This sub-fraction was subjected to another round of SPE chromatography using *n*-hex/CH$_2$Cl$_2$ (from 7:3 to 0:1, *v/v*) and CH$_2$Cl$_2$/MeOH (from 1:0 to 0:1, *v/v*), to provide an additional six sub-fractions (E4A to E4F). The active fraction E4C was submitted to further fractionation through reverse-phase HPLC using a Luna-C18 column (250 mm × 10 mm, 10 µm, 100 Å, Phenomenex, Torrance, CA, USA). The elution was done with a mixture of MeCN/CH$_2$Cl$_2$ (1:1, *v/v*) in a flow of 3 mL/min for 25 min with a continuously polar gradient MeCN/CH$_2$Cl$_2$ (from 3:2 to 1:1, *v/v*). This separation afforded three sub-fractions and, according to the result of zebrafish bioassay, fraction E4C11 was further purified by preparative TLC using precoated silica gel plates with a mixture of MeOH/CH$_2$Cl$_2$ (0:1, *v/v*). The final purification yielded 0.3 mg of compound **2**.

13^2-hydroxy-pheofarnesin a (2): brownish green amorphous solid, HR-ESI-MS *m/z* 817.4522 [M + H]$^+$, calculated for C$_{50}$H$_{64}$N$_4$O$_6$ (816.4825), HR-ESI-MS/MS *m/z* 840.4339 [M + H + Na]$^+$, 609.2697 [M + 2H − farnesyl]$^+$, 591.2604 [M − OH − farnesyl]$^+$, ^{13}C and ^{1}H NMR (600 MHz, CDCl$_3$) data (see Table 1); for NMR and ESI-MS spectra, see Figures S8–S15 (Supplementary Materials).

4.5. Determination of 13^2-hydroxy-pheophytin a by LC–MS

For quantification and confirmation of **1**, HRMS and HRMS/MS data of the extracts were acquired on an Accela HPLC fitted with a Synergi C18 column (4 µm, 80 A, 4.6 mm id × 250 mm, Phenomenex, Torrance, CA, USA), coupled to an Accela PDA detector, Accela autosampler, and Accela 600 pump, and to an LTQ OrbitrapTM XL hybrid spectrometer, controlled by LTQ Tune Plus 2.5.5 and Xcalibur 2.1 (Thermo Scientific). Firstly, 20 µL of each sample was injected and samples were eluted over a gradient of 10% solvent H$_2$O (0.1% *v/v* HCOOH) to reach 100% solvent MeCN (0.1% HCOOH) for 20 min at a flow rate of 0.8 mL/min. The wavelengths were 235, 285, and 650 nm. The LTQ spectrometer was operated in positive ion mode, and the capillary voltage of the electrospray ionization source (ESI) was set to 3.1 kV. The capillary temperature was 300 °C. The sheath gas and auxiliary gas flow rates were at 40 and 10 (arbitrary unit as provided by the software settings). The capillary voltage was 36 V and the tube lens voltage was 85 V. MS data handling software (Xcalibur 2.1.0 QualBrowser software, Thermo Fischer Scientific) was used.

Five different samples were used to assess the production of **1**: *Cyanobium* sp. LEGE07175 was obtained from the LEGEcc (as previously described); *Spirulina* sp. and *Chlorella Vulgaris* were commercially available; leaves of spinach and cabbage were bought from local supermarkets.

Approximately 1.0 g of powder from each sample was dissolved in 70 mL of MeOH (100%) by stirring for 2h twice at room temperature [54]. The supernatants were collected and dried by a rotatory evaporator to obtain crude extracts. Each extract was then prepared at a concentration of 1 mg/mL for LC–MS, and 0.2 mg/mL for MS/MS in MeOH (100%). A standard of **1** at 16 µg/mL (MeOH 100%) was also prepared for comparison with the samples prior to publication.

Xcalibur 2.1.0 software was used to search for **1** using a reference value interval of 887.50–888.50 *m/z*. The PDA chromatogram was analyzed at a wavelength of 428 nm, as it was the maximum of absorption of **1**. Additionally, this software was used to confirm the presence of **1** in the five different samples through comparison of the mass fragmentation pattern (Figure S17, Supplementary Materials).

4.6. Zebrafish Nile Red Fat Metabolism Assay

The lipid-reducing activity of compounds was analyzed with the zebrafish Nile red assay as previously described [43,44]. An approval by an ethics committee was not necessary for the presented work, since chosen procedures are not considered animal experimentation according to the EC Directive 86/609/EEC for animal experiments. In brief, zebrafish embryos were raised from one DPF (days post fertilization) in egg water (60 µg/mL marine sea salt dissolved in distilled H$_2$O) with 200 µM PTU

(1-phenyl-2-thiourea) to inhibit pigmentation. From three DPF to five DPF, zebrafish larvae were exposed to cyanobacterial fractions at a final concentration of 10 μg/mL with daily renewal of water and fractions in a 48-well plate with a density of 6–8 larvae/well (n = 6–8). A solvent control (0.1% DMSO) and positive control (REV, resveratrol, final concentration 50 μM) were included in the assay. Neutral lipids were stained with Nile red overnight at the final concentration of 10 ng/mL. For imaging, the larvae were anesthetized with tricaine (MS-222, 0.03%) for 5 min and fluorescence analyzed with a fluorescence microscope (Olympus, BX-41, Hamburg, Germany). Fluorescence intensity was quantified in individual zebrafish larvae by ImageJ (http://rsb.info.nih.gov/ij/index.html). EC_{50} values of purified compounds and of chlorophyll a (chl a) and b (chl b) analytical standards (Sigma-Aldrich) were determined by dose–response curves in further assays by using a dilution series from 156 ng/mL to 10 μg/mL in seven dilution steps.

4.7. Differentiated Murine Preadipocytes Grown as Spheroids

Murine preadipocytes 3T3-L1 cell line (ATCC, USA) at 50,000 cells/mL were seeded in an Ultra-Low attachment 96-well plate in Dulbecco's modified Eagle medium (DMEM, Invitrogen, Carlsbad, CA) supplemented with 10% fetal bovine serum (FBS), 1% penicillin/streptomycin, and 0.1% amphothericin B, and kept under 37 °C at 5% CO_2 for five days. Differentiation was then induced on the newly formed spheroids of 3T3-L1 with DMEM supplemented with 10 μg/mL insulin (Sigma-Aldrich, St. Louis, USA), 250 nM dexamethasone (Sigma-Aldrich, St. Louis, MO, USA), and 500 μM isobutylmethylxanthine (Sigma-Aldrich) for three days. The differentiation medium was changed to a maintenance medium containing only insulin (10 μg/mL) on DMEM culture medium, for five days. Spheroids were then exposed to **1** and **2** at three different concentrations, 30 μg/mL, 15 μg/mL, and 7.5 μg/mL, over 48 h in two independent assays with six replicates each (n = 6). After exposure, spheroids were stained with Calcein AM (Life Technologies, Carlsbad, CA, USA) 3 μM and Nile red 4 μM (Sigma-Aldrich, St. Louis, USA) for 1h, and then fluorescence was quantified in an Olympus BX41 coupled with an Olympus DP47 camera, and images were analyzed with Cell Profiller software [55] followed by statistical analysis.

4.8. Lipolysis

Lipolysis was evaluated by quantifying the free glycerol content present in 50 μL of the medium where 3T3-L1 organoids were exposed to **1** and **2** over 48 h. Then, 80 μL of free glycerol reagent was added (Sigma-Aldrich, St. Louis, USA), and the mixture was incubated at 37 °C for 5 min. Absorbance was recorded at 540 nm. A calibration curve with glycerol standard (0.052 mg/mL) and blank (deionized water) was performed in order to calculate glycerol content (mg/mL) according to the following equation:

$$(A \text{ sample} - A \text{ blank})/(A \text{ standard} - A \text{ blank}) \times \text{standard concentration.} \tag{1}$$

4.9. Real-Time PCR

Zebrafish larvae were exposed to **1** and **2** at EC_{50} concentration and to a solvent control group (DMSO 0.1%) for 48 h between 3DPF and 5DPF as described above. Eight biological replicates consisting of a pool of 10 zebrafish larvae each were sampled per group. The protocol for RNA extraction, quantification, and further processing for real-time PCR analysis followed the one described in Reference [43]. Target gene expression (fatty-acid synthase (FASN), sirtuin 1 (SIRT1), peroxisome proliferator activated receptor gamma (PPARγ), microsomal triglyceride transfer protein (MTP) was normalized to the combination of reference genes (beta-2 microglobulin, B2M/ elongation factor 1-alpha, EF1A). A multiple reference gene approach was chosen for normalization of mRNA expression in order to avoid quantification bias [56]. Real-time PCR was performed using the iQ5 real-time PCR machine (Bio-Rad) and samples were run as described in Reference [57].

4.10. Statistics

The data from bioactivity quantifications and mRNA expression are represented as box-whisker plots with values in 5–95 percentiles. The Gaussian distribution was tested by a Kolmogorov–Smirnov normality test (p value < 0.05), and homogeneity of variance was determined by Bartlett's test. One-way ANOVA followed by Dunnett post hoc test (parametric distribution) and Kruskal–Wallis followed by Dunn's post hoc test (non-parametric distribution) were used to compare the solvent control group (DMSO) and the fractions. Statistically significant differences were considered with p-values < 0.05.

The data from dose–response curves were used to determine EC_{50} values for bioactivity level. Mean intensity fluorescence data were normalized to the mean values of the solvent control (100%) and to mean values of the 50 μM resveratrol positive control (0%), and concentrations of the compound were log-transformed. A non-linear regression was applied with a variable slope and least square fitting to obtain the dose–response curves.

5. Conclusions

A known and a novel chlorophyll derivative were discovered from marine cyanobacteria with significant lipid-reducing activities in the zebrafish Nile red fat metabolism assay and in MCS of differentiated 3T3-L1 adipocytes. The more potent compound **1** is produced in large quantities in *Spirulina*, which has the GRAS status for human consumption. Lipolysis is not involved in the lipid-reducing activity, but *pparγ* mRNA expression was altered. Regarding its biological properties and sources for production, **1** could be developed as a nutraceutical with lipid reduction activity in the future.

Supplementary Materials: The following are available online at http://www.mdpi.com/1660-3397/17/4/229/s1: Figures S1–S18, the NMR spectra and HR-ESI-MS and HR-ESI-MS/MS chromatograms of compounds **1** and **2**.

Author Contributions: S.F., isolation of compound **1**, bioactivity screening, qPCR, writing; N.G.S., isolation of compound **2**, bioactivity screening, writing; M.L.S., spheroid activity and lipolysis; T.R. and F.R., quantification of compound 1 from different source materials; P.N.L., contribution for isolation and structural elucidation of compound **1**; V.V., funding; M.A.R., contribution for isolation and structural elucidation of compound **2**; R.U., supervision of bioactivity screening, mechanism of action, funding, and writing.

Funding: This research was funded by the European ERA-NET Marine Biotechnology project CYANOBESITY (ERA-MBT/0001/2015), financed by national funds through FCT (Foundation for Science and Technology, Portugal), and by the project INNOVMAR—Innovation and Sustainability in the Management and Exploitation of Marine Resources (reference NORTE-01-0145-FEDER-000035, within the research line NOVELMAR, supported by North Portugal Regional Operational Program (NORTE 2020) under the PORTUGAL 2020 Partnership Agreement through the European Regional Development Fund (ERDF). The research was additionally supported by the FCT strategic fund UID/Multi/04423/2019. Ralph Urbatzka, Pedro Leão, Maria Lígia Sousa, and Sara Freitas were supported by FCT grants SFRH/BPD/112287/2015, IF/01358/2014, SFRH/BD/108314/2015, and SFRH/BD/116009/2016, respectively.

Conflicts of Interest: The herein reported lipid-reducing activity of the two chlorophyll derivatives formed the basis for a patent application (20191000013283, INPI—Instituto Nacional da Propriedade Industrial), in which some of the authors of the present manuscript are co-inventors.

References

1. Fu, C.; Jiang, Y.; Guo, J.; Su, Z. Natural products with anti-obesity effects and different mechanisms of action. *J. Agric. Food Chem.* **2016**, *64*, 9571–9585. [CrossRef] [PubMed]
2. Castro, M.; Preto, M.; Vasconcelos, V.; Urbatzka, R. Obesity: The metabolic disease, advances on drug discovery and natural product research. *Curr. Top. Med. Chem.* **2016**, *16*, 2577–2604. [CrossRef] [PubMed]
3. Fox, C.; Massaro, J.; Hoffmann, U.; Pou, K.; Maurovich-Horvat, P.; Liu, C.; Vasan, R.; Murabito, J.; Meigs, J.; Cupples, L.; et al. Abdominal visceral and subcutaneous adipose tissue compartments: Association Pereira DCR. *Circulation* **2007**, *116*, 39–48. [CrossRef] [PubMed]
4. Kang, J.G.; Park, C.-Y. Anti-Obesity Drugs: A Review about Their Effects and Safety. *Diabetes Obes. Metab.* **2012**, *36*, 13–25. [CrossRef] [PubMed]
5. Daneschvar, H.L.; Aronson, M.D.; Smetana, G.W. FDA-approved anti-obesity drugs in the United States. *Am. J. Med.* **2016**, *129*, e1–e6. [CrossRef]

6. Inuzuka, T.; Yamamoto, K.; Iwasaki, A.; Ohno, O.; Suenaga, K.; Kawazoe, Y.; Uemura, D. An inhibitor of the adipogenic differentiation of 3T3-L1 cells, yoshinone A, and its analogs, isolated from the marine cyanobacterium *Leptolyngbya* sp. *Tetrahedron Lett.* **2014**, *55*, 6711–6714. [CrossRef]

7. Blunt, J.W.; Carrol, A.R.; Copp, B.R.; Davis, R.A.; Keyzers, R.A.; Princep, M.R. Marine natural products. *Nat. Prod. Rep.* **2018**, *35*, 8–53. [CrossRef]

8. Luzzatto-Knaan, T.; Garg, N.; Wang, M.; Glukhov, E.; Peng, Y.; Ackemann, G.; Amir, A.; Duggan, B.M.; Ryazanov, S.; Gerwick, L.; et al. Digitizing mass spectrometry data to explore the chemical diversity and distribution of marine cyanobacteria and algae. *eLife* **2017**, *6*, e24214. [CrossRef]

9. Brito, A.; Gaifem, J.; Ramos, V.; Glukhov, E.; Dorrestein, P.C.; Gerwick, W.H.; Vasconcelos, V.M.; Mendes, M.V.; Tamagnini, P. Bioprospecting portuguese atlantic coast cyanobacteria for bioactive secondary metabolites reveals untapped chemodiversity. *Algal Res.* **2015**, *9*, 218–226. [CrossRef]

10. Sharma, N.K.; Tiwari, S.P.; Tripathi, K.; Rai, A.K. Sustainability and cyanobacteria (blue-green algae): Facts and challenges. *J. Appl. Phycol.* **2011**, *23*, 1059–1081. [CrossRef]

11. Ramos, V.; Morais, J.; Castelo-Branco, R.; Pinheiro, A.; Martins, J.; Regueiras, A.; Pereira, A.L.; Lopes, V.R.; Frazão, B.; Gomes, D.; et al. Cyanobacterial diversity held in microbial biological resource centers as a biotechnological asset: The case study of the newly established LEGE culture collection. *J. Appl. Phycol.* **2018**, *30*, 1437–1451. [CrossRef]

12. Leão, P.N.; Costa, M.; Ramos, V.; Pereira, A.R.; Fernandes, V.C.; Domingues, V.F.; Gerwick, W.H.; Vasconcelos, V.M.; Martins, R. Antitumor Activity of Hierridin B, a Cyanobacterial Secondary Metabolite Found in both Filamentous and Unicellular Marine Strains. *PLoS ONE* **2013**, *8*, e69562. [CrossRef]

13. Leão, P.N.; Nakamura, H.; Costa, M.; Pereira, A.R.; Martins, R.; Vasconcelos, V.; Gerwick, W.H.; Balskus, E.P. Biosynthesis-assisted structural elucidation of the bartolosides, chlorinated aromatic glycolipids from cyanobacteria. *Angew. Chem. Int. Ed. Engl.* **2015**, *54*, 11063–11067. [CrossRef] [PubMed]

14. Afonso, T.B.; Costa, M.S.; Rezende de Castro, R.; Freitas, S.; Silva, A.; Schneider, M.P.C.; Martins, R.; Leão, P.N. Bartolosides E-K from a marine coccoid cyanobacterium. *Nat. Prod.* **2016**, *79*, 2504–2513. [CrossRef] [PubMed]

15. Ribeiro, T.; Lemos, F.; Preto, M.; Azevedo, J.; Sousa, M.L.; Leão, P.N.; Campos, A.; Linder, S.; Vitorino, R.; Vasconcelos, V.; et al. Cytotoxicity of portoamides in human cancer cells and analysis of the molecular mechanisms of action. *PLoS ONE* **2017**, *12*, e0188817. [CrossRef] [PubMed]

16. Nguyen, M.; Yang, E.; Neelkantan, N.; Mikhaylova, A.; Arnold, R.; Poudel, M.K.; Stewart, A.M.; Kalueff, A.V. Developing 'integrative' zebrafish models of behavioral and metabolic disorders. *Behav. Brain Res.* **2013**, *256*, 172–187. [CrossRef]

17. Oka, T.; Nishimura, Y.; Zang, L.; Hirano, M.; Shimada, Y.; Wang, Z.; Umemoto, N.; Kuroyanagi, J.; Nishimura, N.; Tanaka, T. Diet-induced obesity in zebrafish shares common pathophysiological pathways with mammalian obesity. *BMC Physiol.* **2010**, *10*, 21. [CrossRef] [PubMed]

18. Jones, K.S.; Alimov, A.P.; Rilo, H.L.; Jandacek, R.J.; Woollett, L.A.; Penberthy, W.T. A high throughput live transparent animal bioassay to identify non-toxic small molecules or genes that regulate vertebrate fat metabolism for obesity drug development. *Nutr. Metab.* **2008**, *5*, 1–11. [CrossRef]

19. Jerz, G.; Arrey, T.N.; Wray, V.; Du, Q.; Winterhalter, P. Structural characterization of 13²-hydroxy-(13²-*S*)-phaeophytin-a from leaves and stems of *Amaranthus tricolor* isolated by high-speed countercurrent chromatography. *Innov. Food Sci. Emerg. Technol.* **2007**, *8*, 413–418. [CrossRef]

20. Yaacob, N.S.; Yankuzo, H.M.; Devaraj, S.; Wong, J.K.M.; Lai, C.-S. Anti-Tumor Action, Clinical biochemistry profile and phytochemical constituents of a pharmacologically active fraction of *S. crispus* in NMU-Induced Rat Mammary Tumour Model. *PLoS ONE* **2015**, *10*, e0126426. [CrossRef]

21. Lee, T.H.; Lu, C.K.; Kuo, Y.H.; Lo, J.M.; Lee, C.K. Unexpected novel pheophytin peroxides from the leaves of *Biden Pilosa. Helv. Chim. Acta* **2008**, *91*, 79–84. [CrossRef]

22. Li, H.; Li, L.; Zheng, Q.; Kuroda, C.; Wang, Q. Phaeophytin analogues from *Ligularia knorringiana. Molecules* **2012**, *17*, 5219–5224. [CrossRef] [PubMed]

23. Masuda, T.; Fujita, Y. Regulation and evolution of chlorophyll metabolism. *Photochem. Photobiol. Sci.* **2008**, *7*, 1131–1149. [CrossRef]

24. Matsuo, A.; Ono, K.; Hamasaki, K.; Nozaki, H. Phaeophytins from a cell suspension culture of the liverwort *Plagiochila ovalifolia. Phytochemistry* **1996**, *42*, 427–430. [CrossRef]

25. Nakatani, Y.; Ourisson, G.; Beck, J.P. Chemistry and biochemistry of chinese drugs. VII. Cytostatic pheophytins from silkworm excreta, and derived photocytotoxic pheophorbides. *Chem. Pharm. Bull.* **1981**, *29*, 2261–2269. [CrossRef] [PubMed]

26. Desarzens, S.; Liao, W.H.; Mammi, C.; Caprio, M.; Faresse, N. Hsp90 blockers inhibit adipocyte differentiation and fat mass accumulation. *PLoS ONE* **2014**, *9*, e94127. [CrossRef] [PubMed]

27. Aronoff, S. The chlorophylls—An introductory survey. In *The Chlorophylls*; Vernon, L.P., Seely, G.R., Eds.; Academic Press: New York, NY, USA, 1996; pp. 3–20.

28. Scheer, H. Structure and occurrence of chlorophylls. In *Chlorophylls*; Scheer, H., Ed.; CRC Press: Boca Raton, FL, USA, 1991; pp. 3–30.

29. Tanaka, R.; Tanaka, A. Tetrapyrrole biosynthesis in higher plants. *Annu. Rev. Plant Biol.* **2007**, *58*, 321–346. [CrossRef]

30. Vavilin, D.V.; Vermaas, W.F. Regulation of the tetrapyrrole biosynthetic pathway leading to heme and chlorophyll in plants and cyanobacteria. *Physiol. Plant* **2002**, *115*, 9–24. [CrossRef] [PubMed]

31. Kang, Y.-R.; Park, J.; Jung, S.K.; Chang, Y.H. Synthesis, characterization, and functional properties of chlorophylls, pheophytins, and Zn-pheophytins. *Food Chem.* **2018**, *245*, 943–950. [CrossRef]

32. Subramoniam, A.; Asha, V.V.; Nair, S.A.; Sasidharan, S.P.; Sureshkumar, P.K.; Rajendran, K.N.; Karunagaran, D.; Ramalingam, K. Chlorophyll revisited: Anti-inflammatory activities of chlorophyll a and inhibition of expression of TNF-α gene by the same. *Inflammation* **2012**, *35*, 959–966. [CrossRef] [PubMed]

33. Ferruzzi, M.; Böhm, V.; Courtney, P.; Schwartz, S. Antioxidant and antimutagenic activity of dietary chlorophyll derivatives determined by radical scavenging and bacterial reverse mutagenesis assays. *J. Food Sci. Technol.* **2002**, *67*, 2589–2595. [CrossRef]

34. Zhao, Y.; Wang, X.; Wang, H.; Liu, T.; Xin, Z. Two new noroleanane-type triterpene saponins from the methanol extract of *Salicornia herbacea*. *Food Chem.* **2014**, *151*, 101–109. [CrossRef]

35. Wang, S.-Y.; Tseng, C.-P.; Tsai, K.-C.; Lin, C.-F.; Wen, C.-Y.; Tsay, H.-S.; Sakamoto, N.; Tseng, C.-H.; Cheng, J.-C. Bioactivity-guided screening identifies pheophytin a as a potent anti-hepatitis C virus compound from *Lonicera hypoglauca* Miq. *Biochem. Biophys. Res. Commun.* **2009**, *385*, 230–235. [CrossRef] [PubMed]

36. Gomes, R.A.; Teles, Y.C.; Pereira, F.D.; Rodrigues, L.A.; Lima, E.D.; Agra, M.D.; Souza, M.D. Phytoconstituents from *Sidastrum micranthum* (A. St.-Hil.) Fryxell (Malvaceae) and antimicrobial activity of pheophytin a. *Braz. J. Pharm. Sci.* **2015**, *51*, 861–867. [CrossRef]

37. Ina, A.; Hayashi, K.-I.; Nozaki, H.; Kamei, Y. Pheophytin A, a low molecular weight compound found in the marine brown alga *Sargassum fulvellum*, promotes the differentiation of PC12 cells. *Int. J. Dev. Neurosci.* **2007**, *25*, 63–68. [CrossRef]

38. Sharifuddin, Y.; Chin, Y.-X.; Lim, P.-E.; Phang, S.-M. Potential bioactive compounds from seaweed for diabetes management. *Mar. Drugs* **2015**, *13*, 5447–5491. [CrossRef]

39. Semaan, D.G.; Igoli, J.O.; Young, L.; Gray, A.I.; Rowan, E.G.; Marrero, E. In vitro anti-diabetic effect of flavonoids and pheophytins from *Allophylus cominia* Sw. on the glucose uptake assays by HepG2, L6, 3T3-L1 and fat accumulation in 3T3-L1 adipocytes. *J. Ethnopharmacol.* **2018**, *216*, 8–17. [CrossRef]

40. Cheng, H.H.; Wang, H.K.; Ito, J.; Bastow, K.F.; Tachibana, Y.; Nakanishi, Y.; Xu, Z.; Luo, T.Y.; Lee, K.H. Cytotoxic pheophorbide-related compounds from *Clerodendrum calamitosum and C. cyrtophyllum*. *J. Nat. Prod.* **2001**, *64*, 915–919. [CrossRef] [PubMed]

41. Chen, R.; He, J.; Tong, X.; Tang, L.; Liu, M. The *Hedyotis diffusa* Willd. (Rubiaceae): A review on phytochemistry, pharmacology, quality control and pharmacokinetics. *Molecules* **2016**, *21*, 710. [CrossRef]

42. Shu, M.H.; Appleton, D.; Zandi, K.; AbuBakar, S. Anti-inflammatory, gastroprotective and antiulcerogenic effects of red algae *Gracilaria changii* (Gracilariales, Rhodophyta) extract. *BMC Complement. Altern. Med.* **2013**, *13*, 61. [CrossRef]

43. Urbatzka, R.; Freitas, S.; Palmeira, A.; Almeida, T.; Moreira, J.; Azevedo, C.; Afonso, C.; Correia-da-Silva, M.; Sousa, E.; Pinto, M.; et al. Lipid reducing activity and toxicity profiles of a library of polyphenol derivatives. *Eur. J. Med. Chem.* **2018**, *151*, 272–284. [CrossRef] [PubMed]

44. Noinart, J.; Buttachon, S.; Dethoup, T.; Gales, L.; Pereira, J.A.; Urbatzka, R.; Freitas, S.; Lee, M.; Silva, A.M.S.; Pinto, M.M.M.; et al. A new ergosterol analog, a new bis-anthraquinone and anti-obesity activity of anthraquinones from the marine sponge-associated fungus *Talaromyces stipitatus* KUFA 0207. *Mar. Drugs* **2017**, *16*, 15. [CrossRef] [PubMed]

45. Yao, L.; Gerde, J.A.; Lee, S.L.; Wang, T.; Harrata, K.A. Microalgae lipid characterization. *J. Agric. Food Chem.* **2015**, *63*, 1773–1787. [CrossRef] [PubMed]

46. Lim, H.; Park, J.; Kim, H.-L.; Kang, J.; Jeong, M.-Y.; Youn, D.-H.; Jung, Y.; Kim, Y.-I.; Kim, H.-J.; Ahn, K.S.; et al. Chrysophanic acid suppresses adipogenesis and induces thermogenesis by activating AMP-activated protein kinase alpha *in vivo* and *in vitro*. *Front. Pharmacol.* **2016**, *7*, 476. [CrossRef] [PubMed]

47. Klingelhutz, A.J.; Gourronc, F.A.; Chaly, A.; Wadkins, D.A.; Burand, A.J.; Markan, K.R.; Idiga, S.O.; Wu, M.; Potthoff, M.J.; Ankrum, J.A. Scaffold-free generation of uniform adipose spheroids for metabolism research and drug discovery. *Sci. Rep.* **2018**, *8*, 523. [CrossRef]

48. Turner, P.A.; Harris, L.M.; Purser, C.A.; Baker, R.C.; Janorkar, A.V. A surface-tethered spheroid model for functional evaluation of 3T3-L1 adipocytes. *Biotechnol. Bioeng.* **2014**, *111*, 174–183. [CrossRef] [PubMed]

49. Hihi, A.K.; Michalik, L.; Wahli, W. PPARs: Transcriptional effectors of fatty acids and their derivatives. *Cell. Mol. Life Sci.* **2002**, *59*, 790–798. [CrossRef]

50. Fraher, D.; Sanigorski, A.; Mellett, N.A.; Meikle, P.J.; Sinclair, A.J.; Gibert, Y. Zebrafish embryonic lipidomic analysis reveals that the yolk cell is metabolically active in processing lipid. *Cell Rep.* **2016**, *14*, 1317–1329. [CrossRef]

51. Chiarelli, F.; Di Marzio, D. Peroxisome proliferator-activated receptor-γ agonists and diabetes: Current evidence and future perspectives. *Vasc. Health Risk Manag.* **2008**, *4*, 297–304. [CrossRef]

52. Chen, K.; Roca, M. *In vitro* bioavailability of chlorophyll pigments from edible seaweeds. *J. Funct. Foods* **2018**, *41*, 25–33. [CrossRef]

53. Vieira, I.; Chen, K.; Ríos, J.J.; Benito, I.; Pérez-Gálvez, A.; Roca, M. First-Pass Metabolism of Chlorophylls in Mice. *Mol. Nutr. Food Res.* **2018**, *17*, e1800562. [CrossRef] [PubMed]

54. Henriques, M.; Silva, A.; Rocha, J. Extraction and quantification of pigments from a marine microalga: A simple and reproducible method. *Appl. Microbiol.* **2007**, *2*, 586–893.

55. Carpenter, A.E.; Jones, T.R.; Lamprecht, M.R.; Clarke, C.; Kang, I.H.; Friman, O.; Guertin, D.A.; Chang, J.H.; Lindquist, R.A.; Moffat, J.; et al. CellProfiler: Image analysis software for identifying and quantifying cell phenotypes. *Genome Biol.* **2006**, *7*, R100. [CrossRef] [PubMed]

56. Urbatzka, R.; Galante-Oliveira, S.; Rocha, E.; Castro, L.F.; Cunha, I. Normalization strategies for gene expression studies by real-time PCR in a marine fish species, Scophthalmus maximus. *Mar. Genom.* **2013**, *10*, 17–25. [CrossRef] [PubMed]

57. Freitas, S.; Martins, R.; Costa, M.; Leão, P.N.; Vitorino, R.; Vasconcelos, V.; Urbatzka, R. Hierridin B isolated from a marine cyanobacterium alters VDAC1, mitochondrial activity, and cell cycle genes on HT-29 colon adenocarcinoma cells. *Mar. Drugs* **2016**, *14*, 158. [CrossRef] [PubMed]

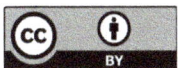

marine drugs

MDPI

Article

Hypolipidemic Effect of *Arthrospira* (*Spirulina*) *maxima* Supplementation and a Systematic Physical Exercise Program in Overweight and Obese Men: A Double-Blind, Randomized, and Crossover Controlled Trial

Marco Antonio Hernández-Lepe [1], Abraham Wall-Medrano [2], José Alberto López-Díaz [2], Marco Antonio Juárez-Oropeza [3], Oscar Iván Luqueño-Bocardo [3], Rosa Patricia Hernández-Torres [4] and Arnulfo Ramos-Jiménez [2,*]

[1] Medicine and Psychology School, Autonomous University of Baja California, Tijuana 22390, Mexico; marco.antonio.hernandez.lepe@uabc.edu.mx
[2] Biomedical Sciences Institute. Autonomous University of Ciudad Juarez, Ciudad Juarez 32310, Mexico; awall@uacj.mx (A.W.-M.); joslopez@uacj.mx (J.A.L.-D.)
[3] Medicine School, National Autonomous University of Mexico, Mexico City 04510, Mexico; majo_ya@yahoo.com.mx (M.A.J.-O.); luqueno@bq.unam.mx (O.I.L.-B)
[4] Physical Culture Sciences School, Autonomous University of Chihuahua, Chihuahua 32310, Mexico; rphernant@yahoo.com
* Correspondence: aramos@uacj.mx; Tel.: +52-656-1679309

Received: 17 April 2019; Accepted: 30 April 2019; Published: 7 May 2019

Abstract: Low-fat diets, lipid-modifying nutraceuticals and a higher level of physical activity are often recommended to reduce dyslipidemia. A double-blind, randomized, crossover, controlled trial was designed to evaluate the independent and synergistic effects of *Arthrospira* (*Spirulina*) *maxima* supplementation (4.5 g·day^{-1}) with or without performing a physical exercise program (*PEP*: aerobic exercise (3 days·week^{-1}) + high-intensity interval training (2 days·week^{-1})) on blood lipids and BMI of 52 sedentary men with excess body weight. During six weeks, all participants were assigned to four intervention treatments (*Spirulina maxima* with PEP (SE), placebo with PEP (Ex), *Spirulina maxima* without PEP (Sm), placebo without PEP (C; control)) and plasma lipids were evaluated spectrophotometrically pre- vs. post intervention in stratified subgroups (overweight, obese and dyslipidemic subjects). Pre/post comparisons showed significant reductions in all plasma lipids in the SE group, particularly in those with dyslipidemia ($p \leq 0.043$). Comparing the final vs. the initial values, BMI, total cholesterol, triglycerides and low-density lipoprotein cholesterol were decreased. High-density lipoprotein cholesterol increased in all treatment groups compared to C. Changes were observed mostly in SE interventions, particularly in dyslipidemic subjects ($p < 0.05$). *Spirulina maxima* supplementation enhances the hypolipidemic effect of a systematic PEP in men with excess body weight and dyslipidemia.

Keywords: *Arthrospira maxima*; dyslipidemia; physical exercise; obesity; double-blind; randomized controlled trial

1. Introduction

Dyslipidemia is an abnormal clinical condition characterized by the altered level of one or more plasma lipids, including but not restricted to total (TC), low-density lipoprotein (LDL-C) and high-density lipoprotein (HDL-C) cholesterol and triglycerides (TG). Dyslipidemias often increase concomitantly with body mass index (BMI) and central adiposity, increasing the risk for metabolic syndrome and cardiovascular diseases (CVD) [1]; its pathophysiology is multifactorial but excess of body weight and sedentarism are two of the most important factors [2]. Effective control measures to stop the pandemic obesity-dyslipidemia consortium are a priority for health systems worldwide [3].

Lifestyle changes aimed to reduce people's sedentarism and the promotion of healthy eating patterns have been widely used to prevent and even treat obesity and dyslipidemias [4,5]. However, moderate physical activity alone is not effective to lose weight or body fat [6] but systematic exercise programs based in high-intensity protocols reduces CVD risk and dyslipidemia [7]. A heart-healthy diet aimed to reduce the intake of saturated/ trans fatty acids and cholesterol, due to their unfavorable metabolic fate, must include functional foods (e.g., plant and marine proteins) and nutraceuticals (e.g., *n*-3 fatty acids, phytosterols and polyphenols) [8,9]. *Arthrospira maxima*, commercially known as *Spirulina maxima* (*S. maxima*), is a cyanobacteria used as a nutritional supplement due to its high content of protein, essential fatty acids, vitamins, polyphenols, carotenoids and phycocyanins [10] with cardio-protective and antioxidant activity. In this regard, Moura et al. [11] reported that *Spirulina* supplementation decreases circulating LDL-C levels more effectively than aerobic training in diabetic Wistar rats while *Spirulina* intake and aerobic physical exercise resulted in even better effects. Mazzola et al. [12] demonstrated that *Spirulina* and physical reduces plasma TG levels in Wistar rats Kata et al. [13] reported reduced levels of TC, TG and LDL-C in hypercholesterolemic rabbits. However, these studies were conducted in animal models and therefore their results cannot be extrapolated to humans, and clinical studies conducted in humans are still very scarce [14].

This study aimed to assess the independent and synergistic effect of *S. maxima* supplementation (4.5 g·day^{-1}) and the practice of systematic physical exercise on plasma lipid levels in young subjects with overweight, obesity or defined dyslipidemia. We hypothesize that *S. maxima* intake with or without a systematic physical exercise program will decrease the BMI while improving plasma lipids in male patients with overweight and obesity.

2. Results

Fifty-two male young (26 ± 5 years) subjects with excess weight (BMI ≥ 25 kg·m^{-2}) were enrolled in the study (Table 1).

Table 1. Baseline characteristics of participants.

	Total	Overweight	Obese
n	52	27	25
Age (years)	26 ± 5	26 ± 4	27 ± 6
Body weight (kg)	90 ± 13	81 ± 8	100 ± 12
Height (m)	1.72 ± 0.1	1.72 ± 0.1	1.73 ± 0.1
BMI (kg·m^{-2})	30.2 ± 4	27.4 ± 1.2	33.3 ± 3.8
Energy intake (kcal·day^{-1})	2054 ± 104	1977 ± 139	2054 ± 151
Total cholesterol (mg·dL^{-1}) *	196 ± 36	177 ± 28	218 ± 30
Triglycerides (mg·dL^{-1})	142 ± 41	136 ± 35	150 ± 46
LDL-C (mg·dL^{-1}) *	134 ± 36	115 ± 27	158 ± 31
HDL-C (mg·dL^{-1})	34 ± 9.6	35.3 ± 8.2	32.5 ± 10.9

Data are expressed as mean ± SD. Asterisk (*) means statistical differences comparing overweight and obese individuals ($p < 0.05$); *n*: Sample size, BMI: body mass index, LDL-C: low-density lipoprotein-cholesterol, HDL-C: high-density lipoprotein-cholesterol.

Baseline characteristics of subjects at day 0 and 56 (wash-out period) did not show differences ($p < 0.05$; see Supplementary File S3). Of all the participants, 52 and 48% were overweight and obese, respectively, while dyslipidemic subjects were distributed as follow: High TC (7 overweight, 8 obese), high TG (11 overweight, 16 obese), high LDL-C (17 overweight, 21 obese) and low HDL-C (17 overweight, 18 obese).

2.1. Diet

The daily energy intake after the six weeks of supplementation showed no statistical differences ($p < 0.05$) for dietary variables at the beginning (2054 ± 104 kcal·day^{-1}) compared with those at the end of the study (2146 ± 98 kcal·day^{-1}). No adverse effects of dietary or *S. maxima* supplementation were reported during the study.

2.2. Intra Group Comparisons (Pre vs. Post) on the Blood Lipid Profile

After 42 days of treatment, there was an improvement ($p < 0.05$) between basal (pre) and final (post) levels of TC, LDL-C and HDL-C in the SE intervention, and by Ex only in LDC-C considering all participants (overweight + obesity, Table 2a). Analysing dyslipidemic participants only, SE presented an improvement for all analysed parameters of blood lipids ($p < 0.05$), Ex on TC, LDL-C and HDL-C, and Sm on TC, TG and HDL-C (Table 2b).

Table 2. Effect of treatments on the blood lipid profile within the total and dyslipidemic participants.

Blood lipid		2a (Overweight and obese subjects)			
		C	SE	Ex	Sm
TC	Basal	190±31	196±35	197±38	201±39
	Final	186±31	163±33	177±36	183±37
	p value (*n*)	0.619 (12)	0.001 (14) *	0.053 (14)	0.103 (12)
TG	Basal	131±31	157±47	139±44	141±37
	Final	125±32	135±37	124±42	127±34
	p value (*n*)	0.517 (12)	0.070 (14)	0.212 (14)	0.176 (12)
LDL-C	Basal	131±32	128±36	137±38	138±37
	Final	127±30	93±34	115±36	117±38
	p value (*n*)	0.680 (12)	0.001 (14) *	0.046 (14) *	0.062 (12)
HDL-C	Basal	35±12	34±9	31±9	35±10
	Final	37±8	42±10	36±9	40±11
	p value (*n*)	0.655 (12)	0.005 (14) *	0.059 (14)	0.071 (12)
Blood lipid		2b (Dyslipidemic subjects)			
		C	SE	Ex	Sm
TC	Basal	219±16	226±22	232±23	233±21
	Final	213±18	189±20	208±28	212±23
	p value (*n*)	0.412 (6)	0.000 (7) *	0.025 (6) *	0.029 (6) *
TG	Basal	160±6	184±40	180±25	167±11
	Final	153±12	156±29	164±21	148±19
	p value (*n*)	0.156 (6)	0.043 (7) *	0.096 (7)	0.004 (7) *
LDL-C	Basal	140±29	141±29	148±33	148±33
	Final	135±27	101±34	124±33	128±32
	p value (*n*)	0.650 (9)	0.001 (10) *	0.030 (10) *	0.060 (9)
HDL-C	Basal	28±8	30±6	28±6	29±6
	Final	31±5	40±10	33±6	35±10
	p value (*n*)	0.172 (7)	0.001 (10) *	0.019 (10) *	0.040 (8) *

Data are expressed as mg·dL^{-1} and mean ± SD. Asterisk (*) means statistical differences between basal and final blood lipid concentration ($p < 0.05$). SE: *Spirulina* and exercise; Ex: Exercise and placebo; Sm: *Spirulina* without exercise; C: Control (Placebo without exercise); TC: total cholesterol, TG: Triglycerides; LDL-C: low density lipoprotein-cholesterol, HDL-C: high density lipoprotein-cholesterol; *n*: Sample size.

2.3. Inter-Group Comparisons of the Blood Lipid Profile

To achieve an objective comparison of the effects of each intervention, absolute changes were calculated (Δ change = *Post* − *Pre* values) for TC and TG (Figure 1; mg·dL^{-1}), LDL-C and HDL-C (Figure 2; mg·dL^{-1}) and BMI (Figure 3; kg·m^{-2}). As compared to C (placebo+no exercise), important reductions in plasma TC levels (Δ change, mg·dL^{-1} [upper; lower quartile]) were observed in overweight (−24 [−43; −17], −17 [−22; −8]) obese (−34 [−44; −24], −23 [−34; −13]) and dyslipidemic (−34 [−43; −29], −25 [−35; −14]) subjects enrolled in SE and Ex. Also, a mild yet significant ($p < 0.05$) reduction in TC level was observed in obese subjects in the Sm treatment (−24 [−34; −18]) and TG level in overweight (−26 [−36; −17]) subjects enrolled in the SE treatment.

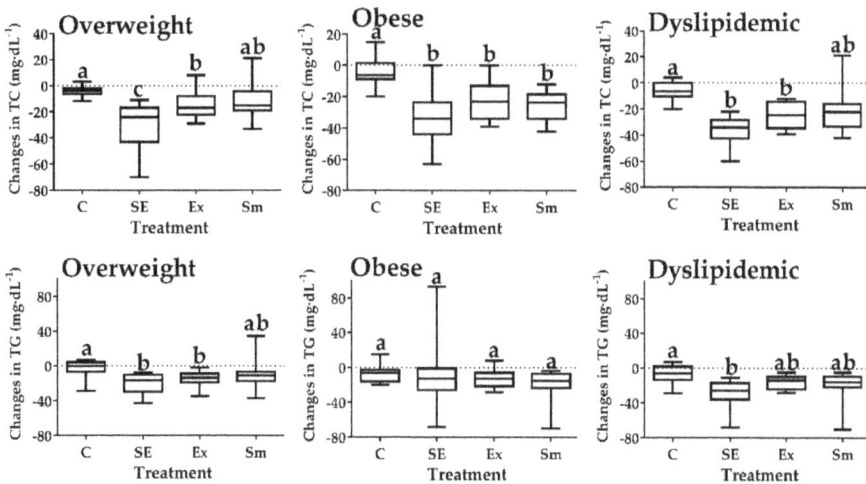

Figure 1. Changes (Δ) in total cholesterol and triglycerides by treatments. SE: *Spirulina* and exercise; Ex: Exercise and placebo; Sm: *Spirulina* without exercise; C: Control (Placebo without exercise); TC: Total cholesterol; TG: Triglycerides. Data presented as box and whisker plots of the median (horizontal line), upper and lower quartiles (box) maximum and minimum (error bars). Different letters indicate statistical difference between treatments ($p < 0.05$), Kruskal-Wallis Test with Dunn's post-hoc for all panels of changes in TC and for changes in TG of overweight and dyslipidemic, ANOVA test for changes in TG of obese subjects.

As compared to C, the LDL-C plasma level (Δ change; mg·dL^{-1}; [upper; lower quartile] Figure 2) in SE, Ex and Sm was lower in overweight (SE (−26 [−49; −19]) > Ex (−19 [−26; −13]) and Sm (−19 [−24; −12])), obese (SE (−33 [−63; −20]) > Ex (−30 [−40; −17]) > Sm (−21 [−31; −17])), and dyslipidemic (SE (−37 [−55; −26]) > Ex (−25 [−30; −16]) > Sm (−19 [−24; −16])) subgroups ($p < 0.05$). On the other hand, HDL−C levels (Δ change, mg·dL^{-1} [upper; lower quartile]) only improved in overweight (+7, [4; 11]) and dyslipidemic (+8, [4; 13]) subjects from the SE treatment.

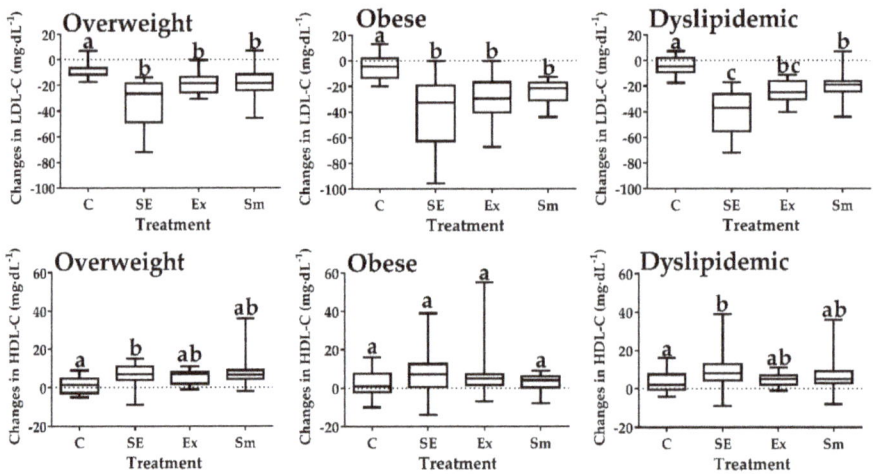

Figure 2. Changes (Δ) in lipoproteins levels by treatments. SE: *Spirulina* and exercise; Ex: Exercise and placebo; Sm: *Spirulina* without exercise; C: Control (Placebo without exercise); LDL-C: Low-density lipoprotein-cholesterol; HDL-C: High-density lipoprotein-cholesterol. Data presented as box and whisker plots of the median (horizontal line), upper and lower quartiles (box) maximum and minimum (error bars). Different letters indicate statistical difference between treatments ($p < 0.05$), Kruskal-Wallis Test with Dunn's post-hoc for all panels of changes in LDL-C and for changes in HDL-C of overweight and dyslipidemic, ANOVA test for changes in HDL-C of obese subjects.

2.4. Inter-Group Comparisons on the Body Mass Index

BMI reduction (Δ change, kg·m^{-2}; [upper; lower quartile]; Figure 3) was only observed in overweight (−0.6 [−1.2; −0.60]; −0.4 [−0.7; −0.3]) and dyslipidemic (−0.7 [−1.3; −0.4]; −0.4 [−0.7; −0.3]) subjects enrolled in SE and Sm treatments. Such reductions in BMI directly correlated with TC ($r = 0.49$; $p < 0.01$), TG ($r = 0.22$; $p < 0.05$), and LDL-C ($r = 0.42$; $p < 0.01$).

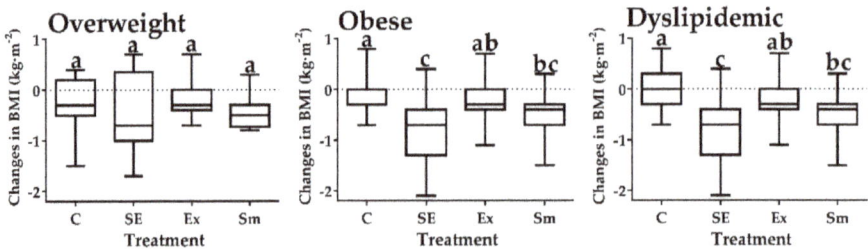

Figure 3. Changes (Δ) in body mass index by treatments. SE: Spirulina and exercise; Ex: Exercise and placebo; Sm: Spirulina without exercise; C: Control (Placebo without exercise); BMI: Body mass index. Data presented as box and whisker plots of the median (horizontal line), upper and lower quartiles (box) maximum and minimum (error bars). Different letters indicate statistical difference between treatments ($p < 0.05$), Kruskal-Wallis test with Dunn's post-hoc for changes in BMI of obese and dyslipidemic, ANOVA test for changes in BMI of overweight subjects.

3. Discussion

The excess of body weight is highly associated with dyslipidemias [15]; the world health care systems yearly boost new initiatives to prevent and treat these and other CVD risks [16]. This study provides unique evidence on the synergistic effects of *S. maxima* supplementation (4.5 g·day^{-1}) and a systematic exercise program on improving blood lipid levels in overweight, obese and dyslipidemic subjects by using a double-blind, randomized, crossover trial design. It is noteworthy that very few studies have been focused on *Spirulina* supplementation on dyslipidemia. However, even without being part of the hypothesis, the main finding of this study was the improvement on blood lipids concentration of dyslipidemic men by six weeks of treatment with *S. maxima* supplementation (4.5 g·day^{-1}) and/or systematic physical exercise practice.

There is no information in the literature about clinical trials using *Spirulina* together with aerobic exercise or high-intensity interval training. Only a few studies have focused on *Spirulina* supplementation effects against dyslipidemia and CVD risk factors. Mani et al. [17] studied the effect of *Spirulina* supplementation (2 g·day^{-1}) during two months on the serum lipid profile of 15 patients affected by type II diabetes mellitus (T2DM), resulting in a significant reduction of TG, TC, LDL-C, and free fatty acid in blood concentrations. By means of a better-structured trial, Lee et al. [18] studied the effect of *Spirulina* supplementation (8 g·day^{-1}) during 12 weeks in 37 patients with T2DM, reporting a significant reduction in TG levels after the intervention.

Many of the beneficial effects of *Spirulina* are attributed to its nutritional content, but its action mechanisms are poorly understood [19]. Our findings corroborate previous investigations in animal models. Some authors suggest that a possible component responsible of the *S. maxima* hypolipidemic effect is C-phycocyanin protein, which improves the blood lipid profile. Iwata et al. [20] studied the effect of a diet containing *Spirulina* compared to a high fructose diet in rats; they reported a decrease in TG concentration after the intervention, and attribute the possible action mechanism to the lipoprotein lipase activity in the lipoprotein metabolism. Other authors suggest that C-phycocyanin increases endogenous enzymes activity, scavenging free radicals [21], and downregulates cofactors in fat metabolism like adenine dinucleotide phosphate [22]. Nagaoka et al. [23] attribute *Spirulina* hypolipidemic effects to the fact that dietary supplementation with the cyanobacteria seems to have decreased the intestinal assimilation of cholesterol, probably because *Spirulina* compounds bind to bile acids in the jejunum, affecting the micellar solubility of cholesterol before suppressing the cholesterol absorption. These biological processes might explain the underlying mechanisms of *S. maxima* involved in the significant improvement on TC, TG, and lipoprotein-associated cholesterol found in this research, but appropriate clinical trials are needed to elucidate this.

Recent studies focus mainly on controlling serum LDL-C concentrations because this lipid is the primary carrier of cholesterol in the blood (60–80% of TC), and when this lipoprotein is decreased, blood TC is also decreased [24]. Although drugs exist against dyslipidemia, they are associated with adverse effects like mild serum creatine kinase level elevations and skeletal muscle complaints, including rhabdomyolysis and myopathy [25], reasons why different alternative treatments are investigated. The main treatment of dyslipidemia is an adequate dietary therapy, including nutraceuticals or functional foods [26], but it is essential to consider all possible factors that trigger this disease, like a sedentary lifestyle.

Actual research focused on physical activity has found that the benefits of aerobic exercise are due to changes in the physical structure of blood-carrier cholesterol proteins, resulting in an improvement of lipid levels [27]. Specifically, systematic exercise increases the activity of lipoprotein lipase that hydrolyzes blood TG, then it acts on lipoprotein particles through the capillaries, releasing free fatty acids that may be taken up by skeletal muscle [28]. Nikolaidis et al. [29] suggest that this degradation of endogenous lipids causes a shrinkage of lipoprotein particles, inducing the transference of lipids between very low-density lipoprotein and the HDL-C.

Tan et al. [30], in a randomized trial, studied the effect of 10 weeks of supervised aerobic exercise (five days per week, one hour per day) in 30 overweight women, resulting in a decrease in body weight, BMI, body fat, and an improvement in the blood lipid profile. Cugusi et al. [31], in an observational study, reported the effect of 12 weeks of an exercise program (50 min a day, 3 days a week) in 18 men affected by type II diabetes mellitus; they report a reduction of TC, TG, and LDL-C. These studies and others [32] support the conclusion that aerobic exercise reduces that blood lipid levels mostly when there exists a decrease in body weight. We previously reported [33] a positive effect of physical exercise and *S. maxima* supplementation on the reduction of body weight and body fat. Type II diabetes mellitus, sedentarism, dyslipidemia, and overweight are all related, a reason why a beneficial effect for any of them can be related to the other ones [34].

The greater synergistic effect of *S. maxima* and systematic physical exercise observed in the obesity group compared with the overweight one was not only due to their elevated BMI and to their dyslipidemia problem. The fact that the participants with obesity that achieved a reduction in BMI showed a difference only in SE compared with control group is not surprising, given that in obesity there exists a lower activity of oxidative enzymes, resulting in an elevated intramuscular lipid content, mostly TG [35]. For that reason, the capacity of obese subjects to use TG-derived fatty acids and circulating LDL-C as fuel during physical activity resulted in a higher lipid oxidation, which can be corroborated with the higher decrease of the blood lipid profile and the BMI in obesity [36].

The individual differences were wide-ranging due to different factors, like genetics [37] or gut microbiota [38]; consequently, it is essential to clarify that our treatment could not be sufficient for reducing cardiovascular risks, but trials of long duration or in different kind of populations can be conducted, measuring not only the blood lipids, but specific markers like creatine kinase, glucose or enzymatic activity to understand better the action mechanism of exercise and/or *S. maxima* intake.

The strong points of the present study were: no missing data, no participants dropped out during the trial, and the double-blind randomized protocol. The beneficial results suggest a synergistic effect of systematic physical exercise and *S. maxima*, resulting in an improvement of the blood lipid profile. Limitations of the study were that only sedentary overweight and obese men were selected, so the results may not be the same in other populations.

4. Materials and Methods

Spirulina maxima was obtained commercially from Alimentos Esenciales para la Humanidad S.A. de C.V. (Mexico City, México) in January 2017, and its chemical/functional characterization and biosafety were evaluated before being used in this clinical trial [33].

4.1. Ethics

The CONSORT checklist (Supplementary File S1) and flow diagram (Supplementary File S2) are available as Supplementary Materials. All participants were informed of the study purpose, physical, clinical and biochemical procedures. Their acceptance was formalized through informed consent, and their anonymity and confidentiality were strictly enforced. The clinical procedures were previously described at ClinicalTrials.gov with trial registration number NCT02837666 (Hypolipidemic and Antioxidant Capacity of *Spirulina* and Exercise Registered 19 July 2016 https://clinicaltrials.gov/ct2/show/NCT02837666?cond= Hypolipidemic+and+Antioxidant+Capacity+of+Spirulina+and+Exercise&rank=1). A detailed protocol for this trial has been published previously [39]. This clinical trial was carried out in accordance with the declaration of Helsinki and was approved by Universidad Autónoma de Ciudad Juárez (UACJ) Review Board: (Reference number: CBE.ICB/062.09-15).

4.2. Participants' Eligibility

Fifty-two sedentary male adults with a BMI over 25 $kg \cdot m^{-2}$ (27 overweight and 25 obese) volunteered to participate from May to September 2017. For the recruitment of participants, an intra-school campaign and personalized interviews were conducted to ensure eligibility. The exclusion criteria of subjects were these: drinking more than 100 mL of alcohol a week, taking drugs and/or diet supplements, presenting chronic disease, and having an impediment to practicing regular physical exercise. The elimination criteria were attendance by the subject of < 80% to the physical exercise sessions. No participants dropped out of the study.

4.3. Baseline Measurements

Initially, each participant visited the exercise physiology laboratory at UACJ with a fasting of 8–10 h before the baseline evaluations. BMI measurements were performed with subjects lightly dressed and barefoot, using an electronic balance (SECA 876, Hamburg, Germany) and the standing height was measured with a stadiometer (SECA 206, Hamburg, Germany). Participants' blood sample was taken by an expert clinician from the antecubital vein.

4.4. Study Design

The clinical trial consisted of *S. maxima* (4.5 g·day^{-1}) or placebo (4.5 g·day^{-1} of a low-calorie saccharine powder) supplementation (both supplements were encapsulated in dark capsules to present the same organoleptic characteristics) during 12 weeks in a randomized, double-blind, placebo-controlled, and counterbalanced crossover trial in a 2 × 2 factorial design.

To avoid study desertion, eligible participants (N = 52) decided whether or not to participate in the systematic physical exercise program (where they stayed during the two treatments of the clinical trial). Then, they were randomly allocated to one of two possible supplementation interventions (*S. maxima* or placebo) divided in four treatments, including physical exercise program with *S. maxima* (SE) supplementation, physical exercise with placebo (Ex) supplementation, *S. maxima* supplementation without physical exercise program (Sm), or placebo supplementation without physical exercise program (C). The crossover was conducted for the supplementation interventions and to assess compliance to the supplement intake. Participants returned each week to the laboratory to receive new capsules and all treatment intake data were recorded on weekly case report forms.

The initial allocation was performed in such way that each group had almost the same proportion of overweight: obese (1:1) individuals using a computer-generated random schedule, stratified by a permuted block design because stratification in small trials confers an adequate balance and slightly more statistical power and precision [40]. Participants' group allocations were performed by an independent researcher, who did not have any other participation during the study (double-blind). The sample size was determined by using the statistical program G*Power [41], selecting a sample of >52 subjects, with $\alpha = 0.05$ and power = 0.85.

The first period of treatment was carried out for six weeks, followed by a two-week wash-out period to avoid any possible delayed effect of *S. maxima* in the organism, and, finally, a further six weeks of treatment for the second intervention groups (Figure 4). Due to the lack of information in the literature, the durations for both the wash-out period (2 weeks) and treatment period (6 weeks) were considered long enough according to a systematic review of clinical trials that used *Spirulina* as treatment [42].

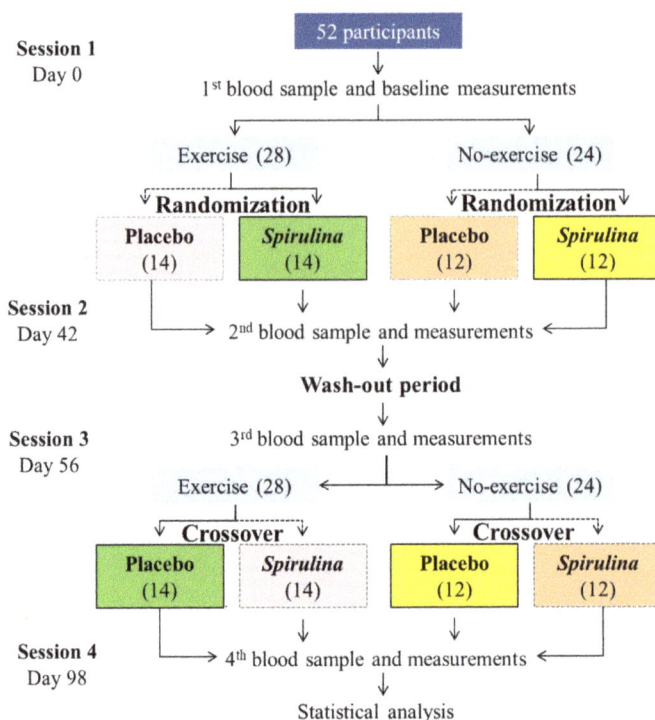

Figure 4. Experimental design for the independent and synergistic effect of *Spirulina maxima* and exercise. The same color means the same group of participants.

4.5. Blood Sample Collection and Biochemical Analysis

Four blood samples were collected during the clinical trial, first on day 0, second on the final of first treatment (day 42), third after the washout period (day 56), and fourth at the end of the second treatment (day 96). Blood samples (8 mL) were collected from the antecubital vein into ethylene diamine tetra acetic acid (EDTA) tubes after 8–10 h of fasting. Plasma from blood samples was obtained by refrigerated centrifugation (4 °C) at 3,000 g for 20 min. Plasma lipid profile (TC, HDL-C, and TG) concentrations were analyzed by using standard enzymatic procedures (Spinreact, Girona, Spain) with a microplate spectrophotometer (Epoch, Biotek, VT, USA) at 505 nm, and LDL-C was calculated with Friedewald's formula [43]. Abnormal cutoffs for TC, TG, LDL-C and HDL-C were >200, >150, >100, and <40 mg·dL^{-1}, respectively.

4.6. Dietary Analysis

All participants were subjected to a nutritional survey to define the daily calories required to establish dietary recommendations. Dietary intake was monitored by two trained nutritionists using three 24 h dietary recalls (semi-quantitative method), on days 0, 42, 56, and 98, and two food frequency questionnaires (qualitative method), on days 0 and 98, according to Nelson's guidelines [44], in order to ensure the independence of both dietary assessment tools. Dietary records were first inspected for missing data (e.g., missing food items or no complete responses) by a nutritionist and then analyzed for total calories, protein, carbohydrate, and fat intake (Diet Analysis Plus, ESHA Research, Salem, OR, USA). Lastly, compliance with the intake of supplements (*S. maxima* or placebo) and diet was monitored weekly by scheduled laboratory visits and carried out by trained nutritionists.

4.7. Systematic Physical Exercise Protocol

Exercise prescription was individual and accorded with the American College of Sports Medicine (ACSM) recommendations for people with overweight and obesity [45]. Participants in SE and Ex exercised for five days a week. The protocol began with a warm-up exercise (5–10 min), followed by muscular endurance exercise (20–30 min), then 20–30 min of cardiovascular exercise (walking, jogging, running, or cycling), and finally, five minutes of stretching. The intensity of cardiovascular exercise was administered as follows: For three of the five days, the intensity was between 50% and 80% of their heart rate reserve, and for the other two days, the intensity was between 80% and 90% of their heart rate reserve, using high-intensity interval training.

Muscular endurance exercise consisted of working all muscle groups (arms, legs, chest, back, and shoulders) once a week, using a medium-resistance repetition protocol divided in four different exercises for each specific muscle group, doing three sets of 12–16 repetitions [45]. The protocol for the high-intensity interval training consisted of 5 to 7 sets of 1 min of running at 80–90% heart rate reserve followed by 3 min of active resting at 50–70% of this heart rate. Heart rate was monitored since it is closely related to the percent of oxygen uptake reserve, making it easier to verify exercise intensity in the exercise prescription program [46]. Subjects performed the physical exercise program in the UACJ gym, always under the technical supervision of a personal trainer.

4.8. Main Physiological Outcomes

The primary outcome of the study was the response of treatments on the TC, TG, LDL-C, and HDL-C blood levels of dyslipidemic overweight and obese subjects, because high levels of blood lipids are of the major risk factors of CVD, and health organizations around the world recommend studies focused on improving these response variables [1].

We included as secondary endpoints the BMI and the blood lipid profile of all the participants of the study, since excess weight has been associated with CVD, regardless of whether dyslipidemia occurs [47].

4.9. Statistical Analysis

All analyses were conducted using the software SPSS 22.0 (SPSS Inc., Chicago, IL, USA) (Supplementary File S3). Data distribution normality was examined by the Shapiro–Wilk test, and the homoscedasticity by the Levene test, for each group. A p-value of less than 0.05 was considered statistically significant. In order to analyze statistical differences among treatments and time, univariate repeated measures ANOVA design with two within-subjects (initial and final values), and four inter-subjects (treatments) factors was used. In addition, initial and final values were compared using paired t-tests. When the variables had a normal distribution ($p > 0.05$) and variances between groups were the same, the Δ was analyzed by one-way ANOVA and Tukey Post-hoc test, but when the variables did not have a normal distribution ($p < 0.05$) and variances between groups were different, the Δ was analyzed by Kruskal-Wallis H and Dunn's Post-hoc test with Bonferroni adjustment for multiple comparisons. To evaluate the associations among variables, a Spearman correlation was performed. Data are presented as the mean ± standard deviation (SD) and, when specified, as the median with lower and upper quartiles.

5. Conclusions

According to the results, *Spirulina maxima* supplementation enhances the effect of a short-term systematic physical exercise program on BMI and blood lipid profile observed in overweight and obese men, but mostly in individuals with dyslipidemia.

Supplementary Materials: The following are available online at http://www.mdpi.com/1660-3397/17/5/270/s1, Supplementary File S1: CONSORT 2010 Checklist of information to include when reporting a randomized trial, Supplementary File S2: CONSORT 2010 Flow Diagram of the progress through the phases of the trial. Supplementary File S3: Statistical analysis.

Author Contributions: The first author, M.A.H.-L., was responsible for the recruitment of participants and led the development of this manuscript. A.R.-J. and M.A.J.-O. designed the study procedures and performed the statistical analyses of the data. R.P.H.-T. conducted the physical exercise program. O.I.L.-B. carried out the biochemical analyses. A.W.-M. and J.A.L.-D. designed the individual dietary recommendations for all the participants of the study. All authors made several critical revisions to the manuscript and approved the final version.

Funding: This research was funded by Programa para el Desarrollo Profesional Docente en Educación Superior (PRODEP).

Acknowledgments: Marco Antonio Hernández-Lepe was supported by a Ph.D. scholarship from the Consejo Nacional de Ciencia y Tecnología (CONACyT).

Conflicts of Interest: All authors have completed the ICMJE uniform disclosure form at http://www.icmje.org/conflicts-of-interest/ and are available on request from the corresponding author. All authors declare that they have no conflicts of interest related to this work.

References

1. Smith, S.C.; Collins, A.; Ferrari, R.; Holmes, D.R.; Logstrup, S.; Vaca, D.; Ralston, J.; Sacco, R.L.; Stam, H.; Taubert, K.; et al. Our time: A call to save preventable death from cardiovascular disease (heart disease and stroke). *J. Am. Coll. Cardiol.* **2012**, *60*, 2343–2348. [CrossRef]

2. D'Adamo, E.; Guardamagna, O.; Chiarelli, F.; Bartuli, A.; Liccardo, D.; Ferrari, F.; Nobili, V. Atherogenic dyslipidemia and cardiovascular risk factors in obese children. *Int. J. Endocrinol.* **2015**, *2015*. [CrossRef] [PubMed]

3. Wall-Medrano, A.; Ramos-Jiménez, A.; Hernández-Torres, R.P.; Villalobos-Molina, R.; Tapia-Pancardo, D.C.; Jiménez-Flores, J.R.; Méndez-Cruz, A.R.; Murguía-Romero, M.; Gallardo-Ortíz, I.A.; Urquídez-Romero, R. Cardiometabolic risk in young adults from northern Mexico: Revisiting body mass index and waist-circumference as predictors. *BMC Public Health* **2016**, *16*, 236. [CrossRef] [PubMed]

4. Ross, R.; Hudson, R.; Stotz, P.J.; Lam, M. Effects of exercise amount and intensity on abdominal obesity and glucose tolerance in obese adults: a randomized trial. *Ann. Intern. Med.* **2015**, *162*, 325–334. [CrossRef] [PubMed]

5. Greene, N.P.; Martin, S.E.; Crouse, S.F. Acute exercise and training alter blood lipid and lipoprotein profiles differently in overweight and obese men and women. *Obesity* **2012**, *20*, 1618–1627. [CrossRef] [PubMed]

6. Shaw, K.A.; Gennat, H.C.; O'Rourke, P.; Del Mar, C. Exercise for overweight or obesity. *Cochrane Db. Syst. Rev.* **2006**, *4*, CD003817. [CrossRef] [PubMed]

7. Shiraev, T.; Barclay, G. Evidence based exercise: Clinical benefits of high intensity interval training. *Aust. Fam. Physician* **2012**, *41*, 960.

8. Chen, G.; Wang, H.; Zhang, X.; Yang, S.-T. Nutraceuticals and functional foods in the management of hyperlipidemia. *Crit. Rev. Food Sci. Nutr.* **2014**, *54*, 1180–1201. [CrossRef]

9. Mimouni, V.; Ulmann, L.; Haimeur, A.; Guéno, F.; Meskini, N.; Tremblin, G. Marine microalgae used as food supplements and their implication in preventing cardiovascular diseases. *OCL* **2015**, *22*, D409. [CrossRef]

10. Tomé-Carneiro, J.; Visioli, F. Polyphenol-based nutraceuticals for the prevention and treatment of cardiovascular disease: Review of human evidence. *Phytomedicine* **2016**, *23*, 1145–1174. [CrossRef]

11. Memije-Lazaro, I.N.; Blas-Valdivia, V.; Franco-Colín, M.; Cano-Europa, E. Arthrospira maxima (Spirulina) and C-phycocyanin prevent the progression of chronic kidney disease and its cardiovascular complications. *J. Funct. Food* **2018**, *43*, 37–43. [CrossRef]

12. Moura, L.P.; Puga, G.M.; Beck, W.R.; Teixeira, I.P.; Ghezzi, A.C.; Silva, G.A.; Mello, M.A.R. Exercise and spirulina control non-alcoholic hepatic steatosis and lipid profile in diabetic Wistar rats. *Lipids Health Dis.* **2011**, *10*, 77. [CrossRef]

13. Mazzola, D.; Fornari, F.; Vigano, G.; Oro, T.; Costa, J.A.V.; Bertolin, T.E. Spirulina platensis Enhances the beneficial effect of exercise on oxidative stress and the lipid profile in rats. *Braz. Arch. Biol. Techn.* **2015**, *58*, 961–969. [CrossRef]

14. Kata, F.S.; Athbi, A.M.; Manwar, E.Q.; Al-Ashoor, A.; Abdel-Daim, M.M.; Aleya, L. Therapeutic effect of the alkaloid extract of the cyanobacterium Spirulina platensis on the lipid profile of hypercholesterolemic male rabbits. *Environ. Sci. Pollut. Res. Int.* **2018**, *25*, 19635–19642. [CrossRef]

15. Must, A.; Spadano, J.; Coakley, E.H.; Field, A.E.; Colditz, G.; Dietz, W.H. The disease burden associated with overweight and obesity. *JAMA* **1999**, *282*, 1523–1529. [CrossRef] [PubMed]

16. Wilborn, C.; Beckham, J.; Campbell, B.; Harvey, T.; Galbreat, M.; La Bounty, P.; Nassar, E.; Wismann, J.; Kreider, R. Obesity: prevalence, theories, medical consequences, management, and research directions. *J. Int. Soc. Sport. Nutr.* **2005**, *2*, 4. [CrossRef] [PubMed]

17. Mani, U.V.; Desai, S.; Iyer, U. Studies on the long-term effect of spirulina supplementation on serum lipid profile and glycated proteins in NIDDM patients. *J. Nutraceuticals Funct. Med. Food* **2000**, *2*, 25–32. [CrossRef]

18. Lee, E.H.; Park, J.E.; Choi, Y.J.; Huh, K.B.; Kim, W.Y. A randomized study to establish the effects of spirulina in type 2 diabetes mellitus patients. *Nutr. Res. Pract.* **2008**, *2*, 295–300. [CrossRef] [PubMed]

19. Kalafati, M.; Jamurtas, A.Z.; Nikolaidis, M.G.; Paschalis, V.; Theodorou, A.A.; Sakellariou, G.K.; Koutedakis, Y.; Kouretas, D. Ergogenic and antioxidant effects of spirulina supplementation in humans. *Med. Sci. Sports Exerc.* **2010**, *42*, 142–151. [CrossRef]

20. Iwata, K.; Inayama, T.; Kato, T. Effects of Spirulina platensis on plasma lipoprotein lipase activity in fructose-induced hyperlipidemic rats. *J. Nutr. Sci. Vitaminol.* **1990**, *36*, 165–171. [CrossRef] [PubMed]

21. Upasani, C.D.; Balaraman, R. Protective effect of Spirulina on lead induced deleterious changes in the lipid peroxidation and endogenous antioxidants in rats. *Phytother. Res.* **2003**, *17*, 330–334. [CrossRef]

22. Sharma, N.K.; Tiwari, S.P.; Tripathi, K.; Rai, A.K. Sustainability and cyanobacteria (blue-green algae): facts and challenges. *Appl. Phycol.* **2011**, *23*, 1059–1081. [CrossRef]

23. Nagaoka, S.; Shimizu, K.; Kaneko, H.; Shibayama, F.; Morikawa, K.; Kanamaru, Y.; Otsuka, A.; Hirahashi, T.; Kato, T. A novel protein C-phycocyanin plays a crucial role in the hypocholesterolemic action of Spirulina platensis concentrate in rats. *J. Nutr.* **2005**, *135*, 2425–2430. [CrossRef]

24. Chen, Z.Y.; Jiao, R.; Ma, K.Y. Cholesterol-lowering nutraceuticals and functional foods. *J. Agric. Food Chem.* **2008**, *56*, 8761–8773. [CrossRef]

25. Thompson, P.D.; Clarkson, P.; Karas, R.H. Statin-associated myopathy. *JAMA* **2003**, *289*, 1681–1690. [CrossRef]

26. Gao, L.; Lin, Z.; Liu, Y.; Wang, X.; Wan, L.; Zhang, L.; Liu, X. Hypolipidemic effect of Fragarianilgerrensis Schlecht. medicine compound on hyperlipidemic rats. *Lipids Health Dis.* **2018**, *17*, 222. [CrossRef]

27. Kraus, W.E.; Houmard, J.A.; Duscha, B.D.; Knetzger, K.J.; Wharton, M.B.; McCartney, J.S.; Bales, C.W.; Henes, S.; Samsa, G.P.; Otvos, J.D.; et al. Effects of the amount and intensity of exercise on plasma lipoproteins. *N. Engl. J. Med.* **2002**, *347*, 1483–1492. [CrossRef]

28. Oscai, L.B.; Essig, D.A.; Palmer, W.K. Lipase regulation of muscle triglyceride hydrolysis. *J. Appl. Physiol.* **1990**, *69*, 1571–1577. [CrossRef]

29. Nikolaidis, M.G.; Paschalis, V.; Giakas, G.; Fatouros, I.G.; Sakellariou, G.K.; Theodorou, A.A.; Koutedakis, Y.; Jamurtas, A.Z. Favorable and prolonged changes in blood lipid profile after muscle-damaging exercise. *Med. Sci. Sports Exerc.* **2008**, *40*, 1483–1489. [CrossRef]

30. Tan, S.; Wang, J.; Cao, L.; Guo, Z.; Wang, Y. Positive effect of exercise training at maximal fat oxidation intensity on body composition and lipid metabolism in overweight middle-aged women. *Clin. Physiol. Funct. Imaging* **2016**, *36*, 225–230. [CrossRef]

31. Cugusi, L.; Cadeddu, C.; Nocco, S.; Orrù, F.; Bandino, S.; Deidda, M.; Caria, A.; Bassareo, P.P.; Piras, A.; Cabras, S.; et al. Effects of an aquatic-based exercise program to improve cardiometabolic profile, quality of life, and physical activity levels in men with type 2 diabetes mellitus. *PM R* **2015**, *7*, 141–148. [CrossRef]

32. Kelley, G.A.; Kelley, K.S.; Tran, Z.V. Aerobic exercise, lipids and lipoproteins in overweight and obese adults: a meta-analysis of randomized controlled trials. *Int. J. Obes.* **2005**, *29*, 881. [CrossRef]

33. Hernández-Lepe, M.; López-Díaz, J.; Juárez-Oropeza, M.; Hernández-Torres, R.P.; Wall-Medrano, A.; Ramos-Jiménez, A. Effect of Arthrospira (Spirulina) maxima Supplementation and a Systematic Physical Exercise Program on the Body Composition and Cardiorespiratory Fitness of Overweight or Obese Subjects: A Double-Blind, Randomized, and Crossover Controlled Trial. *Mar. Drugs* **2018**, *16*, 364. [CrossRef]

34. Nguyen, N.T.; Magno, C.P.; Lane, K.T.; Hinojosa, M.W.; Lane, J.S. Association of hypertension, diabetes, dyslipidemia, and metabolic syndrome with obesity: Findings from the national health and nutrition examination survey, 1999 to 2004. *J. Am. Coll. Surg.* **2008**, *207*, 928–934. [CrossRef]

35. He, J.; Watkins, S.; Kelley, D.E. Skeletal muscle lipid content and oxidative enzyme activity in relation to muscle fiber type in type 2 diabetes and obesity. *Diabetes* **2001**, *50*, 817–823. [CrossRef]

36. Goodpaster, B.H.; Wolfe, R.R.; Kelley, D.E. Effects of obesity on substrate utilization during exercise. *Obes. Res.* **2002**, *10*, 575–584. [CrossRef]

37. Das, U.N.; Rao, A.A. Gene expression profile in obesity and type 2 diabetes mellitus. *Lipids Health Dis.* **2007**, *6*, 35. [CrossRef]

38. Baothman, O.A.; Zamzami, M.A.; Taher, I.; Abubaker, J.; Abu-Farha, M. The role of gut microbiota in the development of obesity and diabetes. *Lipids Health Dis.* **2016**, *15*, 108. [CrossRef]

39. Hernández-Lepe, M.A.; López-Díaz, J.A.; de la Rosa, L.A.; Hernández-Torres, R.P.; Wall-Medrano, A.; Juarez-Oropeza, M.A.; Pedraza-Chaverri, J.; Urquidez-Romero, R.; Ramos-Jiménez, A. Double-blind randomised controlled trial of the independent and synergistic effect of Spirulina maxima with exercise (ISESE) on general fitness, lipid profile and redox status in overweight and obese subjects: Study protocol. *BMJ Open* **2017**, *7*, 013744. [CrossRef]

40. Schulz, K.F.; Grimes, D.A. Generation of allocation sequences in randomised trials: Chance, not choice. *Lancet* **2002**, *359*, 515–519. [CrossRef]

41. Faul, F.; Erdfelder, E.; Lang, A.G.; Buchner, A. G* Power 3: A flexible statistical power analysis program for the social, behavioral, and biomedical sciences. *Behav. Res. Methods.* **2007**, *39*, 175–191. [CrossRef]

42. Hernández-Lepe, M.A.; Wall-Medrano, A.; Juárez-Oropeza, M.A.; Ramos-Jiménez, A.; Hernández-Torres, R.P. Spirulina y su efecto hipolipemiante y antioxidante en humanos: una revisión sistemática. *Nutr. Hosp.* **2015**, *32*, 494–500. [CrossRef]

43. Friedewald, W.T.; Levy, R.I.; Fredrickson, D.S. Estimation of the concentration of low-density lipoprotein cholesterol in plasma, without use of the preparative ultracentrifuge. *Clin. Chem.* **1972**, *18*, 499–502.

44. Nelson, M. The validation of dietary assessment. In *Design Concepts in Nutritional Epidemiology*, 2nd ed.; Margetts, B.M., Nelson, M., Eds.; Oxford University Press: Oxford, UK, 1997; pp. 266–295.

45. American College of Sports Medicine. *ACSM's Guidelines for Exercise Testing and Prescription*, 10th ed.; Lippincott Williams & Wilkins: Philadelphia, PA, USA, 2016; pp. 111–142.

46. Swain, D.P.; Leutholtz, B.C. Heart rate reserve is equivalent to% VO2 reserve, not to% VO2max. *Med. Sci. Sports Exerc.* **1997**, *29*, 410–414. [CrossRef]

47. Meydani, M.; Hasan, S.T. Dietary polyphenols and obesity. *Nutrients* **2010**, *2*, 737–751. [CrossRef]

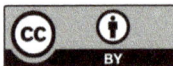

marine drugs

MDPI

Article

Identification of Cyanobacterial Strains with Potential for the Treatment of Obesity-Related Co-Morbidities by Bioactivity, Toxicity Evaluation and Metabolite Profiling

Margarida Costa [1], Filipa Rosa [2], Tiago Ribeiro [2], Rene Hernandez-Bautista [3], Marco Bonaldo [4], Natália Gonçalves Silva [2], Finnur Eiríksson [5], Margrét Thorsteinsdóttir [1], Siegfried Ussar [3] and Ralph Urbatzka [2,*]

[1] Faculty of Pharmaceutical Sciences, University of Iceland, Hofsvallagata 53, 107 Reykjavik, Iceland; costa.anamarg@gmail.com (M.C.); margreth@hi.is (M.T.)
[2] Interdisciplinary Centre of Marine and Environmental Research (CIIMAR/CIMAR), University of Porto, Avenida General Norton de Matos, s/n, 4450-208 Matosinhos, Portugal; frosa@ciimar.up.pt (F.R.); tribeiro@ciimar.up.pt (T.R.); nsilva@ciimar.up.pt (N.G.S.)
[3] RG Adipocyte and Metabolism, Institute for Diabetes and Obesity, Helmholtz Center Munich, 85764 Neuherberg, Germany; rene.hernandez@helmholtz-muenchen.de (R.H.-B.); siegfried.ussar@helmholtz-muenchen.de (S.U.)
[4] INBB, Consorzio Interuniversitario Biosistemi e Biostrutture, 00136 Rome, Italy; marcobonaldo90@libero.it
[5] ArcticMass, Sturlugata 8, 101 Reykjavik, Iceland; finnur@arcticmass.is
* Correspondence: rurbatzka@ciimar.up.pt; Tel.: +351-223-401-818

Received: 13 April 2019; Accepted: 7 May 2019; Published: 10 May 2019

Abstract: Obesity is a complex disease resulting in several metabolic co-morbidities and is increasing at epidemic rates. The marine environment is an interesting resource of novel compounds and in particular cyanobacteria are well known for their capacity to produce novel secondary metabolites. In this work, we explored the potential of cyanobacteria for the production of compounds with relevant activities towards metabolic diseases using a blend of target-based, phenotypic and zebrafish assays as whole small animal models. A total of 46 cyanobacterial strains were grown and biomass fractionated, yielding in total 263 fractions. Bioactivities related to metabolic function were tested in different *in vitro* and *in vivo* models. Studying adipogenic and thermogenic gene expression in brown adipocytes, lipid metabolism and glucose uptake in hepatocytes, as well as lipid metabolism in zebrafish larvae, we identified 66 (25%) active fractions. This together with metabolite profiling and the evaluation of toxicity allowed the identification of 18 (7%) fractions with promising bioactivity towards different aspects of metabolic disease. Among those, we identified several known compounds, such as eryloside T, leptosin F, pheophorbide A, phaeophytin A, chlorophyll A, present as minor peaks. Those compounds were previously not described to have bioactivities in metabolic regulation, and both known or unknown compounds could be responsible for such effects. In summary, we find that cyanobacteria hold a huge repertoire of molecules with specific bioactivities towards metabolic diseases, which needs to be explored in the future.

Keywords: anti-obesity drugs; metabolite profiling; zebrafish Nile red fat metabolism assay; uncoupling protein 1; bioactivity screening; diabetes; fatty liver disease; cyanobacteria

1. Introduction

The worldwide prevalence of obesity as a modern and imminent health hazard is clear and very well documented [1]. If the current growth rates are maintained, 38% of the global adult population will be overweight and 28% obese by 2030 [2]. Obesity is defined by a body mass index (BMI) greater than 30, and associated with complex co-morbidities such as type 2 diabetes, cardiovascular disease and several types of cancer [3–6]. Exercise and healthy nutrition show only limited effects on weight loss and patients tend to get back to or exceed the original weight after only a few years. Furthermore, many anti-obesity drugs have adverse side-effects. One example is Sibutramine, which was withdrawn in 2010 due to cardiovascular events and strokes [7]. In contrast, bariatric surgery is by far the most effective treatment for obesity, however it has significant risk for complications and only a fraction of obese patients is eligible for these operations.

Therefore, new sources of anti-obesity drugs and therapies are urgently needed. A current strategy seems to return to basic natural product drug discovery [8]. Natural products are mostly secondary metabolites from macro- and microorganisms that evolved through time to target specific molecules. The potential of most natural products is still underexplored, in particular in marine environments, and may represent a promising source of new anti-obesity agents, as already reported in a few studies using marine cyanobacteria or marine sponge-associated fungi [9,10].

Cyanobacteria are a group of gram-negative prokaryotes widespread in the planet with numerous biosynthetic routes that lead to structural diverse and biologically active secondary metabolites [11]. The Interdisciplinary Centre of Marine and Environmental Research (CIIMAR) hosts a cyanobacterial culture collection (LEGE-cc) with approx. 400 strains mainly collected in freshwater, estuarine and marine environments [12]. A small part of this chemical diversity was already explored for the identification of anti-cancer activities [13]; however, the anti-obesity potential has not been analyzed before.

The aim of this work was to identify cyanobacterial strains with the potential to produce promising secondary metabolites that have strong bioactivities towards obesity or obesity-related co-morbidities. The screening focused on obesity and obesity-related bioactivities using cellular models *in vitro* and physiologically relevant whole small animal models *in vivo*. Effects on lipid homeostasis were analyzed in zebrafish, while effects on glucose and lipid metabolism were studied in human HepG2 cells and complemented by analysis of compound activity towards adipocyte differentiation and thermogenic gene expression in murine brown adipocytes. Metabolite profiling and toxicity studies further narrowed the selection to the most promising 18 (7%) fractions. Produced metabolites were categorized into known or unknown compounds by data base searches.

2. Results

2.1. Lipid Reducing Activity in Zebrafish Larvae

The library of cyanobacterial fractions was screened for lipid reducing activity using the zebrafish Nile red fat metabolism assay. From the 263 analyzed fractions, 17 (6.5%) reduced the mean fluorescence intensity (MFI) >50%, while 29 (11%) diminished the MFI >30% (Figure 1A,B). The most promising fractions belong to 15 different cyanobacterial strains (12, 23, 130, 131, 141, 144, 161, 180, 187, 193, 196, 226, 232, 250, 256, 259, 262), with the majority from marine ecosystems (73%).

2.2. Anti-Steatosis Activity in HepG2 Cells

HepG2 cells were fed with 62 μM sodium oleate in order to induce the formation of lipid droplets. Fat overloading works similarly in primary hepatocytes and HepG2 cells and is an established *in vitro* model for hepatic steatosis [14]. Reduction of lipids was quantified after 6 h exposure to oleate and individual cyanobacterial fractions. Oleate exposure increased HepG2 lipid content compared to cells cultured in regular cell culture medium (Figure 1C,D). Among the 263 analyzed fractions, 50 (19%) reduced lipid content (mean fluorescence intensity of Nile red; MFI >30%), and 32 (12.2%) reduced the MFI >50%. Taking into account the toxicity of some fractions, as detailed below, the most promising fractions (58, 77, 89, 90, 101, 102, 107, 108, 109, 177, 178, 192, 199, 202, 220, 231, 232) were derived from 11 cyanobacterial strains and 54.4% belong to marine ecosystems.

2.3. Effects on Brown Adipocyte Differentiation and Thermogenic Gene Expression

Uncoupling protein-1 (UCP-1) is a brown adipocyte specific gene, which uncouples the mitochondrial respiratory chain to produce heat instead of ATP. Thus, expression of UCP-1 is an indicator for the thermogenic capacity of brown adipocytes and for distinguishing energy storing white from energy dissipating brown adipocytes. However, gene expression analysis is just an indicator of the functional protein, and hence, future confirmation is necessary. Assessment of UCP-1 gene expression upon treatment with 10 µg mL^{-1} of each individual cyanobacterial fraction during differentiation revealed significantly increased expression after exposure to fractions 168, 228, 229 and 232 (Figure 2A). The cyanobacterial fractions were tested on their effect on brown adipocyte differentiation, as monitored by expression of the key adipogenic transcription factor PPARγ. As shown in Figure 2B, the fractions 139, 141, 142, 155 and 232 significantly increased PPARγ expression, when cells were treated with the individual fractions during the eight-day time course of differentiation.

Correlation analysis of UCP-1/PPARγ expression revealed that 168, 232, 228 and 229 increased both UCP-1 and PPARγ expression. The fractions 139, 142, 143 and 155 resulted in overexpression of PPARγ, but low levels UCP-1 expression. The fractions 18, 37, 80 and 46 reduced both UCP-1 and PPARγ expression. However, reduction on both markers could also indicate toxicity and loss of cells (Figure 2C).

Bright-field images of fully differentiated brown adipocytes at day 8 of differentiation that were treated with cyanobacterial fractions during differentiation are shown in Supplementary Figure S13. Differences in brown adipocyte morphology were observed upon treatment with the fractions. We noticed that the adipocytes treated with fractions that showed an increased expression of UCP1 and PPARγ (fractions 228, 168, 229 and 232) appeared elongated compared to the adipocytes treated with fractions that reduced marker gene expression (fractions 18, 37, 46 and 80). None of the tested fractions induced obvious signs of toxicity resulting in cell loss.

2.4. Glucose Uptake in HepG2 Cells

The library of cyanobacterial fractions was screened for activity on glucose uptake using 2-(*N*-(7-Nitrobenz-2-oxa-1,3-diazol-4-yl)Amino)-2-Deoxyglucose (2-NBDG) in HepG2 cells. From the 263 analyzed fractions, five (1.9%) increased glucose uptake (MFI) >30%, while only one (0.4%) increased glucose uptake >50% (Figure 2D). Most promising fractions, characterized by consistent fluorescence values between replicates and no cytotoxicity, belong to four cyanobacterial strains, two from marine ecosystems (25 and 130) and two from freshwater ecosystems (48 and 77).

2.5. Toxicity Evaluation

Cytotoxicity was accessed in HepG2 cells following the glucose uptake assay using an MTT assay. Seven fractions revealed cytotoxicity higher than 30% (6, 7, 15, 32, 34, 119 and 149) and only one fraction revealed cytotoxicity greater than 50% (229). The remaining fractions did not show any cytotoxicity (Figure 2E). To determine the effect of cyanobacterial fractions on the viability of HepG2 cells, the sulforhodamine B (SrB) assay was performed following the anti-steatosis assay. The viability was reduced more than 30% by 50 of the fractions (19%) (3, 5, 12, 14, 17, 21, 22, 23, 24, 50, 52, 59, 69, 66, 67, 68, 69, 76, 79, 88, 99, 110, 116, 119, 121, 129, 135, 143, 145, 150, 160, 184, 187, 189, 190, 193, 196, 210, 214, 216, 217, 219, 222, 225, 226, 235, 246, 250, 259, 262), while 11 fractions (3.8%) (4, 57, 122, 130, 141, 142, 144, 154, 223, 229, 253) reduced the viability more than 50% (Figure 2F). General toxicity was evaluated in zebrafish larvae during the assessment of lipid homeostasis. Only one fraction (14) led to the death of all zebrafish larvae within 48 h of exposure, while the remaining fractions did not show any toxicity or malformations on the zebrafish larvae at the screening concentration of 10 µg mL^{-1}.

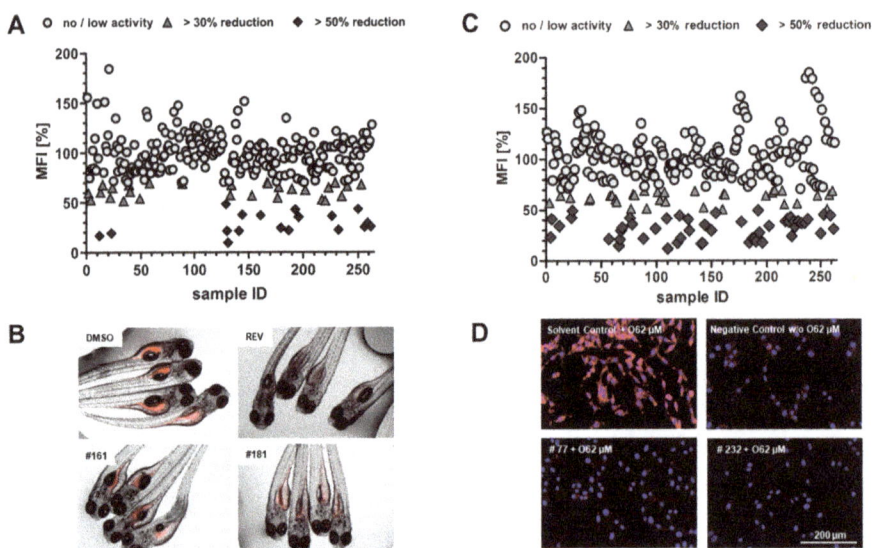

Figure 1. Bioactivity screening using the zebrafish Nile red fat metabolism assay and the anti-steatosis assay in HepG2 cells. (**A**) Data are presented as mean fluorescence intensity (MFI) relative to the solvent control. Zebrafish at 3 days post fertilization (DPF) were exposed for 48 h to 10 µg mL^{-1} cyanobacterial fractions and lipids around the yolk sac and intestine were stained with Nile red. (**B**) Representative images of zebrafish larvae (overlay of brightfield picture and red fluorescence channel). Solvent control, 0.1% dimethyl sulfoxide (DMSO); positive control, 50 µM REV and exposure to fraction #161 and #180. (**C**) Data are presented as MFI relative to solvent control (0.5% DMSO + O62 µM). HepG2 cells were exposed for 6 h to 62 µM sodium oleate (O62 µM) and 10 µg mL^{-1} cyanobacterial fractions. Nile red fluorescence stains neutral lipid reservoirs (red) and Hoechst 33342 the nucleus (blue). (**D**) Representative images of HepG2 cells (overlay of red and blue fluorescence channel). 0.5% DMSO + O62 µM; negative control, 0.5% DMSO; exposure to fraction #77 and #232.

2.6. Metabolite Profiling

The untargeted metabolite profiling of cyanobacterial strains was performed with an UPLC-QTOF MS platform. The different fraction types of cyanobacterial strains (e.g., fractions D) were individually analyzed. A principal component analysis (PCA) was used as the first step to identify metabolites from cyanobacterial fractions that substantially differ from the majority of the other metabolite profiles within the same fraction type. From 263 cyanobacteria fractions, 12 individual PCA's were studied (one for each fraction type), as shown in Table 1. This analysis provided a number of markers ranging from 482 for fractions A to 1228 for fractions G, highlighting the chemical diversity of the fractions. Each of the markers was a single mass peak, characterized by its specific retention time and accurate mass. The first principal component (PC1) accounted from 11% to 27% of the total variance and the second from 9% to 15% for all analyzed fractions. Fraction I had a higher variability, while fractions E and H had the lowest variability. In the PCA's, we searched for fractions that cluster differently compared to the majority of fractions of the same type, which should represent those fractions with the potential to produce different secondary metabolites. A summary of those fractions is given in Table 1, while all the corresponding PCA plots are shown in Supplementary Figures S1–S12.

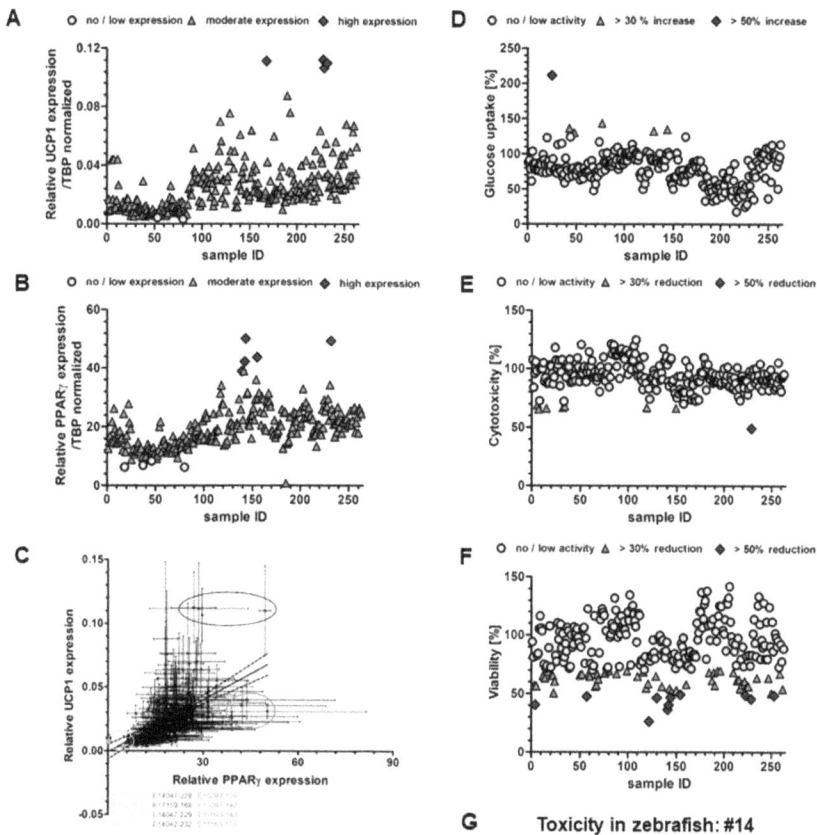

Figure 2. Analysis of mRNA expression of genes involved in (**A**) thermogenesis (uncoupling protein-1 (UCP-1)) and (**B**) adipocyte differentiation (PPARγ) by qPCR in brown adipocytes (*n* = 3). (**C**) Correlation between PPARγ and UCP-1 mRNA expression identifies three different groups (low UCP-1/low PPARγ; low UCP-1/high PPARγ; high UCP-1/high PPARγ). Values are shown as mean ± SEM. (**D**) Glucose uptake assay using 2-(*N*-(7-Nitrobenz-2-oxa-1,3-diazol-4-yl)Amino)-2-Deoxyglucose (2-NBDG) in HepG2 cells. Cells were exposed for 2 h to 10 µg mL^{-1} cyanobacterial fractions. An increase in fluorescence signal indicates higher uptake of the glucose analog 2-NBDG. Data are shown as mean fluorescence increase relative to the solvent control, 0.5% DMSO. (**E**) Cytotoxicity analysis by MTT from HepG2 cells following the glucose uptake assay. Data are presented relative to the solvent control, 0.5% DMSO. (**F**) Cytotoxicity of cyanobacterial fractions on HepG2 cells following the anti-steatosis screening assay. Data are presented in percentage relative to the solvent control (0.5% DMSO) + O62 µM. (**G**) The fraction 14 was the only to induce general toxicity in the zebrafish assay at 10 µg mL^{-1} (100% of mortality after 24/48 h of exposure).

As next step, we matched the obtained information regarding the (i) potential to produce different metabolites with (ii) bioactivity, and (iii) toxicity, in order to narrow the selection of promising fractions. Two examples are shown in Figure 3. The principal component analysis of the metabolite profiling of E fractions from all strains (Figure 3A) showed a central cluster with a relatively uniform distribution. The E fractions of LEGE03283 (#110), LEGE07175 (#130), LEGE07075 (#142) and LEGE06104 (#58) had a different distribution on the plot, but only the LEGE06104 fraction E (#58) showed anti-steatosis activity and no cytotoxicity, while the others did not have any anti-steatosis activity. The analysis of its chromatogram allowed the identification of several possible known compounds, but also contained a few peaks of possible unknown compounds with anti-steatosis activities (Supplementary Table S5). Figure 3B shows the principal component analysis of G fractions. The G fractions of the majority of the strains appeared together in one big cluster, except for LEGE07211 (#69), LEGE06174 (#122) and LEGE00246 (#180). From those three fractions, only fraction G of the LEGE00246 strain (#180) had strong bioactivity in the zebrafish fat metabolism assay and no toxicity. The analysis of the chromatogram revealed a potential for the isolation of new compounds. (Supplementary Table S3). From the total of 263 cyanobacterial fractions, a total of 66 (25% of 263 fractions) were identified with relevant bioactivities. The metabolite profiling and toxicity evaluation allowed the selection of the most promising 18 fractions (7%), which are summarized in Table 2.

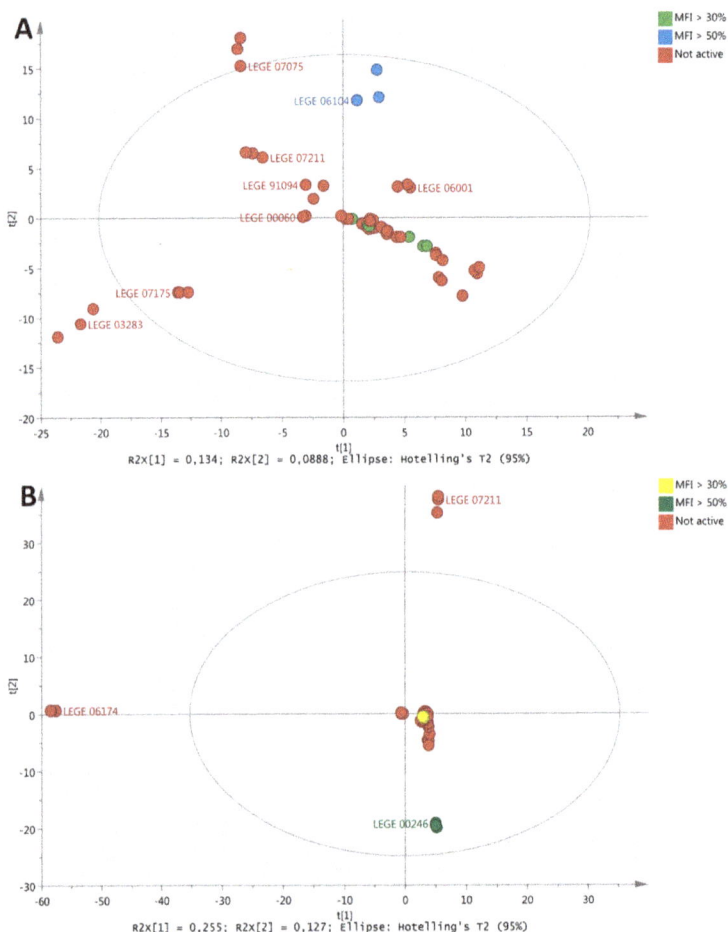

Figure 3. Matching of metabolite profiling with bioactivities for the selection of most promising cyanobacterial fractions. (**A**) PCA scores plot of E fractions colored according to anti-steatosis bioassay in HepG2 cells. Bioactivity is indicated as percentage MFI, mean fluorescence intensity. Strain names are indicated on the plot (e.g., LEGE07211). (**B**) PCA scores plot of G fractions colored according to activity in the zebrafish Nile red fat metabolism assay. The analysis was based on 1002 and 1228 collected markers on fraction E and G, respectively. The fractions were prepared in triplicate, and each replicate was run in triplicate.

Table 1. Summary of principal component analysis (PCA) of the metabolite profiling of cyanobacterial fractions. Each marker was a single mass peak characterized by its specific retention time and accurate mass. Fractions that cluster differently were identified as those with the potential to produce different secondary metabolites, in comparison to fractions that clustered together, which were regarded to produce similar metabolites. IPE, increased polarity extraction; VLC, vacuum liquid chromatography; PC, principal component.

Fraction/Extract	Markers	Variance PC1 (%)	Variance PC2 (%)	Fractions with Potential to Produce Different Metabolites
A (IPE)	485	18	14	201, 216, 225, 228, 234, 240, 243, 249, 255, 258
B (IPE)	1131	19	9	199, 202, 205, 214, 217, 220, 226, 229, 235, 244, 253, 256
C (IPE)	1028	13	13	197, 221, 224, 248, 251, 254, 260
A (VLC)	815	15	11	1, 54, 75, 106
B (VLC)	628	19	11	20, 29, 46, 64, 139
C (VLC)	816	15	14	3, 12, 21, 77, 108
D (VLC)	943	16	10	19, 66, 88, 141
E (VLC)	1002	13	9	23, 40, 58, 67, 110, 130, 142, 160
F (VLC)	914	26	11	80, 121
G (VLC)	1228	26	13	69, 122, 180
H (VLC)	1178	11	10	92, 103, 123, 134, 154, 181
I (VLC)	1105	27	15	83, 164

Table 2. Summary of most promising fractions with relevant bioactivities towards obesity, steatosis, diabetes or thermal energy release.

Bioactivity	Selected Fraction
Zebrafish—Lipid reducing	LEGE07175 H/#134
	LEGE00246 G/#180
	LEGE07172 A/#240
	LEGE07172 C/#242
	LEGE07173 B/#256
HepG2—Anti-steatosis	LEGE07084 D/#48
	LEGE03283 C/#108
	LEGE03283 D/#109
	LEGE07167 B/#199
	LEGE07160 B/#202
	LEGE06134 B/#220
HepG2—Glucose uptake	LEGE06001 G/#25
	LEGE06104 E/#58
	LEGE07212 C/#77
	LEGE07175 E/#130
Brown adipocytes—PPARγ and UCP-1 inducing activities	LEGE00247 D/#168
	LEGE06137 A/#228
	LEGE06097 B/#232

The identification of known and unknown compounds for one fraction of each bioactivity is represented in Figure 4, and the remaining chemical characterizations of promising fractions are shown in the Supplementary Tables S3–S6. By database searches in MarinLit [15], ChemSpider [16] and SciFinder [17], several known and unknown metabolites were identified, and the exact masses of the mass peaks compared to those available in the databases. For example, in Figure 4A, the search in databases resulted in the identification of eryloside T and a xanthin compound amongst several unidentified mass peaks in the fraction LEGE07173B with lipid reducing activity in zebrafish. In Figure 4B, the characterization of mass peaks identified leptosin F and a phaeophytin analogue in the fraction LEGE07167B with anti-steatosis activity.

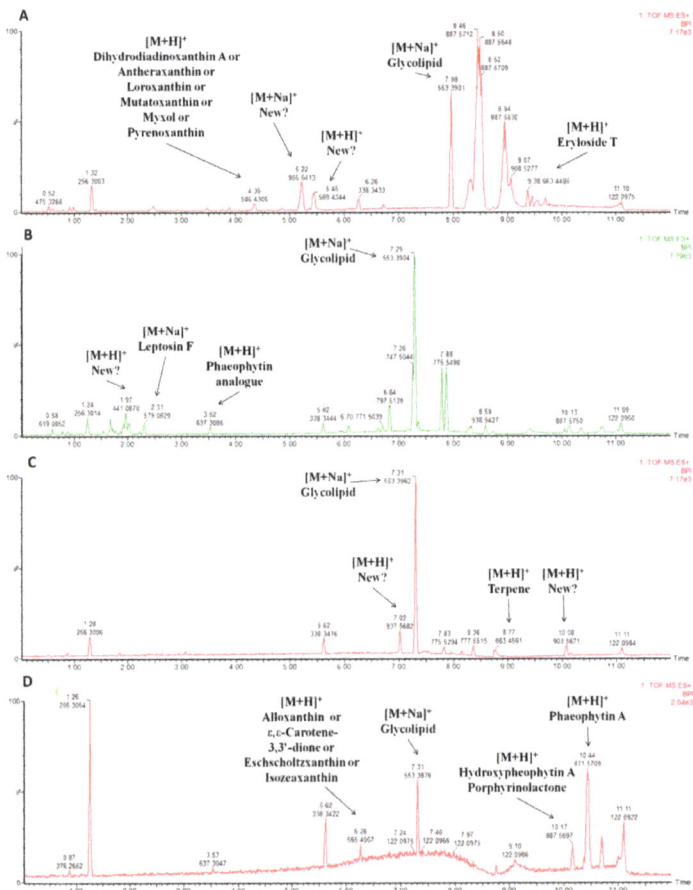

Figure 4. Base peak intensity chromatograms of selected cyanobacterial fractions with a respective identification of the compounds by database searches in MarinLit, ChemSpider and SciFinder. (**A**) Fraction LEGE 07173B (#256) selected based on zebrafish Nile red fat metabolism assay. (**B**) Fraction LEGE 07167B (#199), selected based on anti-steatosis bioassay. (**C**) Fraction LEGE 07172C (#77) selected based on glucose uptake bioassay. (**D**) Fraction LEGE 00247D (#168) selected based on PPARγ/UCP-1 expression levels. More information can be found in Supplementary Tables S3–S6.

3. Discussion

The use of natural products as anti-obesity agents had been discussed in the literature [18,19], however, research in this field is still underexplored. While the striking potential of marine resources as producer of unique chemical structures is largely recognized, the exploration is often limited by the fact that the majority of species are not cultivable, by the lack of sustainable use of resources or by difficulties in chemical synthesis [20]. Phenotypic screening approaches regained the attention of many research groups and pharmaceutical companies [21]. These cell-based systems are efficient in detecting bioactivity of a compound but still poorly predict the *in vivo* characteristics. Small whole animal models were proposed to overcome the current limitation of the cell-based phenotypic assays, by adding a level of complexity to the models and incorporating a rudimentary safety test early in drug discovery [22]. In our study, we applied a blend of phenotypic cellular assays (lipid lowering and glucose uptake in HepG2 cells), target-based assays (adipocyte differentiation, and thermogenic gene expression) and the zebrafish Nile red fat metabolism assay [23] as a whole small animal model *in vivo* for lipid reduction. A total of 15 of the tested cyanobacteria fractions showed the capacity to reduce neutral lipids in zebrafish larvae *in vivo*. The characterization of the most promising fractions with lipid reducing activity led to the identification of the reported compounds eryloside T, pheophorbide A and phaeophytin A. Those compounds are minor peaks of the analyzed fractions and besides the literature reports them as bioactive, no obesity-related bioactivity is described. Phaeophyin A and pheophorbide A are two products of chlorophyll A degradation and were reported as effective anti-proliferative [24,25] and immunomodulatory [26–28] compounds. Those compounds seem to be widespread among the analyzed fractions, representing, in many of them, major peaks. Eryloside T, a minor peak in LEGE07173 B (#256), was previously isolated from the sponge *Erylus goffrilleri* and shown to have toxicity against Ehrlich carcinoma cells [29]. Lipid reducing activity of those compounds was not yet discovered. Other studies described bioactive compounds with lipid reducing potential in zebrafish larvae. *Talaromyces stipitatus*, a sponge-associated fungus, produces several anthraquinones and secalonic acid that show anti-obesity activity in the same animal model [10]. However, future studies will be necessary to study whether those known compounds or other present, unknown compounds in the fractions are responsible for the observed bioactivity.

The liver is the main organ responsible for coordination of energy metabolism and lipid conversion. Non-alcoholic fatty liver disease (NAFLD) commonly appears as a result of excessive body fat gain [30]. As fat overloading works in a similar manner in primary hepatocytes and HepG2 cells, the latter represents a suitable model of hepatic steatosis [14]. A total of 50 fractions had shown anti-steatosis potential, however, many were cytotoxic, and finally, 17 fractions were selected with promising lipid lowering activity. Recent efforts have been made to discover novel molecules for the treatment of NAFLD. Siphonaxanthin, a marine carotenoid, isolated from green algae such as *Codium cylindricum Holmes*, showed a strong *in vitro* inhibitory effect of hepatic lipogenesis on the HepG2 cell line suppressing excessive lipid accumulation [31]. Another carotenoid, fucoxanthin, decreased lipid accumulation in FL83B hepatocytes [32]. Our metabolite profiling approach led to the identification of leptosin F, pheophorbide A, phaeophytin A and chlorophyll A in the promising fractions with anti-steatosis activities. Leptosin F, found as a minor peak, is an inhibitor of DNA topoisomerases I and II, important molecular targets of several potent anticancer agents, and cytotoxic effects in several tumor cell lines [33]. Chlorophyll A promotes similar activities as its degradation products, namely anti-proliferative [24,25] and immunomodulatory [26–28] activities. The pigment was, however, found as a minor peak. Hepatic lipid lowering of these compounds is not known yet.

Hepatic glucose uptake and metabolism are important regulators of glycogen storage and *de novo* lipogenesis. To this end, four cyanobacterial fractions increased glucose uptake in HepG2 cells without any cytotoxicity. The characterization of those fractions identified, once again, chlorophyll A and its degradation products, as well as several carotenoids and terpenes. Carotenoids and terpenes are classes of compounds common in those fractions. Carotenoids are referenced for their diverse bioactivities such as anticancer, anti-inflammatory, cardioprotective, anti-obesity and anti-diabetic activities [34]. Terpenes are described for its health-related activities, such as cytotoxic, anti-microbial or anti-angiogenic [35,36]. These classes were, however, found in minority, when compared to unknown peaks. Similarly to our results, six polyoxygenated steroids, isolated from the marine sponge *Clathria gombawuiensis*, demonstrated a moderate increase in 2-NBDG uptake in 3T3-L1 adipocytes [37]. Other bioassays involving key macromolecules in DTM2 disease are more frequently applied, such as the activity of the tyrosine phosphatase 1B (PTP1B). PTP1B is a negative regulator of the insulin signalling pathway and considered a potential target to treat diabetes. Many compounds isolated from algae, like bromophenols, phlorotannins and sterols have shown strong inhibitory activity [38]. A bisabolane-related metabolite, isolated from the marine sponge *Axinyssa* sp., showed potent inhibitory effect of PTP1B [39].

The effect of the cyanobacterial fractions was also tested on brown adipocyte differentiation and thermogenic gene expression. For this purpose, a clonal brown preadipocyte cell line was used, selected for high differentiation capacity and robust expression of the mitochondrial uncoupling protein 1 (UCP-1), which mediates heat production through mitochondrial uncoupling. PPARγ is the key transcription factor promoting adipogenic differentiation and a well-established marker to assess adipogenesis [40]. UCP-1 gene expression was selected as indicator of thermogenesis (heat production), however, a confirmation by other methodologies will be necessary in the future to prove the positive effects on thermogenesis. Four fractions increased UCP-1 mRNA expression, and the metabolite profiling identified pheophorbide A, phaeophytin A, several terpenes and carotenoids, already identified in the previous fractions. The pattern seen before remains, and chlorophyll degradation products represent, in some cases, major peaks, but the other classes are minor. Several major peaks correspond to unidentified compounds that can represent novel structures. The low expression levels of UCP-1 and high expression of PPARγ upon treatment with four fractions were indicative for a shift of the treated cells towards a more energy-storing white adipocyte-like phenotype, while the reduction in both markers could indicate an inhibitory effect on adipogenesis in general. The previously mentioned fucoxanthin was described to induce UCP-1 expression in white adipose tissue [41]. Indeed, rats fed with the marine microalgae *Tisochrysis lutea* showed increased levels of both UCP-1 and PPARγ [42].

Metabolite profiling is an excellent tool to identify and select fractions/extracts for lead identification, as this technique is based on chemical profiling [43]. Due to the high amount of data acquired during metabolomic studies, statistical and multidimensional analysis are crucial for data mining and visualization. Principal component analysis (PCA) compares the variance between different samples. When applied to the cyanobacterial fractions, this technique allowed selecting the ones with a differentiating factor, representing different metabolites compared to the other samples. PCA, allied to metabolite profiling, has successfully resulted in the identification of several secondary metabolites, such as the 3-Alkyl Pyridine Alkaloids found in the sponge *Haliclona rosea* [44], or in the isolation of those metabolites, as N-Acyl-Taurine Geodiataurine, isolated from the polar sponge *Geodia macandrewi* [45]. In our study, the use of metabolite profiling and toxicity evaluation allowed to reduce the list of bioactive fractions to a handful of fractions with promising properties. Those properties have (i) relevant bioactivity towards diverse metabolic function, (ii) no toxicity *in vitro* and *in vivo*, (iii) the potential to produce novel compounds. After careful analysis of the compounds present in the cyanobacterial fractions, we expect that unknown compounds are causative for the tested obesity-related bioactivities. Although the activities for the identified compounds have never been studied in this context, they are only present as minor chromatographic peaks. Chlorophyll A and its degradation products could, however, be responsible for some of the reported activities. Future work is necessary in order to identify those compounds and to decipher the underlying molecular mechanism.

4. Materials and Methods

4.1. Growth of Cyanobacteria and Construction of Screening Library

Cyanobacterial strains used in this study were selected from Blue Biotechnology and Ecotoxicology Culture Collection [12] and are listed in Supplementary Table S1. All cyanobacteria were grown under a light/dark cycle of 14/10 h at 25 °C and a photon irradiance of approximately 30 μmol.m^{-2} s^{-1}. Freshwater and estuarine strains were cultured in Z8 medium [46]. Marine strains were cultured in Z8 medium supplemented with 25 g L^{-1} NaCl and 20 μg L^{-1} vitamin B12. At the exponential growth phase, cells were harvested by centrifugation and freeze-dried. Lyophilized biomass was fractionated to obtain a screening library for the different bioassays. Two different approaches were used: vacuum liquid chromatography (VLC) fractionation or increasing polarity extraction.

4.1.1. Vacuum Liquid Chromatography Fractionation

Lyophilized biomass was repeatedly extracted by percolation with a warm (<40 °C) mixture of dichloromethane:methanol (CH$_2$Cl$_2$:MeOH, 2:1 *v/v*) (VWR, Radnor, PA, USA). The resulting crude organic extract was separated using VLC with silica gel 60 (0.015–0.040 mm, Merck KGaA, Darmstadt, Germany) as stationary phase and a step-wise mobile phase gradient from 100% *n*-hexane (VWR) to 100% ethyl acetate (EtOAc) (VWR) and then to 100% methanol (MeOH) (VWR), yielding 10 fractions [47].

4.1.2. Increasing Polarity Extraction

Lyophilized biomass was sequentially extracted with *n*-hexane, EtOAc and MeOH, with three extraction steps for each solvent. Briefly, each solvent was added to the biomass, and placed for 30 s in the ultrasonic bath, followed by 1 min in the vortex. Centrifugation at 4600 rpm for 15 min was performed and the supernatant collected. Three fractions were obtained, one for each solvent extraction. The fractions were dried and resuspended in dimethyl sulfoxide (DMSO) (VWR international, Radnor, PA, USA) at 10 mg mL^{-1} and stored at $-20\,^{\circ}$C.

4.2. Zebrafish Nile Red Fat Metabolism Assay

Lipid reducing activity was analyzed by the zebrafish Nile red fat metabolism assay [10,23]. Approval by an ethics committee was not necessary as chosen procedures are not considered animal experimentation according to the EC Directive 86/609/EEC for animal experiments. In brief, zebrafish embryos were raised from 1-day post fertilization (DPF) on in egg water (60 μg mL^{-1} marine sea salt) with 200 μM 1-phenyl-2-thiourea (PTU) to inhibit pigmentation. From 3 to 5 DPF, zebrafish larvae were exposed to cyanobacterial fractions at a final concentration of 10 μg mL^{-1} with daily renewal of water and fractions in a 48-well plate with a density of 6–8 larvae/well (*n* = 6–8). A solvent control (0.1% DMSO) and positive control (REV, resveratrol, 50 μM) were included in the assay. Neutral lipids were stained with 10 ng mL^{-1} Nile red overnight. The larvae were anesthetized with tricaine (MS-222, 0.03%) for 5 min before imaging on a fluorescence microscope (Olympus, BX-41, Hamburg, Germany). Fluorescence intensity was quantified in individual zebrafish larvae by ImageJ [48].

4.3. Cell Culture

HepG2 cells were purchased from American Type Culture Collection (ATCC) (Manassas, VA, USA) and cultured in Dulbecco Modified Eagle Medium (DMEM) (Gibco, Thermo Fisher Scientific, Waltham, MA, USA). Cells were grown in DMEM supplemented with 10% (*v/v*) fetal bovine serum (Biochrom, Berlin, Germany), 1% penicillin/streptomycin (100 IU mL^{-1} and 10 mg mL^{-1}, respectively) (Biochrom) and 0.1% amphotericin (GE Healthcare, Little Chalfont, UK). HepG2 cells were incubated in a humidified atmosphere with 5% CO$_2$, at 37 °C. A clonal cell line was derived from an SV40 large T immortalized brown preadipocytes, derived from the brown adipose tissue of a male C57Bl/6 mouse [49], based on high UCP-1 induction upon differentiation. Brown preadipocyte clones were cultured in normal growth medium (DMEM + GlutaMAXTM, 4.5 g L^{-1} D-glucose, pyruvate, 10% Fetal Bovine Serum (FBS) and 1% penicillin/streptomycin).

4.4. Anti-Steatosis Assay in HepG2 Cells and Sulforhodamine B (SRB) Assay

The anti-steatosis assay was adapted from [50] and [14]. Cells were seeded at 10^4 cells/well in 96-well plates and adhered overnight. The medium was changed to DMEM supplemented with 62 μM sodium oleate (Sigma-Aldrich, St. Louis, MO, USA) and fractions were added at 10 μg mL^{-1}. DMSO and 0.5% MeOH were used as solvent control, 62 μM sodium oleate as a negative control (maximum lipid accumulation) and resveratrol (REV) (Santa Cruz Biotechnology, Santa Cruz, CA, USA) as a positive control. After 6 h, cells were stained with 75 ng mL^{-1} Nile Red (Sigma-Aldrich) and 10 μg mL^{-1} Hoechst 33342 (HO-33342) (Sigma Aldrich) in Hanks Buffered Salt Solution (HBSS) (0.137 M NaCl, 5.4 mM KCl, 0.25 mM Na$_2$HPO$_4$, 0.44 mM KH$_2$PO$_4$, 1.3 mM CaCl$_2$, 1.0 mM MgSO$_4$, 4.2 mM NaHCO$_3$, glucose free). After incubating at 37 °C for 10 min and in the absence of light, cells were washed twice with HBSS. Fluorescence was read in a Synergy HT Multi-detection microplate reader (Biotek, Bad Friedrichshall, Germany) at 485/572 nm excitation/emission for Nile red and 360/460 nm for HO-33342 [51].

Cytotoxicity of the fractions was tested on HepG2 cell line using the SRB (MP Biomedicals, LLC, Illkirch-Graffenstaden, France) colorimetric assay. Following the anti-steatosis assay, cells were fixed for 1 h at 4 °C, in the dark, adding 50% (*w/v*) ice-cold trichloroacetic acid (TCA) (Fisher Scientific, Loughborough, UK) to the culture medium. Cells were washed four times with deionized water and the plates air-dried. Then, 0.4% (*w/v*) SRB in 1% acetic was added to each well for 15 min, followed by five washes with 1% acetic acid. The plates were again air-dried and 10 mmol L^{-1}, pH 10.5 Tris–HCl (VWR international, Gen-Apex) was added to each well. Absorbance was read at 492 nm with reference at 650 nm on a Synergy HT Multi-detection microplate reader (Biotek, Bad Friedrichshall, Germany).

4.5. Glucose Uptake Assay in HepG2 Cells and MTT Assay

To evaluate the potential for diabetes of the library fractions, the uptake of 2-(*N*-(7-Nitrobenz-2-oxa-1,3-diazol-4-yl)Amino)-2-Deoxyglucose (2-NBDG) (Life Technologies, Thermo Fischer Scientific) was measured as described in [52]. Briefly, HepG2 cells were seeded in 96-well plates at a concentration of 10^5 cells/well. Then, 24 h after seeding, cells were starved on Hank's Buffered Salt Solution (HBSS) for 16 h. Cells were then exposed to the fractions at 10 µg mL^{-1}. Then, 0.5% DMSO was used as solvent control and Emodin (TargetMol, Boston, Massachusetts, USA) as positive control. After 2 h of incubation, 100 µM 2-NBDG was added to each well for 1 h. Cells were then washed twice with ice-cold HBSS and the fluorescence was measured at 485/535 nm (excitation/emission) at Fluoroskan Ascent CF (MTX Lab Systems, Bradenton, FL, USA).

The MTT assay (3-(4,5-Dimethylthiazol-2-yl)-2,5-Diphenyltetrazolium Bromide) was used to assess the cytotoxicity of the fractions on the HepG2 cells following the glucose uptake screening. Cells were exposed to 0.2 mg mL^{-1} MTT and incubated at 37 °C for 2 h. The medium was removed and 100 µL DMSO added to each well. The absorbance was read at 570 nm on Synergy HT Multi-detection microplate reader.

4.6. Brown Adipocyte Differentiation

Differentiation of brown pre-adipocytes was induced by adding DMEM containing 10% FBS, 1% penicillin and streptomycin, 500 µM IBMX, 5 µM dexamethasone, 125 µM indomethacin, 1 nM Triiodothyronine (T3), 100 nM insulin and 1 µM rosiglitazone. After two days, the induction medium was replaced by freshly prepared differentiation medium (DMEM containing 10% FBS, 1% penicillin and streptomycin, 1 nM T3 and 100 nM insulin and until day 4, 1 µM rosiglitazone). The differentiation medium was changed every other day until the cells were fully differentiated at day 8. To study the effects of cyanobacterial fractions on brown adipocyte differentiation, preadipocytes were differentiated, as described above, in the presence of 10 µg mL^{-1} cyanobacterial fractions from the day 0 until day 6. Cell cultures were tested regularly negative for mycoplasm. Live cells were imaged with a Keyence (America Inc.; BZ-9000 BioRevo, Chicago, IL, USA) microscope, using a Nikon Plan- Apochromatic 20x/0.75 objective (Nikon, Japan). Bright field images were captured using 'Multi-color image capturing software' built in the BZ-9000 system.

PPARγ and UCP-1 mRNA Expression by Real-Time PCR

For mRNA expression analyses, RNA from differentiated brown adipocytes was isolated using the QuickExtractTM RNA extraction kit (Epicentre Biotechnologies, Madison, WI, USA,), following the manufacturer's instructions. Synthesis of cDNA was performed in a Thermo Cycler by using the high-Capacity cDNA reverse transcription kit (Applied Biosystem, Foster City, CA, USA), according to the manufactures protocol. Real-time PCR with SYBR green was performed using iTaqTM Universal SYBR® Green Supermix (BIO-RAD, Hercules, CA, USA) in a CFX384 Touch Real-Time PCR Detection System (BIO-RAD). Relative mRNA expression was calculated after normalization by TATA-binding protein (Tbp) expression. Primer sequences are listed in the Supplementary Table S2. Differential expression levels were calculated via the ΔΔCt method [53].

4.7. Metabolite Profiling

The metabolic profiling of cyanobacterial extracts was performed using a Waters ACQUITY UPLC system (Waters, Milford, MA, USA), coupled to a Waters Synapt G1 mass spectrometer equipped with electrospray ionization (ESI) probe (Waters, Wilmslow, UK). The analytical column ACQUITY UPLC BEH C18 (2.1×100 mm, 1.7 μm) (Waters, Milford, MA, USA) was used for separation and was maintained at 60 °C. Mobile phase A was water with 0.1% formic acid and mobile phase B was acetonitrile with 0.1% formic acid. The flow was maintained at 0.45 mL min^{-1}. A linear gradient was used from 65% to 100% B during the first 8 min, followed by a column clean up at 100% B for 0.5 min and reconditioning at the initial conditions for 1.5 min. The total chromatographic run time was 12 min. The sample manager was maintained at 10 °C. The samples were analyzed in positive ionization mode and the ionization source parameters were kept as follows: capillary voltage 3.5 kV; cone voltage 42 V; source temperature 125 °C; desolvation temperature 450 °C, at a flow rate of 700 L h^{-1} (N$_2$); cone gas flow rate 50 L h^{-1}. Data acquisition was carried out using MassLynx 4.1 and MarkerLynx XS was used for peak picking, alignment and identification of markers (Waters, Milford, MA, USA). Markers between 100 and 1500 Da were collected with an intensity threshold of 100 counts and retention time and mass windows of 0.10 min and 0.050 Da, respectively. The noise level was set to 5.00. Statistical analysis of the data was done using EZinfo 3.0 (Sartorius Stedim Biotech, Umea, Sweden) and SIMCA 15 (Sartorius Stedim Biotech).

5. Conclusions

This work demonstrates the potential of marine, estuarine and freshwater species of cyanobacteria, to produce secondary metabolites with relevant bioactivities towards several metabolic functions. The combination of screening assays with metabolite profiling and toxicity evaluation allowed the selection of a few, very promising fractions. Within such fractions, several known and unknown secondary metabolites were identified, however, major mass peaks corresponded to unknown compounds. In the future, the compounds responsible for the bioactivities will be isolated and structures elucidated, before exploring their role for the treatment of metabolic diseases.

Supplementary Materials: The following are available online at http://www.mdpi.com/1660-3397/17/5/280/s1. Table S1: List of the cyanobacterial strains used; Table S2: List of the qPCR primers used in the bioactivity screening; Figures S1–S12: PCA plots of all cyanobacterial fractions; Figure S13: Representative images of brown adipocytes; Tables S3–S6 Identification of the compounds present on each fraction.

Author Contributions: R.U., S.U. and M.T. designed the experiments. M.C. performed the metabolite profiling and statistical data analysis transversal to all bioactivities. F.R. and N.G.S. identified known compounds from mass spectrometry. F.R. performed the anti-steatosis assay. T.R. performed the glucose uptake assay. R.H.-B. performed PPARγ and UCP1 assay. F.E., M.T. supervised the metabolite profiling. S.U. supervised the PPARγ/UCP-1 bioassay. R.U. and M.B. performed the lipid reducing assay, R.U. supervised the assays for lipid reducing, anti-steatosis and glucose uptake activities. M.C., T.R. and R.U. wrote the manuscript. All the authors read and revised the manuscript.

Funding: This work was financed by national funds through FCT (Portugal), BMBF (Germany), Rannis (Iceland) and Formas (Sweden), within the framework of the European ERA-NET Marine Biotechnology project "CYANOBESITY—Cyanobacteria as a source of bioactive compounds with effects on obesity and obesity-related co-morbidities". The research was additionally supported by the FCT strategic fund UID/Multi/04423/2019. Ralph Urbatzka and Tiago Ribeiro were supported by FCT grants SFRH/BPD/112287/2015 and SFRH/BD/139131/2018 respectively. SU received additional funding from the project Aging and Metabolic Programming (AMPro).

Conflicts of Interest: The authors declare no conflict of interest.

References

1. Collaboration, N.R.F. Trends in adult body-mass index in 200 countries from 1975 to 2014: a pooled analysis of 1698 population-based measurement studies with 19.2 million participants. *Lancet* **2016**, *387*, 1377–1396.
2. Kelly, T.; Yang, W.; Chen, C.S.; Reynolds, K.; He, J. Global burden of obesity in 2005 and projections to 2030. *Int. J. Obes.* **2008**, *32*, 1431. [CrossRef] [PubMed]

3. Nguyen, N.T.; Magno, C.P.; Lane, K.T.; Hinojosa, M.W.; Lane, J.S. Association of Hypertension, Diabetes, Dyslipidemia, and Metabolic Syndrome with Obesity: Findings from the National Health and Nutrition Examination Survey, 1999 to 2004. *J. Am. Coll. Surg.* **2008**, *207*, 928–934. [CrossRef] [PubMed]
4. Berger, N.A. Obesity and cancer pathogenesis. *Ann. N. Y. Acad. Sci.* **2014**, *1311*, 57–76. [CrossRef]
5. Abdelaal, M.; le Roux, C.W.; Docherty, N.G. Morbidity and mortality associated with obesity. *Ann. Transl. Med.* **2017**, *5*, 161. [CrossRef] [PubMed]
6. Apovian, C.M.; Gokce, N. Obesity and cardiovascular disease. *Circulation* **2012**, *125*, 1178–1182. [CrossRef]
7. Kang, J.G.; Park, C.-Y. Anti-Obesity Drugs: A Review about Their Effects and Safety. *Diabetes Metab.* **2012**, *36*, 13–25. [CrossRef]
8. Thomford, N.E.; Senthebane, D.A.; Rowe, A.; Munro, D.; Seele, P.; Maroyi, A.; Dzobo, K. Natural Products for Drug Discovery in the 21st Century: Innovations for Novel Drug Discovery. *Int. J. Mol. Sci.* **2018**, *19*, 1578. [CrossRef]
9. Koyama, T.; Kawazoe, Y.; Iwasaki, A.; Ohno, O.; Suenaga, K.; Uemura, D. Anti-obesity activities of the yoshinone A and the related marine γ-pyrone compounds. *J Antibiot.* **2016**, *69*, 348–351. [CrossRef]
10. Noinart, J.; Buttachon, S.; Dethoup, T.; Gales, L.; Pereira, J.A.; Urbatzka, R.; Freitas, S.; Lee, M.; Silva, A.M.S.; Pinto, M.M.M.; et al. A New Ergosterol Analog, a New Bis-Anthraquinone and Anti-Obesity Activity of Anthraquinones from the Marine Sponge-Associated Fungus Talaromyces stipitatus KUFA 0207. *Mar. Drugs* **2017**, *15*, 139. [CrossRef] [PubMed]
11. Dittmann, E.; Gugger, M.; Sivonen, K.; Fewer, D.P. Natural Product Biosynthetic Diversity and Comparative Genomics of the Cyanobacteria. *Trends Microbiol.* **2015**, *23*, 642–652. [CrossRef]
12. Ramos, V.; Morais, J.; Castelo-Branco, R.; Pinheiro, Â.; Martins, J.; Regueiras, A.; Pereira, A.L.; Lopes, V.R.; Frazão, B.; Gomes, D.; et al. Cyanobacterial diversity held in microbial biological resource centers as a biotechnological asset: the case study of the newly established LEGE culture collection. *J. Appl. Phycol.* **2018**, *30*, 1437–1451. [CrossRef]
13. Costa, M.; Garcia, M.; Costa-Rodrigues, J.; Costa, M.S.; Ribeiro, M.J.; Fernandes, M.H.; Barros, P.; Barreiro, A.; Vasconcelos, V.; Martins, R. Exploring bioactive properties of marine cyanobacteria isolated from the Portuguese coast: high potential as a source of anticancer compounds. *Mar. Drugs* **2013**, *12*, 98–114. [CrossRef]
14. Gómez-Lechón, M.J.; Donato, M.T.; Martínez-Romero, A.; Jiménez, N.; Castell, J.V.; O'Connor, J.-E. A human hepatocellular in vitro model to investigate steatosis. *Chem. Biol. Interact.* **2007**, *165*, 106–116. [CrossRef]
15. MarineLit. Available online: http://pubs.rsc.org/marinlit/ (accessed on 10 January 2019).
16. Royal Society of Chemistry. ChemSpider. Available online: http://www.chemspider.com/ (accessed on 4 March 2019).
17. Society, A.C. SciFinder. Available online: https://scifinder.cas.org/ (accessed on 4 March 2019).
18. Yun, J.W. Possible anti-obesity therapeutics from nature—A review. *Phytochemistry* **2010**, *71*, 1625–1641. [CrossRef]
19. Castro, M.; Preto, M.; Vasconcelos, V.; Urbatzka, R. Obesity: The Metabolic Disease, Advances on Drug Discovery and Natural Product Research. *Curr. Top. Med. Chem.* **2016**, *16*, 2577–2604. [CrossRef]
20. Molinski, T.F.; Dalisay, D.S.; Lievens, S.L.; Saludes, J.P. Drug development from marine natural products. *Nat. Rev. Drug Discov.* **2008**, *8*, 69. [CrossRef]
21. Zheng, W.; Thorne, N.; McKew, J.C. Phenotypic screens as a renewed approach for drug discovery. *Drug Discov. Today* **2013**, *18*, 1067–1073. [CrossRef]
22. Giacomotto, J.; Ségalat, L. High-throughput screening and small animal models, where are we? *Br. J. Pharmacol.* **2010**, *160*, 204–216. [CrossRef]
23. Urbatzka, R.; Freitas, S.; Palmeira, A.; Almeida, T.; Moreira, J.; Azevedo, C.; Afonso, C.; Correia-da-Silva, M.; Sousa, E.; Pinto, M.; et al. Lipid reducing activity and toxicity profiles of a library of polyphenol derivatives. *Eur. J. Med. Chem.* **2018**, *151*, 272–284. [CrossRef]
24. Hibasami, H.; Kyohkon, M.; Ohwaki, S.; Katsuzaki, H.; Imai, K.; Nakagawa, M.; Ishi, Y.; Komiya, T. Pheophorbide a, a moiety of chlorophyll a, induces apoptosis in human lymphoid leukemia molt 4B cells. *Int. J. Mol. Med.* **2000**, *6*, 277–279. [CrossRef] [PubMed]
25. Tang, P.M.-K.; Chan, J.Y.-W.; Au, S.W.-N.; Kong, S.-K.; Tsui, S.K.-W.; Waye, M.M.-Y.; Mak, T.C.-W.; Fong, W.-P.; Fung, K.-P. Pheophorbide a, an active compound isolated from *Scutellaria barbata*, possesses photodynamic

activities by inducing apoptosis in human hepatocellular carcinoma. *Cancer Biol. Ther.* **2006**, *5*, 1111–1116. [CrossRef] [PubMed]

26. Subramoniam, A.; Asha, V.V.; Nair, S.A.; Sasidharan, S.P.; Sureshkumar, P.K.; Rajendran, K.N.; Karunagaran, D.; Ramalingam, K. Chlorophyll Revisited: Anti-inflammatory Activities of Chlorophyll a and Inhibition of Expression of TNF-α Gene by the Same. *Inflammation* **2012**, *35*, 959–966. [CrossRef] [PubMed]

27. Park, S.; Choi, J.J.; Park, B.-K.; Yoon, S.J.; Choi, J.E.; Jin, M. Pheophytin a and chlorophyll a suppress neuroinflammatory responses in lipopolysaccharide and interferon-γ-stimulated BV2 microglia. *Life Sci.* **2014**, *103*, 59–67. [CrossRef] [PubMed]

28. Bui-Xuan, N.-H.; Tang, P.M.-K.; Wong, C.-K.; Chan, J.Y.-W.; Cheung, K.K.Y.; Jiang, J.L.; Fung, K.-P. Pheophorbide a: A photosensitizer with immunostimulating activities on mouse macrophage RAW 264.7 cells in the absence of irradiation. *Cell. Immunol.* **2011**, *269*, 60–67. [CrossRef] [PubMed]

29. Afiyatullov, S.S.; Kalinovsky, A.I.; Antonov, A.S.; Ponomarenko, L.P.; Dmitrenok, P.S.; Aminin, D.L.; Krasokhin, V.B.; Nosova, V.M.; Kisin, A.V. Isolation and Structures of Erylosides from the Carribean Sponge Erylus goffrilleri. *J. Nat. Prod.* **2007**, *70*, 1871–1877. [CrossRef] [PubMed]

30. Hwang, Y.-J.; Wi, H.-R.; Kim, H.-R.; Park, K.W.; Hwang, K.-A. Pinus densiflora Sieb. et Zucc. Alleviates Lipogenesis and Oxidative Stress during Oleic Acid-Induced Steatosis in HepG2 Cells. *Nutrients* **2014**, *6*, 2956–2972. [CrossRef] [PubMed]

31. Zheng, J.; Li, Z.; Manabe, Y.; Kim, M.; Goto, T.; Kawada, T.; Sugawara, T. Siphonaxanthin, a Carotenoid From Green Algae, Inhibits Lipogenesis in Hepatocytes via the Suppression of Liver X Receptor α Activity. *Lipids* **2018**, *53*, 41–52. [CrossRef]

32. Chang, Y.-H.; Chen, Y.-L.; Huang, W.-C.; Liou, C.-J. Fucoxanthin attenuates fatty acid-induced lipid accumulation in FL83B hepatocytes through regulated Sirt1/AMPK signaling pathway. *Biochem. Biophys. Res. Commun.* **2018**, *495*, 197–203. [CrossRef]

33. Yanagihara, M.; Sasaki-Takahashi, N.; Sugahara, T.; Yamamoto, S.; Shinomi, M.; Yamashita, I.; Hayashida, M.; Yamanoha, B.; Numata, A.; Yamori, T.; et al. Leptosins isolated from marine fungus Leptoshaeria species inhibit DNA topoisomerases I and/or II and induce apoptosis by inactivation of Akt/protein kinase B. *Cancer Sci.* **2005**, *96*, 816–824. [CrossRef]

34. Chuyen, H.V.; Eun, J.-B. Marine carotenoids: Bioactivities and potential benefits to human health. *Crit. Rev. Food Sci. Nutr.* **2017**, *57*, 2600–2610. [CrossRef] [PubMed]

35. Elissawy, A.M.; El-Shazly, M.; Ebada, S.S.; Singab, A.B.; Proksch, P. Bioactive Terpenes from Marine-Derived Fungi. *Mar. Drugs* **2015**, *13*, 1966–1992. [CrossRef] [PubMed]

36. Ebel, R. Terpenes from Marine-Derived Fungi. *Mar. Drugs* **2010**, *8*, 2340–2368. [CrossRef] [PubMed]

37. Woo, J.-K.; Ha, T.K.Q.; Oh, D.-C.; Oh, W.-K.; Oh, K.-B.; Shin, J. Polyoxygenated Steroids from the Sponge Clathria gombawuiensis. *J. Nat. Prod.* **2017**, *80*, 3224–3233. [CrossRef]

38. Ezzat, S.M.; Bishbishy, M.H.E.; Habtemariam, S.; Salehi, B.; Sharifi-Rad, M.; Martins, N.; Sharifi-Rad, J. Looking at Marine-Derived Bioactive Molecules as Upcoming Anti-Diabetic Agents: A Special Emphasis on PTP1B Inhibitors. *Molecules* **2018**, *23*, 3334. [CrossRef] [PubMed]

39. Abdjul, D.B.; Kanno, S.-I.; Yamazaki, H.; Ukai, K.; Namikoshi, M. A dimeric urea of the bisabolene sesquiterpene from the Okinawan marine sponge Axinyssa sp. inhibits protein tyrosine phosphatase 1B activity in Huh-7 human hepatoma cells. *Bioorg. Med. Chem. Lett.* **2016**, *26*, 315–317. [CrossRef]

40. Villarroya, F.; Iglesias, R.; Giralt, M. PPARs in the Control of Uncoupling Proteins Gene Expression. *PPAR Res.* **2007**, *2007*, 74364. [CrossRef]

41. Maeda, H. Nutraceutical effects of fucoxanthin for obesity and diabetes therapy: a review. *J. Oleo Sci.* **2015**, *64*, 125–132. [CrossRef]

42. Bigagli, E.; Cinci, L.; Niccolai, A.; Biondi, N.; Rodolfi, L.; D'Ottavio, M.; D'Ambrosio, M.; Lodovici, M.; Tredici, M.R.; Luceri, C. Preliminary data on the dietary safety, tolerability and effects on lipid metabolism of the marine microalga Tisochrysis lutea. *Algal Res.* **2018**, *34*, 244–249. [CrossRef]

43. Wu, C.; Kim, H.K.; van Wezel, G.P.; Choi, Y.H. Metabolomics in the natural products field – a gateway to novel antibiotics. *Drug Discov. Today Technol.* **2015**, *13*, 11–17. [CrossRef]

44. Einarsdottir, E.; Magnusdottir, M.; Astarita, G.; Köck, M.; Ögmundsdottir, H.; Thorsteinsdottir, M.; Rapp, H.; Omarsdottir, S.; Paglia, G. Metabolic Profiling as a Screening Tool for Cytotoxic Compounds: Identification of 3-Alkyl Pyridine Alkaloids from Sponges Collected at a Shallow Water Hydrothermal Vent Site North of Iceland. *Mar. Drugs* **2017**, *15*, 52. [CrossRef]

45. Olsen, E.K.; Soderholm, K.L.; Isaksson, J.; Andersen, J.H.; Hansen, E. Metabolomic Profiling Reveals the N-Acyl-Taurine Geodiataurine in Extracts from the Marine Sponge Geodia macandrewii (Bowerbank). *J. Nat. Prod.* **2016**, *79*, 1285–1291. [CrossRef]

46. Kotai, J. *Instructions for Preparation of Modified Nutrient Solution Z8 for Algae Norwegian*; Institute for Water Research, Blindern: Oslo, Norway, 1972; Volume B-11/69, p. 5.

47. Costa, M.S.; Rego, A.; Ramos, V.; Afonso, T.B.; Freitas, S.; Preto, M.; Lopes, V.; Vasconcelos, V.; Magalhães, C.; Leão, P.N. The conifer biomarkers dehydroabietic and abietic acids are widespread in Cyanobacteria. *Sci. Rep.* **2016**, *6*, 23436. [CrossRef]

48. ImageJ. Available online: https://imagej.nih.gov/ij/index.html (accessed on 1 March 2019).

49. Pramme-Steinwachs, I.; Jastroch, M.; Ussar, S. Extracellular calcium modulates brown adipocyte differentiation and identity. *Sci Rep.* **2017**, *7*, 8888. [CrossRef]

50. Donato, M.T.; Tolosa, L.; Jiménez, N.; Castell, J.V.; Gómez-Lechón, M.J. High-Content Imaging Technology for the Evaluation of Drug-Induced Steatosis Using a Multiparametric Cell-Based Assay. *J. Biomol. Screen.* **2011**, *17*, 394–400. [CrossRef]

51. Dave, T.; Tilles, A.W.; Vemula, M. A Cell-Based Assay to Investigate Hypolipidemic Effects of Nonalcoholic Fatty Liver Disease Therapeutics. *SLAS Discov.* **2018**, *23*, 274–282. [CrossRef]

52. Hassanein, M.; Weidow, B.; Koehler, E.; Bakane, N.; Garbett, S.; Shyr, Y.; Quaranta, V. Development of High-Throughput Quantitative Assays for Glucose Uptake in Cancer Cell Lines. *Mol. Imaging Biol.* **2011**, *13*, 840–852. [CrossRef]

53. Plaffl, M.W. A new mathematical model for relative quantification in real-time RT-PCR. *Nucleic Acids Res.* **2001**, *29*, e45.

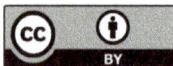

marine drugs

MDPI

Article

Application of Bioactive Thermal Proteome Profiling to Decipher the Mechanism of Action of the Lipid Lowering 13²-Hydroxy-pheophytin Isolated from a Marine Cyanobacteria

Ana Carrasco del Amor [1], Sara Freitas [2], Ralph Urbatzka [2], Olatz Fresnedo [3] and Susana Cristobal [1,4,*

[1] Department of Clinical and Experimental Medicine, Cell Biology, Faculty of Medicine, Linköping University, 581 85 Linköping, Sweden; ana.carrasco@liu.se
[2] CIIMAR, Interdisciplinary Centre of Marine and Environmental Research, 4450-208 Matosinhos, Portugal; freitas.srf.09@gmail.com (S.F.); rurbatzka@ciimar.up.pt (R.U.)
[3] Department of Physiology, Faculty of Medicine and Nursing, University of the Basque Country UPV/EHU, 48940 Leioa, Spain; olatz.fresnedo@ehu.eus
[4] Department of Physiology, Ikerbasque, Faculty of Medicine and Nursing, University of the Basque Country UPV/EH, 48940 Leioa, Spain
* Correspondence: susana.cristobal@liu.se

Received: 24 April 2019; Accepted: 15 June 2019; Published: 21 June 2019

Abstract: The acceleration of the process of understanding the pharmacological application of new marine bioactive compounds requires identifying the compound protein targets leading the molecular mechanisms in a living cell. The thermal proteome profiling (TPP) methodology does not fulfill the requirements for its application to any bioactive compound lacking chemical and functional characterization. Here, we present a modified method that we called bTPP for bioactive thermal proteome profiling that guarantees target specificity from a soluble subproteome. We showed that the precipitation of the microsomal fraction before the thermal shift assay is crucial to accurately calculate the melting points of the protein targets. As a probe of concept, the protein targets of 13²-hydroxy-pheophytin, a compound previously isolated from a marine cyanobacteria for its lipid reducing activity, were analyzed on the hepatic cell line HepG2. Our improved method identified 9 protein targets out of 2500 proteins, including 3 targets (isocitrate dehydrogenase, aldehyde dehydrogenase, phosphoserine aminotransferase) that could be related to obesity and diabetes, as they are involved in the regulation of insulin sensitivity and energy metabolism. This study demonstrated that the bTPP method can accelerate the field of biodiscovery, revealing protein targets involved in mechanisms of action (MOA) connected with future applications of bioactive compounds.

Keywords: thermal proteome profiling; mechanisms of action; bioactive compound; label-free quantitative proteomics; marine biodiscovery

---

1. Introduction

The identification of protein targets from novel bioactive compounds is one of the biggest challenges of the field of biodiscovery. The function of those proteins would define the MOA of any bioactive compound, predicting the mode of action at the cellular level, as well as possible secondary or harmful effects. Phenotypic screening was the principal strategy for drug and bioactive compound discovery until the 80s. This methodology has attracted renewed interest in connection with biodiscovery programs for terrestrial natural sources [1]. As an alternative, targeted screening had offered enormous success in drug discovery, but requires a preliminary rational approach to

MOA and an extensive screening of compound libraries against specific purified proteins used as targets [2]. Therefore, target selection should be restricted to proteins that can be expressed, purified, and adapted for interaction assays. Those limitations are introducing an intrinsic bias in the research. Moreover, considering that an average proteomic analysis from an homogenous cell could identify around 2000 proteins [3], and that over 700 proteins have been estimated to be targeted by current drugs [4], the traditional targeted screening approach faces difficulties to offer complete responses to drug–target opportunities.

The target engagement of a bioactive compound in cells and tissue depends on its local concentration, which is governed by parameters such as absorption, distribution, metabolism and excretion; and its affinity, which is also regulated by structural factors, including activation state of the protein target, co-factors, and post-translational modifications [5]. The challenge of evaluating those parameters in the cellular environment was solved by the development of the cellular thermal shift assay (CETSA) [6]. The biophysical principle of increase of thermal stability to unfolding of proteins in complexes compared to individual soluble proteins was the basis of CETSA [7]. The next step, extending the resolution power of this methodology to any possible protein targets within a cell, is offered by the TPP method [8]. The TPP method enables the analysis of the thermal stability of a proteome by applying quantitative mass spectrometry based on isobaric tandem mass tag 10-plex reagents. The method has been applied to study drug–target interaction [9,10], protein–substrate interaction in complex samples [11], and protein degradation [12].

The aim of biodiscovery is to understand the MOA of an array of newly discovered chemical compounds with possible bioactivity, limited structural characterization, and absence of any mechanistic knowledge. Identifying protein targets capable of interacting with the compound inside the cells is a huge challenge. In marine biodiscovery, cyanobacteria are recognized as being an interesting resource for obtaining novel compounds with applications in the field of human health. Cyanobacteria synthesize a wide variety of bioactive compounds with antimicrobial, antiviral and anticancer activity, among other things. Most secondary metabolites of cyanobacteria are lipopeptides, amino acids, fatty acids, macrolides, and amides. Although small compounds of cyanobacterial origin have been revealed to have activities of interest for application in pharmacology or as nutraceuticals, the strategies for elucidating MOA are still based on methods with low resolution [13].

In this study, we propose that implementation of the TPP methodology is applicable to novel bioactive compounds. The key implementation aims to gain in specificity and sensitivity for compound with limited chemical characterization. It should be considered that the TPP method was targeted to well-characterized drugs or druggable compounds. As phenotypic screening is the most common strategy for selecting positive candidates for bioactivity, chemical characterizations are not available at the early stages. The hydrophilic or hydrophobic nature of a new compound could compromise its interaction with biological membranes such as microsomes as a result of cellular lysis and fractionation. We evaluate the initial centrifugation step that determines the subproteome subjected to thermal shift analysis. Here, we present a method named bioactive thermal proteome profiling (bTPP). This is an improvement of the TPP method enabling sensitive analysis of protein targets across a proteome in any novel bioactive compound. To demonstrate the applicability of bTPP to the field of biodiscovery, we studied the protein targets of 13^2-hydroxy-pheophytin a, a chlorophyll derivative with novel lipid-reducing activities that has recently been isolated from a marine cyanobacteria [14]. Given that this molecule is produced in high quantities in *Spirulina*, and is approved for human consumption, it is possible that a nutraceutical with anti-obesity activity may be developed in the future [14]. The identification of the direct targets of 13^2-hydroxy-pheophytin a (hpa) in HepG2 liver cells and the discussion of possible MOA will provide important information in terms of its applicability.

2. Results

2.1. Implementation of the Novel Methodology, bTPP

We presented the bTPP method which is a TPP-based method able to identify the protein targets that interact with a bioactive compound. In particular, this method does not require preliminary knowledge of the chemical structure or function of a bioactive compound (Figure 1).

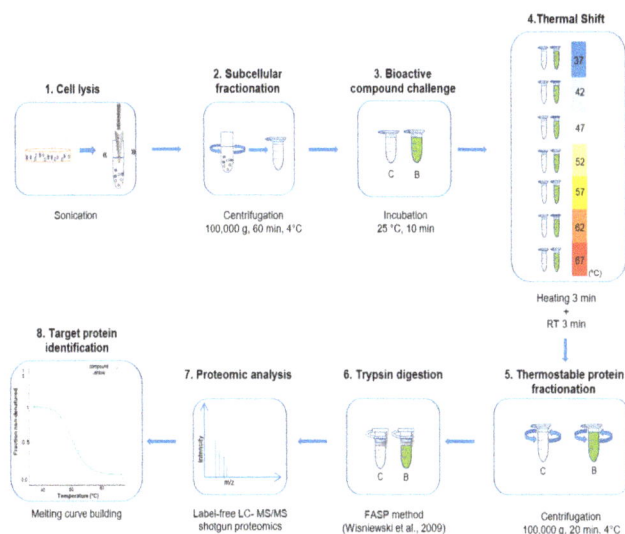

Figure 1. Outline of the bTPP workflow. (**1**) Cell lysis: performed using sonication with a vertical tip in the cell suspension. (**2**) Subcellular fractionation: soluble subproteome was collected in the supernatant after centrifugation at 100,000 g, for 60 min at 4 °C. (**3**) Bioactive compound challenge: the soluble protein was incubated with compound or vehicle at 25 °C for 10 min. (**4**) Thermal shift assay: performed at 7 temperatures between 37 °C and 67 °C for 3 min, and at RT for 3 min. (**5**) Thermostable protein fractionation: the studied sample was collected after centrifugation at 100,000 g for 20 min at 4 °C. (**6**) Trypsin digestion: the FASP method was applied. (**7**) Proteomic analysis: the peptides were separated by label-free LC-MS/MS and analysis by shotgun proteomic. (**8**) Target protein identification: protein data analysis was used to fit the melting curves of each protein.

We attempted to apply the TPP method as described for drug discovery [8]. We utilized ö, which has lipid-reducing activity and was extracted from marine cyanobacteria, as the test compound; it exhibited a green color in solution. The compound was dissolved in dimethyl sulfoxide (DMSO) due to its hydrophobicity. The first visual observation was the accumulation of hpa in the pellet following thermal shift assay centrifugation, which is defined in the TPP method as 100,000 g for 20 min (Figure 2). We hypothesized that, with the thermal shift incubation, the hydrophobic compound would be accumulated in the microsomes that were present in the soluble fraction. It has been described in the literature that the sedimentation of microsomes requires a centrifugation force at least equivalent to 100,000 g for 60 min [15–17]. Nevertheless, the TPP method applies only 100,000 g for 20 min to define the soluble fraction, and this fraction therefore contains insoluble microsomal vesicles [18]. The TPP method contains a second centrifugation step of 100,000 g for 20 min after the thermal shift assay, which would also precipitate additional microsomal vesicles. The TPP method is not able to discriminate, based on centrifugation, between an increase in protein instability caused by thermal effects and microsomal membranes precipitated with their sedimentation coefficient (Figure 2A). Thus, the first parameter to be modified is the definition of soluble subproteomes as a soluble protein free from microsomes obtained after centrifugation at 100,000 g for 60 min [15].

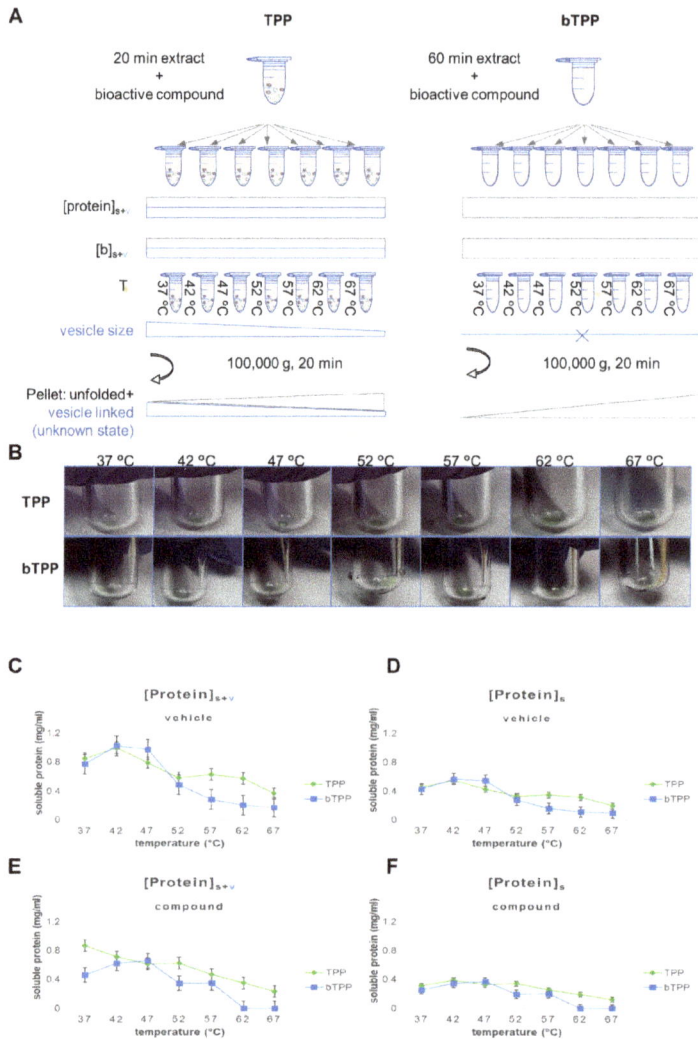

Figure 2. Characterization of the differences between the soluble subproteomes utilized in TPP and bTPP. (**A**) Schema summarizing the variation in the parameters: concentration of soluble protein, vesicular-associated protein, and bioactive compound in response to the thermal shift assay using both methodologies. (**B**) Pictures of the pellets after thermal shift assay centrifugation. (**C,E**) Representation of the total protein concentration from the supernatant of TPP and bTPP for each temperature after the second centrifugation step. (**D,F**) Representation of total protein concentration by % of soluble protein (obtained by Gene ontology (GO) classification) and divided by 100 for each temperature in TPP and bTPP.

The second modification aimed to reduce the time, cost and processing efforts without compromising the robustness of the method. Our new temperature scale still covered the range from

37 °C to 67 °C, as with the original method, but we selected only 7 temperatures, including: 37 °C, 42 °C, 47 °C, 52 °C, 57 °C, 62 °C and 67 °C (Figure 1).

The final modification involved applying label-free quantitative mass spectrometry instead of multiplexed labelled quantitative mass spectrometry. This modification fits the purpose of the bTPP method, gaining the flexibility to be applied to several compounds in parallel and facilitating comparative analysis for more extended biodiscovery studies over extended periods of time.

2.2. Comparative Analysis of Protein Targets Applying TPP and bTPP

To validate our hypothesis, we compared the TPP and bTPP methods with a cell culture model of HepG2 cell homogenates and hpa as the bioactive compound. All of the thermal shift assays were performed at fixed concentrations of the protein and the bioactive compound. First, we deconvoluted the theoretical adjustment of the parameters protein, and bioactive compound, along with the thermal shift assay. This included changing the quality and quantity of the studied subproteome, as well as the availability of the bioactive compound (Figure 2A).

In the TPP method, the concentration of the protein during the thermal shift incubation assay was distributed between the soluble fraction and the microsomal vesicles in the solution. The concentration ratio between both protein fractions is likely to remain constant at different temperatures. On the other hand, the concentration of the bioactive compound was distributed between soluble compound and compound embedded in the microsomes, as observed in the pellets following thermal shift assay centrifugation (Figure 2B). The concentration of the bioactive compound decreased to below the ideal concentration for the assay. Moreover, a temperature-dependent decrease was expected in the size of the vesicles. The concentration of protein in the vesicular fraction should be constant, but a higher number of smaller vesicles are expected at higher temperatures. Finally, the thermal shift assay centrifugation will cause the precipitation of unfolded soluble proteins along with the microsomes. Vesicular fractions would be precipitated depending on their specific sedimentation coefficient. An increase in temperature would reduce the vesicular size, and a higher sedimentation coefficient would be required to precipitate the smaller vesicles. Therefore, increase in temperature is associated with a decrease in the precipitation of the protein from the vesicular fraction (Figure 2A,B for TPP).

For the bTPP method, the schema shows that the concentration of protein or bioactive compound remains constant with the increase of temperature, a fact which constitutes the conceptual basis of any TPP-based method. In our method, only the protein is soluble, as the vesicular fraction has already been sedimented through the cellular fractionation. The proteins accumulated in the pellets after the thermal assay correspond to thermal unfolded proteins (Figure 2A,B for bTPP).

The experimental data confirm this theoretical prediction. In the control samples, the decrease in protein concentration is temperature dependent in the bTPP for both total protein (soluble and vesicular fraction) and soluble protein, whereas a bimodal solubility pattern is observed for TPP (Figure 2C,D). In the presence of the compound, the protein thermostability limits are higher for TPP than for bTPP. This is most likely a consequence of the variation in the concentration of the bioactive compound when the TPP method is applied (Figure 2E). Both TPP and bTPP show a similar thermostability profile when exclusively comparing the soluble fraction that is available to interact with the compound (Figure 2F).

The analysis of the soluble proteomes utilized in both methods showed different patterns in the heatmaps. For the TPP method, the map indicates a higher precipitation of membrane-associated proteins at lower temperatures. For the bTPP method, there was a greater abundance of soluble proteins at lower temperatures (Figure 3A). Both TPP and bTPP followed a sigmoidal trend, making it possible to calculate the melting curves that were fitted with the best R^2 (Figure 3B). Target identification is based on the shift in melting temperature (Tm) induced by the ligand, and is dependent on the steep slope of the curve. At least 77% of all proteins showed curves with steep slopes in both methodologies (Figure 4A). Examples of melting curves with steep and shallow slopes are displayed in Figure 4B.

A

B

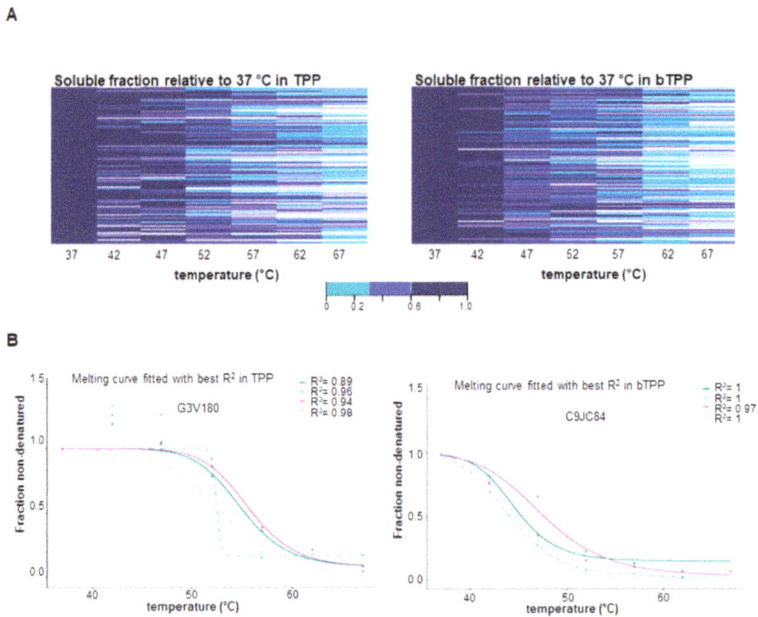

Figure 3. Thermal proteome profiling using TPP and bTPP. (**A**) Heat map of the protein thermostability in TPP, and bTPP. The colors show the range of protein abundance of the soluble fractions normalized to the soluble fraction at the lowest temperature. The soluble fraction here is composed of soluble protein after thermal shift assay and centrifugation. (**B**) Examples of melting curves fitted with the best R^2 in both sets; the filter criterion was $R^2 > 0.8$.

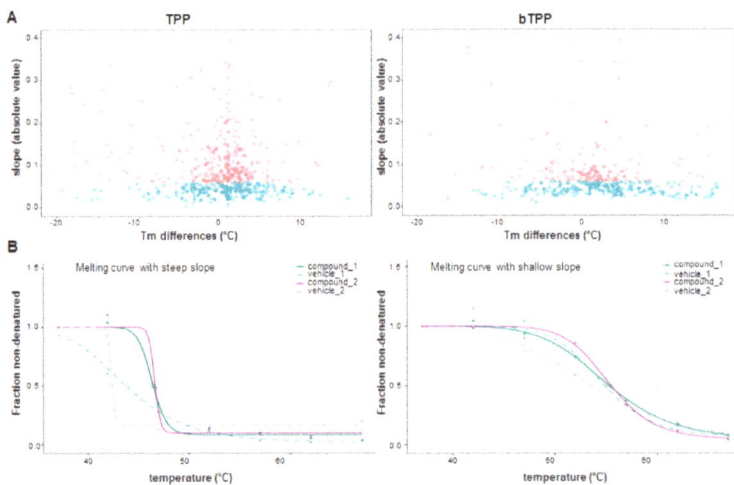

A

B

Figure 4. Differences in melting point between TPP and bTPP. (**A**) Volcano plots shown melting point differences between the two vehicle conditions versus the absolute slopes for the two vehicles and the two compound data sets. Proteins with an absolute slope below 0.06 are plotted in blue. (**B**) Example of a melting curve with a steep slope (left) and one with a shallow slope (right). Melting point reproducibility is dependent on the slope of the melting curve, with shallow slopes indicating less reproducibility.

The number of identified and quantified proteins were similar in both methods, at approximately 2500 proteins. The protein identification confirms that both datasets were associated with different subproteomes. The number of soluble proteins was lower in the subproteome that was utilized for the TPP method than in that used for the bTPP method. The sets of target proteins obtained using both methods differed in number and type of targets, with 19 proteins by TPP and 9 proteins by bTPP (Tables 1 and 2).

Table 1. Protein targets based on the bTPP method. Melting temperatures (Tm) and *p*-values calculated based on non-parametric analysis of response curves (NPARC).

Accession Name	Protein Name	Tm Control 1 (°C)	Tm Treatment 1 (°C)	Tm Control 2 (°C)	Tm Treatment 2 (°C)	*p*-Value
P08865 *	40S Ribosomal protein SA	45.74	47.16	45.32	49.00	0.0385
C9JC84	Fibrinogen gamma chain	44.09	45.32	44.74	47.63	0.1800
O75874	Isocitrate dehydrogenase [NADP] cytoplasmic	47.49	48.86	48.00	49.23	0.6307
P04792 *	Heat shock protein beta-1	45.23	49.82	47.94	51.40	0.0099
P17980	26S proteasome regulatory subunit 6A	44.67	47.01	44.18	46.65	0.1239
P30837	Aldehyde dehydrogenase X, mitochondrial	44.34	44.97	44.19	46.96	0.6788
P60953	Cell division control protein 42 homolog	46.93	47.70	47.09	51.92	0.6179
P68363 *	Tubulin alpha-1B chain	42.59	45.12	42.85	47.43	0.0242
Q9Y617	Phosphoserine aminotransferase	49.03	49.78	49.49	54.35	0.2253

* Proteins that passed quality criteria and *p*-values < 0.05.

Table 2. Protein targets based on TPP method. Melting temperatures (Tm) and *p*-values calculated based on NPARC.

Accession Name	Protein Name	Tm Control 1 (°C)	Tm Treatment 1 (°C)	Tm Control 2 (°C)	Tm Treatment 2 (°C)	*p*-Value
Q00341	Vigilin	47.04	50.62	46.91	47.60	0.2204
P42330 *	Aldo-keto reductase family 1-member C3	47.64	52.02	48.57	52.08	0.0001
G3V180	Dipeptidyl peptidase 3	52.55	55.30	53.01	56.06	0.6632
O14980	Exportin-1	47.84	49.29	49.28	51.48	0.1985
P00558	Phosphoglycerate kinase 1	53.07	53.91	53.03	54.06	0.9584
P07339 *	Cathepsin D	50.68	51.78	50.47	51.73	0.0045
P07814	Bifunctional glutamate/proline–tRNA ligase	43.83	46.51	42.48	46.70	0.2816
P08133	Annexin A6	52.45	53.03	52.99	55.30	0.9961
P09327	Villin-1	49.20	51.33	48.06	50.58	0.3429
P13674	Prolyl 4-hydroxylase subunit alpha-1	51.29	54.34	52.04	54.96	0.0954
P15559	NAD(P)H dehydrogenase [quinone] 1	49.21	50.48	49.08	49.30	0.8192
P30038	Delta-1-pyrroline-5-carboxylate dehydrogenase, mitochondrial	42.97	44.66	42.77	43.22	0.9284
P45954	Short/branched chain specific acyl-CoA dehydrogenase, mitochondrial	45.27	47.28	44.85	46.52	0.7475
P60709 *	Actin, cytoplasmic 1	44.10	48.42	41.84	45.14	0.0455
Q06210	Glutamine–fructose-6-phosphate aminotransferase [isomerizing] 1	47.31	48.12	47.14	47.55	0.9119
Q13347	Eukaryotic translation initiation factor 3 subunit I	46.89	48.21	46.64	46.91	0.6253
Q9NR45	Sialic acid synthase	53.17	53.41	53.22	54.67	0.4993
Q9Y490	Talin-1	49.93	51.85	51.75	53.92	0.1579
Q9Y696	Chloride intracellular channel protein 4	56.78	57.32	56.63	56.85	0.7306

* Proteins that met quality criteria with *p*-values < 0.05.

2.3. Deciphering the MOAs for 13^2-Hydroxypheophytine a by bTPP

The bTPP method was our method of choice for revealing the protein targets in our test compound, 13^2-hydroxypheophytine a. Although the compound was characterized in parallel with its analysis by bTPP, neither chemical nor functional characterization are presumed or required prior to bTPP analysis. The melting curves of the proteins that met all of the quality criteria for both biological replicates were defined as the target proteins. From approximately 2500 proteins analyzed, only 9 target proteins were determined (Figure 5A). These proteins include: 40S ribosomal protein SA (RPSA), which is involved in a wide variety of biological processes including cell adhesion, differentiation, migration, signaling, neurite outgrowth and metastasis; fibrinogen gamma chain (FGG), which is a signaling binding receptor; isocitrate dehydrogenase (IDH1), which is a peroxisomal matrix protein, the enzyme of which catalyzes the reversible oxidative decarboxylation of isocitrate to yield α-ketoglutarate; heat shock protein beta-1 (HSPB1), which is a molecular chaperone and plays a role in stress resistance and actin organization; 26S proteasome regulatory subunit 6A (PSMC3), which is part of the ATP-dependent degradation of ubiquitinated proteins; aldehyde dehydrogenase X (ALDH1B1), which is the enzyme participating in the metabolism of corticosteroids, biogenic amines, neurotransmitters, and lipid peroxidation; the cell division control protein 42 homolog (CDC42), which participates in the regulation of the cell cycle; tubulin alpha-1B chain (TUBA1B), which is a structural protein in the cell; and phosphoserine aminotransferase (PSAT1), which is involved in amino acid synthesis. The targets resulting from the bTPP analysis were investigated for any implications on molecular pathways and cellular functions that might offer initial clues to deciphering the MOA of this compound after interaction with liver cells. The most relevant pathways discussed include serine oxidation, NADPH regeneration, and ethanol oxidation (Figure 5B).

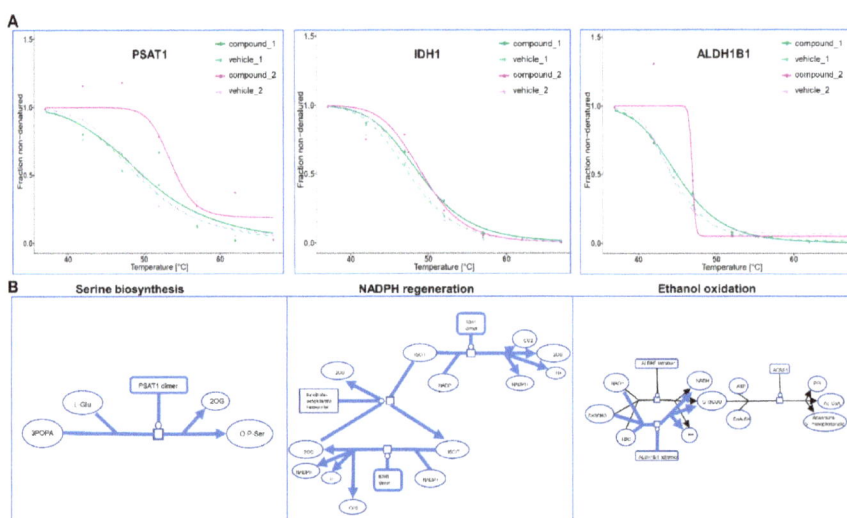

Figure 5. Target proteins and mechanism of actions based on bTPP analysis. (**A**) Melting curves of 3 of the target proteins. (**B**) Pathways of phosphoserine aminotransferase (left), isocitrate dehydrogenase (middle) and aldehyde dehydrogenase X (right).

3. Discussion

We present a TPP-based method that could provide an unbiased identification of target proteins in bioactive compounds without any preliminary information about chemical, functional or phenotypical characterization. The development of the method was specifically oriented towards novel compounds found in the course of biodiscovery. Here, we present a proof-of-concept by applying the novel method to a compound that has recently been isolated from a marine cyanobacteria due to its lipid-reducing activities [14]. The compound is a chlorophyll derivative, 13^2-hydroxy-pheophytine a, which is present in marine and terrestrial organisms. The high rate of production of this molecule in *Spirulina* may enable the development of a future nutraceutical [14], and the identification of its protein targets will be an important step towards this aim.

The TTP is a thermal proteome profiling method, a high-throughput approach that makes it possible to examine an entire soluble proteome for its capability to interact with a drug in a single analytical experiment. Thermal shift-based methods have gained attention in the field of drug biodiscovery since the introduction of proteome analysis and protein target detection on the basis of mass spectrometry [8]. The improved method presented here, named bTPP, differs from the previous TPP methods developed for drug discovery in terms of the definition of the soluble fraction. This fraction is the subproteome analyzed by the thermal shift assay and is a pillar of the method. The robustness of the method and the reproducibility of its results would greatly depend on subjecting a single well-defined soluble proteome and compound to a series of incubations at range of increasing temperatures. If those parameters are modified by the methodological constraints, and the concentrations of the soluble proteins and the compound are variable, the proteomic analyses obtained by the thermal shift assays will not be able to be compiled in order to obtain target identification.

By reviewing theoretical concepts in the field of cellular fractionation in connection with our findings, we determined that the sedimentation force applied to differentiate the soluble proteins from the vesicle-associated proteins using the TPP method [18] did not reach the minimal sedimentation force required to remove microsomal vesicles- by centrifugation [15,17]. The definition of the protein composition of a soluble fraction is not a universal concept. Rather, it is dependent on factors intrinsic to the sample: cell type, composition of the extraction solution, and the method applied for cellular homogenization. No less important are the extrinsic factors, including differential centrifugation, which aim to differentiate soluble from membrane-associated proteins. The soluble fraction is frequently obtained after applying 20,000 g for 20 min [8], or 100,000 g for 20 min of centrifugation [15,17,18]. These processes would barely be sufficient to clarify homogenized cells from the unbroken cells and the nuclear fraction. This type of soluble fraction still contains an abundant portion of organellar fractions such as mitochondria, lysosomes, peroxisomes and microsomal vesicles from the vesicular transport or plasma membrane. Proteins from these vesicle-rich fractions are semi-stable in solution, and would easily become unstable and have their precipitation prompted by the application of the additional steps of centrifugation force required to reach their specific centrifugation coefficients. This is the situation encountered by the TPP soluble fraction when a second centrifugation step at 100,000 g for 20 min is added in order to separate the unfolded proteins from the soluble proteins [18]. Therefore, in the TPP method, the classical microsomal fraction is part of the soluble fraction that is incubated with a bioactive compound. The presence of vesicle-associated proteins in the studied subproteome interferes with the expected results at different levels.

First, the TPP method is based on the incubation of the soluble sample at a fixed concentration that is close to the IC$_{50}$ of the compound at a series of increasing temperatures. The semi-stable soluble proteins after 20 min centrifugation contain vesicle-associated proteins. Those vesicles can potentially interact with hydrophobic compounds and entrap them within the membranes. This was the case for our test compound. The first consequence of this is that the concentration of the compound available for direct interaction with soluble proteins would shift away from the IC$_{50}$, and the concentration would therefore be unknown. On the other hand, the compound inserted into the membranes could also interact with the soluble proteins, potentially leading to precipitation in association with the membrane.

Secondly, the fraction of the compound remaining in the solution would interact with the soluble proteins as predicted by TPP but would also interact with the membrane proteins in the vesicles that were not able to be evaluated using the method. Such interactions would further reduce the opportunities for interaction with the soluble proteins, which are the only proteins under evaluation. This is a second mechanism that modifies both the predicted concentration of the proteins during incubation and the predicted concentration of the compound.

Thirdly, the increasing temperature of successive incubations would affect the vesicles and their fluidity. It should at least be considered that the heterogeneity of the population of microsomal membranes would vary. At higher temperatures, there is expected to be an increase in the proportion of smaller vesicles. Smaller vesicles require a higher sedimentation force than bigger ones. Therefore, at higher temperatures, it is expected that there will be smaller vesicles in the solution and a reduction in the precipitation of the microsomal fraction compared to that observed at lower temperatures.

This parameter is a variable that will affect the precipitation independently from the thermal shift factor or the total time of the centrifugation, and it will vary from temperature to temperature. In summary, applying the concept of the thermal shift to a soluble fraction obtained below the sedimentation coefficient for microsomal membranes will add many new variables to the system that are not considered by the method. Our results showed that this reduces the specificity and sensitivity required for an unbiased identification of the protein targets of our chosen test compound. Therefore, we developed the bTPP by modifying the criterion for protein solubility to require a centrifugation step of 100,000 *g* for 60 min, which is equivalent to the classical criterion for the precipitation of a microsomal fraction.

The bTPP method was our method of choice for revealing the protein targets of our test compound following confirmation that the parameters affecting the thermal shift analysis by bTPP were exclusively dependent on the interaction capability of the studied bioactive compound with the subproteome of the soluble proteins, and that the incubation at the different temperatures would not interfere with or cause variation in the concentration of the compound or the soluble protein. Here, we applied the bTPP method for our test compound without considering any preliminary information regarding its chemical structure, or evaluation or interpretation of the data from any functional assays. Nine proteins were assigned as its cellular targets in hepatocytes. In making a first attempt to discover any functional application of the compound, these targets were integrated in a map of functional pathways.

PSAT1 has already been described as a promising target for anticancer therapy [19]. This enzyme, which is involved in serine biosynthesis, has been associated with the metabolism of cancer, as extracellular serine may be sufficient to maintain cancer cell proliferation [20]. It has been proposed to be an oncogene with a significant role in cancer progression, inducing up-regulation of cyclin D1 via GSK3beta/beta-catenin pathway, leading to the acceleration of the cell cycle [21]. From a physiological perspective focusing on obesity and its related metabolic diseases, hepatic PSAT1 has revealed a novel function in the regulation of insulin sensitivity. The involvement of the nonessential amino acid serine in the regulation of insulin sensitivity opened lines of research into the targeting of PSAT1 for treatment of insulin resistance and type 2 diabetes in mice [22]. These effects on insulin-related disorders such as obesity and type 2 diabetes are also connected to two other protein targets, as revealed by bTPP with our test compound. For instance, ALDHs and their family of enzymes play a protective role in diseases related with obesity. ALDH2 has a role in the protection against diabetic cardiomyopathy, possibly via an Akt-GSK3b-mediated route, lending ALDH2 therapeutic promise in the management of diabetic complications [23]. Yu et al. [24] showed that the activation of the PKCε-ALDH2 regulatory axis may be a therapeutic target for treating obesity and type 2 diabetes in mice. Nonalcoholic fatty liver disease (NAFLD) is the most frequent chronic liver disease; alcohol dehydrogenase and aldehyde dehydrogenase collectively showed altered expression and function in the progression of nonalcoholic steatohepatitis (NASH) patients, which may also lead to significant alterations in the pharmacokinetics of substrate drugs. This information could be useful in making appropriate dosing adjustments for NAFLD patients taking drugs that are metabolized by these pathways [25].

Looking into IDHs, this target protein catalyzes the oxidative decarboxylation of isocitrate to α-ketoglutarate and reduces $NAD(P)^+$ to NAD(P). IDH2 has been suggested as a potential therapeutic target in the treatment of type 2 diabetes and obesity due to its major role in modulating both insulin sensitivity and fuel metabolism in mice [26]. Moreover, Koh et al. [27] reported for the first time that cytosolic $NADP^+$-dependent isocitrate dehydrogenase (IDPc) plays a critical role in fat and cholesterol biosynthesis, showing that transgenic mice with overexpressed IDPc exhibited fatty liver, hyperlipidemia, and obesity without an increase in caloric intake or change in diet composition, converting IDPc into a potential therapeutic target for abnormal fat synthesis. In summary, these 3 target proteins of 13^2-hydroxy-pheophytine a are associated with beneficial properties towards obesity and obesity-related comorbidities. The next steps for progressing towards future application as a possible nutraceutical would be the carrying out of further research in order to validate the targets *in vivo* in a more complex organismal context. However, this study demonstrates that this methodology is able to accelerate the process between the biodiscovery of novel bioactive compounds to the revelation of protein targets involved in MOA of interest for intervention and application.

4. Materials and Methods

4.1. Reagents and Cell Culture

Reagents and medium were purchased from Sigma-Aldrich (Sant Louis, MO, USA), unless otherwise noted. PBS was purchased from Trevigen (Gaithersburg, MD, USA) and supplemented with 10 µL of ProteoGuard™ EDTA-Free Protease Inhibitor Cocktail (Takara Bio USA, Inc., Mountain View, CA, USA) per 1 mL. HepG2 cells were grown in EMEM medium supplemented with 8% fetal bovine serum (ATTC), 1675 mM L-glutamine, 85 U/mL penicillin, 85 µg/mL streptomycin of 80% confluence. Cells were harvested and centrifugated at 340 *g* for 2 min at 4 °C and resuspended in 50 mL PBS. After a second wash step, the cells were resuspended in 10 mL ice-cold PBS and centrifugated again at 340 *g* for 2 min at 4 °C. Washed pellets were either used directly or snap frozen in liquid nitrogen and stored at −80 °C until lysis.

4.2. Selection of 13^2-Hydroxypheophytine a as Test Compound

The compound selected for the proof-of-concept was 13^2-hydroxy-pheophytin a (*hpa*), isolated from the marine cyanobacterial strain LEGE 07175 due to its lipid-reducing activity. The purity was estimated to ~99% by HR-ESI-MS and ^{1}H-NMR analysis (Figure S1). The growth conditions of the cyanobacteria, as well as the chemical isolation methodology, are detailed in Freitas et al., 2019 [14].

4.3. Thermal Proteome Profiling Experiments in Cellular Protein Extracts

The experiments following the TPP method were performed as described in Franken et al. [18] with some modifications. Briefly, cells were resuspended in ice-cold PBS. The cells were homogenized in a Labsonic P disintegrator (B. Braun Biotech International, Göttingen, Germany) with an ultrasonic probe of 3 mm at 25% intensity and 0.5 cycles, with manual switches of 10 s on/5 s off, maintaining the sample in an ice bath. The sample was centrifugated at 100,000 *g* for 20 min at 4 °C [12]. The supernatant from this ultracentrifugation rendered the soluble subproteome that was applied in the TPP method. For the bTPP method, the homogenized sample was centrifugated at 100,000 *g* for 60 min at 4 °C. Protein concentration was determined by Bradford assay (Thermo Fisher Scientific, Waltham, MA, USA) [28]. From this point on, the process in both methods is identical. Two sets of thermal shift assays were performed using each methodology. The samples were incubated for 10 min at 25 °C. For the studied compound, incubation was performed at the compound IC_{50}, and for the control, in the presence of the compound vehicle (DMSO). Seven aliquots of 100 µg of protein were individually heated for 3 min at different temperatures: 37 °C, 42 °C, 47 °C, 52 °C, 57 °C, 62 °C and 67 °C, followed by 3 min at room temperature. Subsequently, the samples were centrifugated at 100,000 *g* for 20 min at 4 °C. The supernatants were analyzed by label-free liquid chromatography-tandem mass spectrometry (nLC-MS/MS) (Thermo Fisher Scientific, Waltham, MA, USA). In accordance with the TPP method, two biological replicates for each set of the thermal shift assay were performed [18].

4.4. Filter Aided Sample Preparation (FASP)

Protein samples were prepared according to Wiśniewski et al. (2012) [29]. The sample was diluted with 200 µL of 8 M urea in 0.1M Tris/HCl, pH 8.5 (UA) in 30 kDa microcon centrifugal filter unit (Merck Millipore, # MRCF0R030, Burlington, MA, USA). The centrifugal filters were centrifugated at 14,000× *g* at 20 °C for 15 min. The concentrates were diluted with 200 µL of UA and centrifugated at 14,000× *g* at 20 °C for 15 min. After discharging the flow-through, 100 µL of 0.05 M iodoacetamide was added to the column, mixed for 1 min at 600 rpm on a thermo-mixer (Eppendorf thermo mixer comfort, Hamburg, Germany), and incubated static for 20 min in dark. The solution was drained by spinning the columns at 14,000 *g* for 10 min. The columns were washed three times with 100 µL buffer UA and centrifugated at 14,000 *g* for 15 min. The columns were washed three times with 100 µL of 50 mM ammonium bicarbonate. Endopeptidase trypsin (Trypsin sequencing grade, Roche # 03708985001, Sigma-Aldrich, Sant Louis, MO, USA) solution in the ratio 1:100 was prepared with 50 mM ammonium bicarbonate (40 µL), dispensed and mixed at 600 rpm in the thermomixer for 1 min. These units were then incubated in a wet chamber at 37 °C for about 18 h to achieve effective trypsination. After 18 h of incubation, the filter units were transferred into new collection tubes. To recover the digested peptides, the tubes were centrifugated at 14,000 *g* for 10 min. Peptide recovery was completed by rinsing the filters with 50 µL of 0.5 M NaCl and collected by centrifugation. The samples were acidified with 10% formic acid (56302 Fluka, Sigma-Aldrich, Sant Louis, MO, USA) to achieve a pH between 3 and 2. Desalting was done using reverse-phase C18 top tips (TT2C18.96, Glygen, Columbia, MD, USA) using acetonitrile (ACN) (60% *v/v*) with formic acid (FA) (0.1% *v/v*) for elution, and vacuum dried (Savant SPD 1010, Thermo Fisher Scientific, Waltham, MA, USA) to be stored at −80 °C until further analysis.

4.5. Nano LC-MS/MS Analysis

The desalted peptides were reconstituted with 0.1% formic acid in ultra-pure milli-Q water, and the concentration was measured using a Nanodrop (ND 2000, Thermo Fisher Scientific, Waltham, MA, USA). The peptides were analyzed using a reverse phase nano-LC (liquid chromatography, Thermo Fisher Scientific, Waltham, MA, USA) coupled to a hybrid LTQ Orbitrap Velos Pro mass spectrometer (Thermo Fisher Scientific, Waltham, MA, USA). Each of the samples was separated using an Agilent 1200 Easy nLC (Agilent Technologies, Santa Clara, CA, USA) system with a nano-electrospray ion source (Thermo Fisher Scientific, Waltham, MA, USA). The peptides were trapped on a pre-column (NS-MP-10-C18-Biosphere, 5 µm particle size, 120 Å, 100 µm × 20 cm) and separated on an analytical column (NS-AC-10-C18-Biosphere, 5 µm particle size, 120 Å, 75 µm × 10.2 cm). A linear gradient of 2 to 40% buffer B (0.1% formic acid in acetonitrile) against buffer A (0.1% formic acid in water) was carried out with a constant flow rate of 300 nL/min, for a 90 min gradient. Full scan MS spectra were acquired in the positive mode electrospray ionization with an ion spray voltage of 2.4 KV, an RF lens voltage of 69, and a capillary temperature of 235 °C. This was acquired over an *m/z* of 380–2000 Da at a resolution of 30,000, and the 20 most intense ions were selected for MS/MS under an isolation width of 1 *m/z* units. Collision energy of 35 was used to fragment the ions in the collision-induced dissociation mode.

4.6. Peptide and Protein Identification and Quantification

Proteome Discoverer (v2.1, Thermo Fisher Scientific, Waltham, MA, USA) was used for protein identification and quantification. The MS/MS spectra (.raw files) were searched by Sequest HT against the human database from Uniprot (73,928 entries). A maximum of 2 tryptic cleavages were allowed, the precursor and fragment mass tolerance were 10 ppm and 0.6 Da, respectively. Peptides with a false discovery rate (FDR) of less than 0.01 and validation based on q-value were used as identified. The minimum peptide length considered was 6, and the false discovery rate (FDR) was set to 0.1. Proteins were quantified using the average of the top three peptide MS1-areas, yielding raw protein abundances. Common contaminants like human keratin and bovine trypsin were also included in the database during the searches in order to minimize false identifications. The mass spectrometry proteomics data have been deposited in the ProteomeXchange Consortium via the PRIDE [30] partner repository with the dataset identifier PXD013227.

4.7. Analysis of TPP Experiments

Melting curves were calculated using a sigmoidal fitting approach with the R package TPP, as described in Franken et al. [18], with modifications. The fold changes were changed to correspond to the 7 temperatures, and the filter criteria for normalization were adjusted to this number of temperatures.

The melting curves were fitted after normalization following the equation described in Savitski et al. [8], computed in R:

$$f(T) = \frac{1 - plateau}{1 + e^{-(\frac{a}{T} - b)}} + plateau$$

where T is the temperature, and a, b and "plateau" are constants. The value of $f(T)$ at the lowest temperature T_{min} was fixed at 1. The melting point of a protein is defined as the temperature T_m at which half of the amount of the protein has been denatured. The quality criteria for filtering the sigmoidal melting curves were: (i) fitted curves for both vehicle- and compound-treated conditions had an R^2 of >0.8; (ii) the vehicle curve had a plateau of <0.3; (iii) the melting point differences under both the control and the treatment conditions were greater than the melting point difference between the two controls; and (iv) in each biological replicate, the steepest slope of the protein melting curve in the paired set of vehicle- and compound-treated conditions was below −0.06. The NPARC of the R package was used to detect significant changes in the temperature-dependent melting behavior of each protein due to changes in experimental conditions [18]. The significance threshold was set at $p < 0.05$.

4.8. Pathway Analysis and Visualization

Pathway analysis was performed using Reactome Pathway analysis [31].

5. Conclusions

We have demonstrated that the thermal shift assay cannot be applied to a subproteome that contains soluble and vesicular fractions. We have deconvoluted the effects of a vesicular fraction in the protein sample, altering the concentration of protein and compound during the assay. These variations introduce uncertainties that challenge the principles of this methodology. Therefore, we presented an improved TPP method named bTPP based on a different postulate for protein solubility. The improvements guarantee that the concentration of proteins and compounds available for a raw thermal shift assay remains constant at any temperature. Finally, in a proof-of-concept experiment, we identified the protein targets in liver cells of 13^2-hydroxy-pheophytine a, a compound recently isolated from a marine cyanobacteria due to its lipid-reducing activities. Three of these proteins have known regulations of insulin sensitivity and energy metabolism.

Supplementary Materials: The following are available online at http://www.mdpi.com/1660-3397/17/6/371/s1, Figure S1: Spectrum of the 13^2-hydroxy-pheophytine a, isolated from a marine cyanobacteria (LEGE07175) of the CIIMAR cyanobacterial culture collection (LEGE-CC), Figure S2: Melting curves from protein targets from bTPP.

Author Contributions: S.C. designed and supervised the experiments, and performed the initial TPP experiments; O.F. implemented the experimental design with scientific advice, and performed the cell lab experiments on the protein extracts and the initial TPP experiments; A.C.d.A. performed most of the TPP experiments, performed the mass spectrometry analysis, implemented the bioinformatic tools for TPP analysis, and performed the TPP analysis; S.F. and R.U. isolated and produced the test compound. A.C.d.A., O.F. and S.C. wrote the manuscript. All authors revised the manuscript.

Funding: This project received funding from the ERA-NET Marine Biotechnology project CYANOBESITY that it is cofounding from FORMAS, Sweden grant nr. 2016-02004 (SC), FCT Foundation of Science and Technology, Portugal, grant number ERA-MBT/0001/2015 (RU). This work has also been funded by IKERBASQUE (SC), Basque Government grant IT-971-16 (SC and OF), and FCT grants SFRH/BPD/112287/2015, SFRH/BD/116009/2016, FCT strategic fund (UID/Multi/04423/2019) (RU and SF).

Acknowledgments: We thank to all the members of ERA-NET MB Cyanobesity consortium for the fruitful scientific discussions. All the mass spectrometry analysis has been performed with instrumentation at the LiU MS facility.

Conflicts of Interest: The authors declare no conflict of interest.

Abbreviations

TPP	thermal proteome profiling
MOA	mechanisms of action
CETSA	cellular thermal shift assay

bTPP	bioactive thermal proteome profiling
Tm	melting temperature
hpa	132-hydroxy-pheophytin a
DMSO	dimethyl sulfoxide
PBS	phosphate buffered saline
nLC-MS/MS	nano liquid chromatography-tandem mass spectrometry
FASP	filter aided sample preparation
RPSA	40S ribosomal protein SA
FGG	fibrinogen gamma chain
IDH1	isocitrate dehydrogenase
HSPB1	heat shock protein beta-1
PSMC3	26S proteasome regulatory subunit 6A
ALDH1B1	aldehyde dehydrogenase X
CDC42	cell division control protein 42 homolog
TUBA1B	tubulin alpha-1B chain
PSAT1	phosphoserine aminotransferase
NPARC	non-parametric analysis of response curves

References

1. Moffat, J.G.; Vincent, F.; Lee, J.A.; Eder, J.; Prunotto, M. Opportunities and challenges in phenotypic drug discovery: An industry perspective. *Nat. Rev. Drug Discov.* **2017**, *16*, 531–543. [CrossRef] [PubMed]

2. Lindsay, M.A. Target discovery. *Nat. Rev. Drug Discov.* **2003**, *2*, 831–838. [CrossRef] [PubMed]

3. Kuruvilla, J.; Bayat, N.; Cristobal, S. Proteomic Analysis of Endothelial Cells Exposed to Ultrasmall Nanoparticles Reveals Disruption in Paracellular and Transcellular Transport. *Proteomics* **2019**, *19*, 1800228. [CrossRef] [PubMed]

4. Hopkins, A.L.; Groom, C.R. The druggable genome. *Nat. Rev. Drug Discov.* **2002**, *1*, 727–730. [CrossRef] [PubMed]

5. Ruiz-Garcia, A.; Bermejo, M.; Moss, A.; Casabo, V.G. Pharmacokinetics in drug discovery. *J. Pharm. Sci.* **2008**, *97*, 654–690. [CrossRef] [PubMed]

6. Martinez Molina, D.; Jafari, R.; Ignatushchenko, M.; Seki, T.; Larsson, E.A.; Dan, C.; Sreekumar, L.; Cao, Y.; Nordlund, P. Monitoring drug target engagement in cells and tissues using the cellular thermal shift assay. *Science* **2013**, *341*, 84–87. [CrossRef] [PubMed]

7. Kurganov, B.I.; Rafikova, E.R.; Dobrov, E.N. Kinetics of thermal aggregation of tobacco mosaic virus coat protein. *Biochemistry* **2002**, *67*, 525–533.

8. Savitski, M.M.; Reinhard, F.B.; Franken, H.; Werner, T.; Savitski, M.F.; Eberhard, D.; Martinez Molina, D.; Jafari, R.; Dovega, R.B.; Klaeger, S.; et al. Tracking cancer drugs in living cells by thermal profiling of the proteome. *Science* **2014**, *346*, 1255784. [CrossRef]

9. Becher, I.; Werner, T.; Doce, C.; Zaal, E.A.; Togel, I.; Khan, C.A.; Rueger, A.; Muelbaier, M.; Salzer, E.; Berkers, C.R.; et al. Thermal profiling reveals phenylalanine hydroxylase as an off-target of panobinostat. *Nat. Chem. Biol.* **2016**, *12*, 908–910. [CrossRef]

10. Azimi, A.; Caramuta, S.; Seashore-Ludlow, B.; Bostrom, J.; Robinson, J.L.; Edfors, F.; Tuominen, R.; Kemper, K.; Krijgsman, O.; Peeper, D.S.; et al. Targeting CDK2 overcomes melanoma resistance against BRAF and Hsp90 inhibitors. *Mol. Syst. Biol.* **2018**, *14*, e7858. [CrossRef]

11. Turkowsky, D.; Lohmann, P.; Muhlenbrink, M.; Schubert, T.; Adrian, L.; Goris, T.; Jehmlich, N.; von Bergen, M. Thermal proteome profiling allows quantitative assessment of interactions between tetrachloroethene reductive dehalogenase and trichloroethene. *J. Proteom.* **2019**, *192*, 10–17. [CrossRef] [PubMed]

12. Savitski, M.M.; Zinn, N.; Faelth-Savitski, M.; Poeckel, D.; Gade, S.; Becher, I.; Muelbaier, M.; Wagner, A.J.; Strohmer, K.; Werner, T.; et al. Multiplexed Proteome Dynamics Profiling Reveals Mechanisms Controlling Protein Homeostasis. *Cell* **2018**, *173*, 260–274.e25. [CrossRef] [PubMed]

13. Mi, Y.; Zhang, J.; He, S.; Yan, X. New Peptides Isolated from Marine Cyanobacteria, an Overview over the Past Decade. *Mar. Drugs* **2017**, *15*, 132. [CrossRef] [PubMed]

14. Freitas, S.; Silva, N.G.; Sousa, M.L.; Ribeiro, T.; Rosa, F.; Leao, P.N.; Vasconcelos, V.; Reis, M.A.; Urbatzka, R. Chlorophyll Derivatives from Marine Cyanobacteria with Lipid-Reducing Activities. *Mar. Drugs* **2019**, *17*, 229. [CrossRef] [PubMed]

15. Cristobal, S.; Ochoa, B.; Fresnedo, O. Purification and properties of a cholesteryl ester hydrolase from rat liver microsomes. *J. Lipid Res.* **1999**, *40*, 715–725. [PubMed]

16. Morgenstern, R.; Guthenberg, C.; Depierre, J.W. Microsomal glutathione S-transferase. Purification, initial characterization and demonstration that it is not identical to the cytosolic glutathione S-transferases A, B and C. *Eur. J. Biochem.* **1982**, *128*, 243–248. [CrossRef] [PubMed]

17. Duve, C. Exploring cells with a centrifuge. *Science* **1975**, *189*, 186–194. [CrossRef] [PubMed]

18. Franken, H.; Mathieson, T.; Childs, D.; Sweetman, G.M.; Werner, T.; Togel, I.; Doce, C.; Gade, S.; Bantscheff, M.; Drewes, G.; et al. Thermal proteome profiling for unbiased identification of direct and indirect drug targets using multiplexed quantitative mass spectrometry. *Nat. Protoc.* **2015**, *10*, 1567–1593. [CrossRef] [PubMed]

19. Liu, B.; Jia, Y.; Cao, Y.; Wu, S.; Jiang, H.; Sun, X.; Ma, J.; Yin, X.; Mao, A.; Shang, M. Overexpression of Phosphoserine Aminotransferase 1 (PSAT1) Predicts Poor Prognosis and Associates with Tumor Progression in Human Esophageal Squamous Cell Carcinoma. *Cell. Physiol. Biochem.* **2016**, *39*, 395–406. [CrossRef]

20. Mattaini, K.R.; Sullivan, M.R.; Vander Heiden, M.G. The importance of serine metabolism in cancer. *J. Cell Biol.* **2016**, *214*, 249–257. [CrossRef]

21. Gao, S.; Ge, A.; Xu, S.; You, Z.; Ning, S.; Zhao, Y.; Pang, D. PSAT1 is regulated by ATF4 and enhances cell proliferation via the GSK3beta/beta-catenin/cyclin D1 signaling pathway in ER-negative breast cancer. *J. Exp. Clin. Cancer Res.* **2017**, *36*, 179. [CrossRef] [PubMed]

22. Yu, J.; Xiao, F.; Guo, Y.; Deng, J.; Liu, B.; Zhang, Q.; Li, K.; Wang, C.; Chen, S.; Guo, F. Hepatic Phosphoserine Aminotransferase 1 Regulates Insulin Sensitivity in Mice via Tribbles Homolog 3. *Diabetes* **2015**, *64*, 1591–1602. [CrossRef] [PubMed]

23. Zhang, Y.; Babcock, S.A.; Hu, N.; Maris, J.R.; Wang, H.; Ren, J. Mitochondrial aldehyde dehydrogenase (ALDH2) protects against streptozotocin-induced diabetic cardiomyopathy: Role of GSK3beta and mitochondrial function. *BMC Med.* **2012**, *10*, 40. [CrossRef] [PubMed]

24. Yu, Y.H.; Liao, P.R.; Guo, C.J.; Chen, C.H.; Mochly-Rosen, D.; Chuang, L.M. PKC-ALDH2 Pathway Plays a Novel Role in Adipocyte Differentiation. *PLoS ONE* **2016**, *11*, e0161993. [CrossRef] [PubMed]

25. Li, H.; Toth, E.; Cherrington, N.J. Alcohol Metabolism in the Progression of Human Nonalcoholic Steatohepatitis. *Toxicol. Sci.* **2018**, *164*, 428–438. [CrossRef] [PubMed]

26. Lee, S.J.; Kim, S.H.; Park, K.M.; Lee, J.H.; Park, J.W. Increased obesity resistance and insulin sensitivity in mice lacking the isocitrate dehydrogenase 2 gene. *Free Radic. Biol. Med.* **2016**, *99*, 179–188. [CrossRef] [PubMed]

27. Koh, H.J.; Lee, S.M.; Son, B.G.; Lee, S.H.; Ryoo, Z.Y.; Chang, K.T.; Park, J.W.; Park, D.C.; Song, B.J.; Veech, R.L.; et al. Cytosolic NADP+-dependent isocitrate dehydrogenase plays a key role in lipid metabolism. *J. Biol. Chem.* **2004**, *279*, 39968–39974. [CrossRef] [PubMed]

28. Bradford, M.M. A rapid and sensitive method for the quantitation of microgram quantities of protein utilizing the principle of protein-dye binding. *Anal. Biochem.* **1976**, *72*, 248–254. [CrossRef]

29. Wisniewski, J.R.; Zougman, A.; Nagaraj, N.; Mann, M. Universal sample preparation method for proteome analysis. *Nat. Methods* **2009**, *6*, 359–362. [CrossRef] [PubMed]

30. Vizcaino, J.A.; Csordas, A.; del-Toro, N.; Dianes, J.A.; Griss, J.; Lavidas, I.; Mayer, G.; Perez-Riverol, Y.; Reisinger, F.; Ternent, T.; et al. 2016 update of the PRIDE database and its related tools. *Nucleic Acids Res.* **2016**, *44*, D447–D456. [CrossRef]

31. Fabregat, A.; Sidiropoulos, K.; Garapati, P.; Gillespie, M.; Hausmann, K.; Haw, R.; Jassal, B.; Jupe, S.; Korninger, F.; McKay, S.; et al. The Reactome pathway Knowledgebase. *Nucleic Acids Res.* **2016**, *44*, D481–D487. [CrossRef] [PubMed]

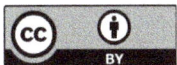

marine drugs

MDPI

Article

New Aromatic Bisabolane Derivatives with Lipid-Reducing Activity from the Marine Sponge *Myrmekioderma* sp.

Margarida Costa [1],*, Laura Coello [2], Ralph Urbatzka [3], Marta Pérez [2] and Margret Thorsteinsdottir [1]

[1]   Faculty of Pharmaceutical Sciences, University of Iceland, Hofsvallagata 53, 107 Reykjavik, Iceland; margreth@hi.is

[2]   Research & Development Department, PharmaMar S.A., Pol. Ind. La Mina Norte, Avda. de los Reyes 1, 28770 Colmenar Viejo (Madrid), Spain; lcoello@pharmamar.com (L.C.); mperez@pharmamar.com (M.P.)

[3]   Interdisciplinary Centre of Marine and Environmental Research (CIIMAR/CIMAR), University of Porto, Avenida General Norton de Matos, s/n, 4450-208 Matosinhos, Portugal; ralph.urbatzka.ciimar@gmail.com

*   Correspondence: costa.anamarg@gmail.com; Tel.: +354-659-1222

Received: 24 March 2019; Accepted: 17 June 2019; Published: 22 June 2019

Abstract: The previously reported 1-(2,4-dihydroxy-5-methylphenyl)ethan-1-one (**1**), (1′Z)-2-(1′,5′-dimethylhexa-1′,4′-dieny1)-5-methylbenzene-1,4-diol (**2**), and 1,8-epoxy-1(6),2,4,7,10-bisaborapentaen-4-ol (**5**) together with four new structures of aromatic bisabolane-related compounds (**3**, **4**, **6**, **7**) were isolated from the marine sponge *Myrmekioderma* sp. Compounds **1**, **2**, and **5** were identified based on spectral data available in the literature. The structures of the four new compounds were experimentally established by 1D and 2D-NMR and (−)-HRESIMS spectral analysis. Cytotoxic and lipid-reducing activities of the isolated compounds were evaluated. None of the isolated compounds were active against the tested cancer cell lines; however, lipid-reducing activity was found for compounds **2–5** and **7** in the zebrafish Nile red fat metabolism assay. This class of compounds should be further explored for their suitability as possible agents for the treatment of lipid metabolic disorders and obesity.

Keywords: marine sponges; natural compounds; bisabolane-related compounds; bioactivity; obesity; whole small animal models

---

1. Introduction

Marine organisms are exposed to continuous and strong selection pressures due to the huge variations in predation, temperature, pressure, and light. For these reasons, they are known to produce secondary metabolites as a mechanism of defense [1]. These secondary metabolites represent an impressive source of structurally diverse molecules with biological activities which can lead to major advances in the field of medicinal chemistry [2,3].

Among marine organisms, sponges represent a prolific source of a vast number of diverse molecules with potential applications for human health. The numbers of compounds isolated from sponges have been increasing every year [4]. Among these compounds, marine sesquiterpenes are recognized as an important class with great structural diversity and a wide range of bioactivities such as anti-HIV, antitumor, antibiotic, antiviral, cytotoxic, insecticidal, antifeedant, and antifungal activities [5,6]. Bisabolane compounds constitute a class of sesquiterpene bioactive metabolites that have been identified from both terrestrial plants and marine invertebrates [7,8]. Several bioactivities are associated with this class of compounds, such as cytotoxicity [9,10] and antifungal [10] properties. Furthermore, their suitability for use as biodiesel is also under investigation [11].

Obesity is increasing at epidemic rates and new therapeutics are needed in order to prevent and control this disorder [12]. Scientists have been working hard to find new compounds from different natural sources, both terrestrial and marine, that show anti-obesity activity [13–15]. Several marine secondary metabolites with anti-obesity properties have already been reported, such as the 5-alkylpyrrole-2-carboxaldehyde derivatives, isolated from the sponge *Mycale lissochela*, which have protein-tyrosine phosphatase 1B (a recognized target for obesity) inhibitory activity [6]. Also, citreorosein and questinol, isolated from the marine sponge-associated fungus *Talaromyces stipitatus* KUFA 0207, decreased the neutral lipids in the zebrafish Nile red fat metabolism assay [16].

As a part of our on-going screening program for the discovery of new secondary metabolites from marine sponges, the study of an organic extract of *Myrmekioderma* sp. resulted in the isolation of seven natural compounds: three known compounds 1-(2,4-dihydroxy-5-methylphenyl)ethan-1-one (**1**), (1′Z)-2-(1′,5′-dimethylhexa-1′,4′-dieny1)-5-methylbenzene-1,4-diol (**2**), 1,8-epoxy-1(6),2,4,7,10-bisaborapentaen-4-ol (**5**), and four new bisabolane derivatives (**3, 4, 6** and **7**). Their planar structures were fully elucidated using spectroscopic and spectrometric techniques. All compounds were tested for their cytotoxic and lipid-reducing activities. Compounds **2**, **5**, and **7** were highly active in the zebrafish Nile red fat metabolism assay and compounds **3** and **4** showed moderate activity in the same bioassay. Cytotoxic activity in the four cancer cell lines tested was not observed for any of the isolated compounds.

2. Results and Discussion

Isolation and Structure Elucidation

The sponge *Myrmekioderma* sp. was collected by hand while scuba diving in Boano (Indonesia). The specimen was repeatedly extracted using dichloromethane:methanol (1:1 v/v). The crude organic extract was subsequently partitioned between *n*-hexane, ethyl acetate, *n*-butanol, and water. The *n*-hexane and ethyl acetate fractions, after vacuum liquid chromatography (VLC) and semi-preparative reverse-phase HPLC separations, led to the isolation of the seven pure compounds shown in Figure 1.

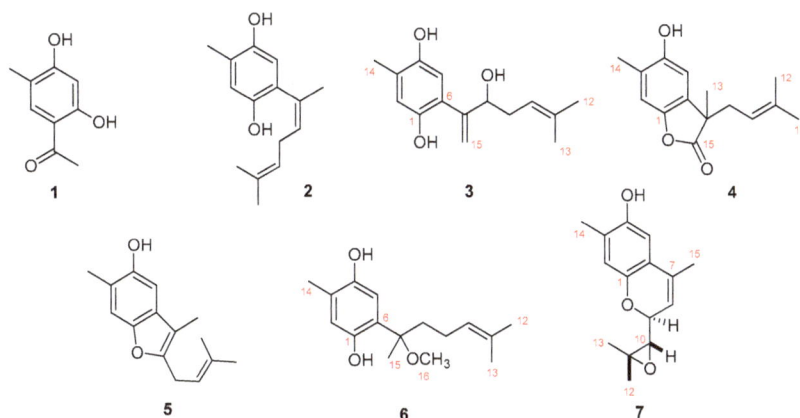

Figure 1. Chemical structures of the compounds **1–7** isolated from *Myrmekioderma* sp.

Compound **1** was isolated as a dark-brown oil. It was identified as 1-(2,4-dihydroxy-5-methylphenyl)ethan-1-one, as shown in Figure 1, based on spectral data available in the literature [17].

Also based on spectral data available in the literature, compound **2** was identified as (1′Z)-2-(1′,5′-dimethylhexa-1′,4′-dieny1)-5-methylbenzene-1,4-diol [18].

Compound **3** was isolated as a yellow amorphous solid. The molecular formula $C_{15}H_{20}O_3$ was established based on the (−)-HRESIMS molecular ion m/z 247.1344 $[M − H]^-$ (calculated 247.1334), which imposed six degrees of unsaturation. The ^{13}C-NMR spectrum of **3**, compiled in Table 1, confirmed the presence of fifteen carbon signals which were assigned, by DEPT and HMQC spectral analysis, to two tertiary (δ_C 26.1, 18.1) and one secondary (δ_C 15.8) methyls, two methylenes (δ_C 120.3, 34.3) of which one was double bonded (δ_C 120.3), two aromatic (δ_C 118.8, 117.2), one double-bonded (δ_C 118.8), and one hydroxylated (δ_C 76.7) methine and six non-protonated carbons (δ_C 148.0, 147.5, 147.0, 136.9, 125.4, 124.2). From the listed non-protonated carbons, two were hydroxylated (δ_C 148.0, 147.5). In accordance, the ^{1}H-NMR spectrum exhibited three methyl singlets (δ_H 2.20, 1.71, 1.53), two splitting methylenes (δ_H 5.43 and 5.24, 2.30, and 2.15), the first two suggesting a double bond, and four methines (δ_H 6.68, 6.50, 5.06, 4.40). Based on COSY and HMBC spectral data, as shown in Figure 2, a simple sesquiterpene structure was proposed for this compound. ^{1}H and ^{13}C data, together with the H-2 HMBC correlations with C-1 and C-5 revealed the presence of a tetrasubstituted benzene ring. C-1 and C-4 deshielded carbon resonances (δ_C 147.5, 147.0) indicated the presence of a benzene-1,4-diol. Me-14 was assigned based on the HMBC correlation Me-14/C-4 and C-6 substitution based on the correlations H-5/C-7 and H_2-15/C-6. The double bond, suggested by H_2-15 resonances (δ_C 120.3, δ_H 5.43, 5.24), was elucidated based on the previously described HMBC correlation of H_2-15/C-6 with the hydroxylated C-8 (δ_C 76.7). The COSY correlations H-8/H_2-9 and H_2-9/H-10 allowed assignment of the methylene and $\Delta^{10(11)}$ double bond. The HMBC cross signals of the methyl groups Me-12 and Me-13 with each other and of both of them with C-10 and C-11 completed the structure. Unfortunately, a paucity of material prevented the assignment of the C-8 absolute stereochemistry. Thus, the structure of **3** was elucidated as the curcuhydroquinone derivative shown in Figure 1: 6-(3-hydroxy-6-methyl-1,5-heptadien-2-yl)-3-methylbenzene-1,4-diol.

Table 1. ^{1}H and ^{13}C-NMR (400 and 100 MHz, respectively) for compounds **3** and **4**. The experiments were performed in CDCl$_3$.

Position	Compound 3		Compound 4	
	δ_C, Type	δ_H, mult (*J* in Hz)	δ_C, Type	δ_H, mult (*J* in Hz)
1	147.5, C		146.4, C	
2	118.8, CH	6.68, s	112.5, CH	6.87, s
3	125.4, C		123.9, C	
4	147.0, C		150.4, C	
5	117.2, CH	6.50, s	110.0, CH	6.64, s
6	124.2, C		130.4, C	
7	148.0, C		48.1, C	
8	76.7, CH	4.40, dd (8.6, 5.4)	37.4, CH$_2$	2.42, dd (14.1, 7.9) 2.58, dd (14.1, 8.3)
9	34.3, CH$_2$	α 2.30, m β 2.15, m	117.2, CH	4.85, dddd (9.7, 5.5, 2.8, 1.4)
10	118.8, CH	5.06, m	136.5, C	
11	136.9, C		18.0, CH$_3$	1.56, s
12	26.1, CH$_3$	1.71, s	25.8, CH$_3$	1.60, s
13	18.1, CH$_3$	1.53, s	23.5, CH$_3$	1.44, s
14	15.8, CH$_3$	2.20, s	16.2, CH$_3$	2.26, s
15	120.3, CH$_2$	α 5.43, d (1.3) β 5.24, d (1.6)	180.8, C	
OH-1		8.02, br s		
OH-4		4.48, br s		4.65, br s
OH-8		3.27, br s		

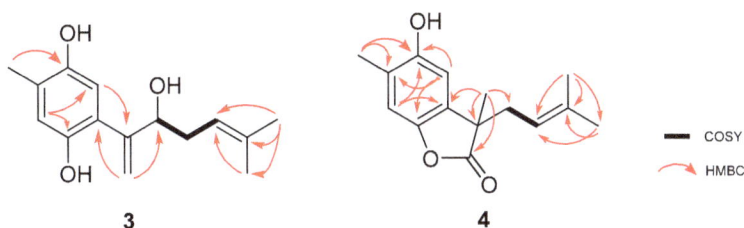

Figure 2. Key ^{1}H-^{1}H COSY and HMBC correlations of compounds 3 and 4.

Compound **4** was isolated as a yellow amorphous powder. The molecular formula $C_{15}H_{18}O_3$ was calculated based on the (−)-HRESIMS *m/z* 245.1126 [M − H]$^-$ (calculated 245.1177) molecular ion peak indicating the existence of seven degrees of unsaturation. Compound **4** ^{1}H and ^{13}C-NMR spectral data, compiled in Table 1, resembled those of compounds **2** and **3**. The ^{13}C-NMR spectrum confirmed the presence of fifteen carbon signals which were assigned, by DEPT and HMQC spectral analysis, to four methyls (δ_C 25.8, 23.5, 18.0, 16.2), one methylene (δ_C 37.4), two aromatic (δ_C 112.5, 110.0), and one olefinic (δ_C 117.2) methines and seven non-protonated carbons (δ_C 180.8, 150.4, 146.4, 136.5, 130.4, 123.9, 48.1), of which two were hydroxylated (δ_C 150.4, 146.4) and one an ester (δ_C 180.8). In accordance, the ^{1}H-NMR spectrum showed four singlet methyls (δ_H 2.26, 1.60, 1.56, 1.44), one splitting methylene (δ_H 2.58, 2.42), two aromatic (δ_H 6.87, 6.64), and one olefinic (δ_H 4.85) methine. The same tetrasubstituted benzene ring found in compounds **2** and **3** was also proposed for compound **4** due to the similarity of the ^{1}H and ^{13}C-NMR data. The HMBC correlations H-2/C-4, H-2/C-6, H-5/C-1, H-5/C-3, and H-5/C-4 confirmed the proposed sub-structure. Further HMBC correlations Me-14/C-3 and Me-14/C-4 corroborated the assignment of this methyl group. The most notable new features of compound **4** were the carbonyl resonance (δ_C 180.8) and a non-protonated alkane carbon (δ_C 48.1). Allocation of these was accomplished based on the HMBC correlations of Me-13 with C-6, C-7, C-8, and C-15, confirming a lactone sub-structure. The COSY correlation H$_2$-8/H-9 allowed assignment of the methylene and the $\Delta^{9(10)}$ double bond, which was linked to the non-protonated C-10 based on the HMBC correlations of Me-11 and Me-12 with both C-9 and C-10. As a result, the structure of compound **4** was elucidated as the sesquiterpene shown in Figure 1: 4-hydroxy-3,7-dimethyl-7-(3-methylbut-2-en-1-yl)benzofuran-15-one.

Compound **5** was isolated as a yellow amorphous powder. Spectral data available in the literature allowed its identification as 1,8-epoxy-1(6),2,4,7,10-bisaborapentaen-4-ol [19].

Compound **6** was isolated as dark-brown oil. The molecular formula $C_{16}H_{24}O_3$ was established based on the (−)-HRESIMS *m/z* molecular ion peak 263.1610 [M − H]$^-$ (calculated 263.1647), indicating five degrees of unsaturation. Both ^{1}H and ^{13}C-NMR indicated structural similarities with compounds **2–5** (Table 2). The same tetrasubstituted hydroquinone ring found in compounds **2** and **3** was suggested for compound **6**. The HMBC correlations H-5/C-1, H-5/C-3, and H-5/C-4, represented in Figure 3, confirmed the proposed hydroquinone ring. The methyl-14 substitution was assigned based on HMBC correlations of this group with C-2, C-3, and C-4. The C-6 substitution was confirmed based on the HMBC correlations H-5/C-7, Me-15/C-6, and Me-15/C-7. The last correlation, together with Me-16/C-7, provided the key to methyl groups -15 and -16. The ^{13}C-NMR and DEPT data suggested the presence of two methylenes (δ_C 39.8, 22.8), consistent with a side chain one carbon longer than found previously. Me-12 and Me-13 were assigned based on their HMBC correlations between each other and with C-10 and C-11. The COSY correlation H-10/H-9 allowed completion of this second sub-structure.

The configuration of the chiral center present in compound **6** could not be clearly elucidated with the material available and the physio-chemical information obtained for this compound. Thus, the structure of **6** was elucidated as the curcuhydroquinone derivative 6-(2-methoxy-6-methylhept-5-en-2-yl)-3-methylbenzene-1,4-diol (Figure 1).

Table 2. ^{1}H and ^{13}C-NMR (400 and 100 MHz, respectively) for compounds **6** and **7**. Experiments with compound **6** were done in CD$_3$OD and with compound **7** in CDCl$_3$.

Position	Compound 6		Compound 7	
	δ_C, Type	δ_H, mult (*J* in Hz)	δ_C, Type	δ_H, mult (*J* in Hz)
1	149.5, C		146.7, C	
2	118.9, CH	6.63, s	116.9, CH	6.70, s
3	124.5, C		125.1, C	
4	146.7, C		148.1, C	
5	114.2, CH	6.48, s	110.3, CH	6.62, s
6	126.0, C		132.1, C	
7	82.4, C		122.0, C	
8	39.8, CH$_2$	1.84, m	118.7, C	5.36, dd (3.8, 1.5)
9	22.8, CH$_2$	α 2.00, m β 1.89, m	75.6, CH	4.51, ddt (8.3, 3.9, 1.5)
10	123.9, CH	5.04, t (6.6, 6.5)	63.8, CH	3.06, d (8.3)
11	132.0, C		57.7, C	
12	17.7, CH$_3$	1.51, m	25.1, CH$_3$	1.33, s
13	25.8, CH$_3$	1.65, s	19.4, CH$_3$	1.35, s
14	15.6, CH$_3$	2.18, s	15.9, CH$_3$	2.19, s
15	22.4, CH$_3$	1.55, s	18.3, CH$_3$	2.01, t (1.5)
16	50.5, OCH$_3$	3.21, s		
OH-1		8.28, br s		
OH-4		8.28, br s		3.49, br s

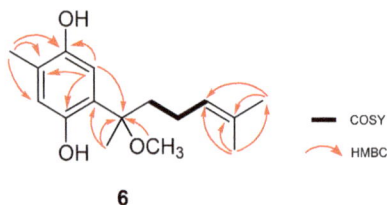

6

Figure 3. Key ^{1}H-^{1}H COSY, HMBC, and TOCSY correlations of compound **6**.

Compound **7** was isolated as a green crystal. The (−)-HRESIMS showed the molecular ion peak *m/z* 245.1126 [M − H]$^-$ (calculated 245.1177), very similar to the one reported for compound **4**. As for compound **4**, C$_{15}$H$_{18}$O$_3$ was the calculated molecular formula, indicating the existence of seven degrees of unsaturation. Analysis of the ^{1}H and ^{13}C-NMR spectral data, compiled in Table 2, and a comparison with of the data for the previously elucidated compounds revealed the presence of the phenolic part of the structure, but with considerable modifications in the side chain. As seen in Figure 4a, the HMBC correlations Me-15/C-6 and Me-15/C-7, together with the deshielded resonance of C-7 (δ_C 122.0) allowed assignment of this methyl group and the Δ$^{7(8)}$ double bond. Based on the COSY correlations between H-8, H-9, and H-10, a spin system was defined. Chemical shifts of the positions 9 (δ 4.51/55.6) and 10 (δ 3.06/63.8) indicated they were bearing an oxygen atom. The HMBC correlations between Me-15 with C-7/C-8/C-9 and H-10 C-11/Me-12/Me-13 allowed us to establish the position of the side chain. Furthermore, the chemical shift of the quaternary C-11 (δC 57.7) indicated that it was also oxygenated. This fact, along with the molecular formula, suggests cyclization of the phenol OH to the C-9 position and an epoxide between C-10 and C-11. Additionally, the chemical shift of the epoxide positions supported the proposed structure when compared to other related epoxide fragments described in the literature [20,21]. Finally, the MS fragmentation pattern showing the *m/z* fragments 230.1421, 165.0497, and 122.0332 (see Supplementary Materials Figure S45) reinforced this proposal.

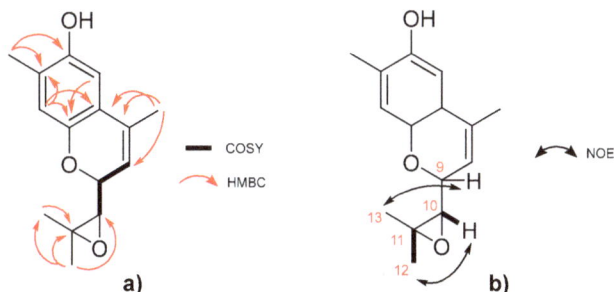

Figure 4. Key correlations for the elucidation of compound 7. (a) ^{1}H-^{1}H COSY and HMBC. (b) NOESY (partial structure).

A comparison of the resonances, together with a large coupling constant between H-9 and H-10 (8.3 Hz), allowed the relative configuration at C-9/C-10 to be determined as anti [22]. Furthermore, the NOE correlations H-12/H-10 and H-13/H-9, represented in Figure 4b, confirmed this configuration. Thus, the structure of **7** was elucidated as the curcuphenol derivative shown in Figure 1: 9-(3,3-dimethyloxiran-2-yl)-1,7-dimethyl-7-chromen-4-ol.

Several bisabolane-type sesquiterpenoids have been reported from different marine organisms, such as the marine sponge *Halichondria* sp. [18], the gorgonians *Pseudopterogorgia* spp. [7] or the red algae *Laurencia scoparia* [23]. The isolation of bisabolane-related compounds from microorganisms, such as the marine-derived fungus *Aspergillus* sp. [24], has been used to suggest that these compounds are produced by microbial-associated organisms and not directly by the host. In this work, we were able to isolate four new bisabolane-related compounds. For these new compounds from this work, no assumptions can be made as to whether the producer is the sponge or possible associated microorganisms since the metabolites were extracted indistinctly.

Bisabolane-like compounds have previously been isolated from marine sponges [9,10]. However, to the best of our knowledge, this work represents the first report of this class of compounds from *Myrmekioderma* sp. Besides belonging to a known class of compounds, the four new isolated bisabolane-related metabolites show novel structural features. Cyclic bisabolane and metabolites bearing oxo functionality are both uncommon among this group of compounds, highlighting the importance of these discoveries.

From the biosynthetic point of view, bisabolane-related compounds have already been described as a result of the combination of the shikimic and mevalonic acid pathways [25,26] and the same routes are proposed for the described compounds. Compound **4**, however, has a migrated carbon relative to the curcuphenol skeleton, a feature that can be found in other related-compounds [27]. Compound **4** is, therefore, proposed to be obtained from tetraketide 3-methyl-orsellinic acid [27,28]. As such, there is strong evidence that the compounds originate from a fungi-associated strain. All seven isolated compounds were tested for their cytotoxic activity against A-549 human lung carcinoma cells, MDA-MB-231 human breast adenocarcinoma cells, HT-29 human colorectal carcinoma, and PSN1 human pancreatic adenocarcinoma cells. Compounds **1–7** were inactive (IC$_{50}$ > 20 µM) in all the cancer cell lines tested.

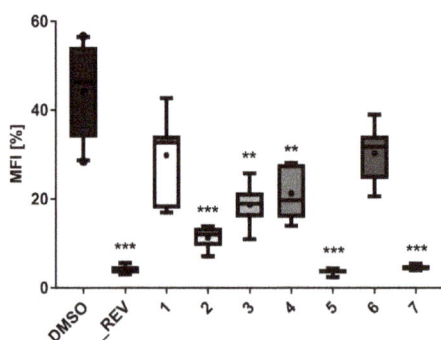

Figure 5. Lipid-reducing activity of compounds **1–7** in zebrafish Nile red fat metabolism assay. MFI represents the mean fluorescence intensity, indicative of neutral lipids. A solvent control with 0.1% DMSO was included in the bioassay, together with the positive control 50 µM resveratrol (REV). Per treatment, 6–8 individual zebrafish larvae were used. ** $p < 0.01$, *** $p < 0.001$.

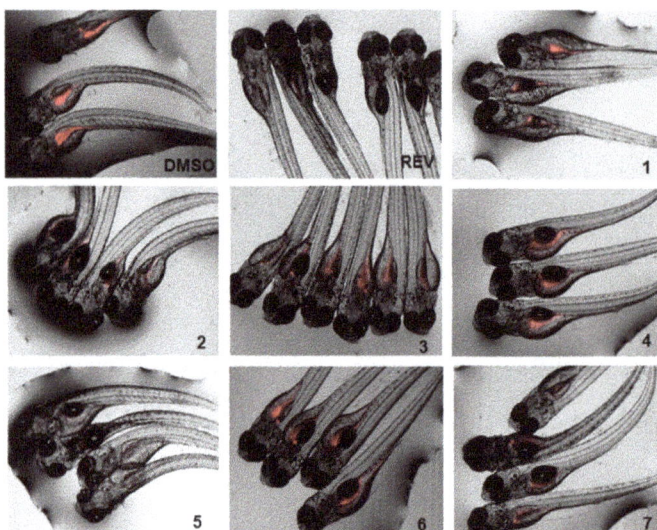

Figure 6. Representative images of the zebrafish Nile red assay. Images show the overlay of the fluorescence and bright field images; 0.1% DMSO was used as solvent control and 50 µM resveratrol (REV) as positive control.

The lipid-reducing activity of compounds **1–7** was also tested using the zebrafish Nile red fat metabolism assay (Figures 5 and 6). This whole small animal model was already successfully used in the discovery of lipid-reducing compounds from fungus [16], chemically modified polyphenols [29] and cyanobacteria [30], and offers higher physiological relevance compared to commonly used cellular in vitro models. Furthermore, it was previously shown that zebrafish larvae responded similarly to humans if challenged with known lipid regulator drugs [31]. The results showed that compounds **2**, **5**, and **7** have potent lipid-reducing activity (IC$_{50}$ = 1.78, 0.84, and 1.22 µM, respectively), reducing significantly the zebrafish Nile red fluorescence intensity, which is indicative of the total amount of neutral lipids. Compounds **3** and **4** also showed moderate lipid-reducing activity (IC$_{50}$ = 7.89, 12.61 µM, respectively). None of the compounds **1–7** had any general toxicity on zebrafish larvae and additionally did not cause any malformations. It is interesting to observe that all the active compounds are bisabolane-related, while compound **1** did not show activity. The structural differences between compounds **2** or **3** compared to compound **6** caused the inactivation of the compound, but cyclizing the side chain (compound **7**) did not. Therefore, more studies are needed in order to understand the relationship between the chemical structure and its lipid-reducing activity.

3. Materials and Methods

3.1. General Experiments

Optical rotations were measured on a Jasco P-1020 polarimeter. The UV spectra were measured using an Agilent 8453 UV-vis spectrometer. The IR spectra were recorded on a Nicolet iZ10 (ThermoFisher Scientific) FTIR spectrophotometer. The NMR experiments were performed on a Bruker 400 spectrometer at 400/100 MHz (^{1}H/^{13}C). Chemical shifts were reported in ppm using residual CD$_3$OD (δ 3.31 for ^{1}H and 49.0 for ^{13}C) and CDCl$_3$ (δ 7.26 for ^{1}H and 77.2 for ^{13}C) as internal references. The HRESIMS was performed on a Waters Synapt G1 UPLC-QTOF mass spectrometer in negative ionization mode.

3.2. Biological Sample

The *Myrmekioderma* sp. sponge was collected by hand while scuba diving in Boano (Indonesia). The sponge was immediately frozen and kept under these conditions until extraction. The specimen was identified by María Jesús Uriz at CEAB, Blanes, Spain. A voucher specimen (ORMA135834) is deposited at PharmaMar facilities (Madrid, Spain).

3.3. Extraction and Isolation

The frozen sponge specimen (320 g) was repeatedly extracted using dichloromethane: methanol (CH$_2$Cl$_2$:MeOH 1:1 v/v). The extract was concentrated under vacuum to yield 25.91 g of crude extract. This crude extract was dissolved in 300 mL of water and subsequently extracted with *n*-hexane (3 × 300 mL), ethyl acetate (EtOAc) (3 × 300 mL), and butanol (*n*-BuOH) (2 × 250 mL). The *n*-hexane extract (6.11 g) was subjected to reversed phase VLC over RP-18 silica gel with a stepped gradient from H$_2$O:MeOH (3:1 v/v) to dichloromethane (CH$_2$Cl$_2$). Fraction 1 (95.6 mg), eluted with H$_2$O:MeOH (3:1 v/v), was subjected to semi-preparative HPLC (Gemini-NX C18 110A, Phenomenex, 5μ, 10.0 × 250 mm, gradient H$_2$O:MeCN 60:40 v/v to 50:50 v/v, in 15 min, 3 mL/min) to yield compound **1** (6.4 mg) at 10 min. Fraction 3 (1640.7 mg), eluted with pure MeOH, was initially separated by preparative HPLC (Luna C18 100A, Phenomenex, 5 μ, 21.20 × 250 mm, gradient H$_2$O:MeCN (25:75 v/v) to 0:100, in 30 min, 6 mL/min), yielding HPLC Fraction 2 at 14 minutes (444.2 mg). This fraction was again separated by preparative HPLC (Luna C18 100A, Phenomenex, 5 μ, 21.20 × 250 mm, gradient H$_2$O:MeCN 50:50 v/v to 40:60 v/v, in 25 min, 10 mL/min), yielding compound **2** (98.6 mg) at 21 minutes and HPLC Fraction 4 at 24 minutes (146.6 mg). The HPLC Fraction 4 was submitted to a final semi-preparative HPLC separation (Gemini-NX C18 110A column, 5 μ, Phenomenex, 10.0 × 250 mm, gradient H$_2$O:MeCN 50:50 v/v to 30:70 v/v, in 35 min, 2.3 mL/min) to yield compounds **3** (1.3 mg) at 11 min, **4** (4.9 mg) at 21 min and **5** (9.4 mg) at 34 min. The EtOAc extract from the original liquid/liquid extraction was also subjected to reversed phase VLC over RP-18 silica gel with a stepped gradient from H$_2$O:MeOH (3:1 v/v) to CH$_2$Cl$_2$. Fraction 2 (1021.7 mg) eluted with H$_2$O:MeOH (1:3 v/v) and was further separated by preparative HPLC (Luna C18 100A, Phenomenex, 5 μ, 21.20 × 250 mm, gradient H$_2$O:MeCN (50:50 v/v) to 20:80 v/v, in 30 min, 8 mL/min), to yield compounds **6** (46.5 mg) at 28 min and **7** (23.3 mg) at 19 min.

1-(2,4-dihydroxy-5-methylphenyl)ethan-1-one (1): Dark-brown oil; IR (neat) ν_{max} 3314 (br), 2971, 2853, 1652, 1406, 1038 cm^{-1}; UV/Vis (MeOH) λ_{max} 194, 210, 232, 265, 360 nm. HRESIMS: *m/z* 165.0552 [M − H]$^-$ (calcd for C$_9$H$_9$O$_3$, 165.0552).

(1′Z)-2-(1′,5′-dimethylhexa-1′,4′-dieny1)-5-methylbenzene-1,4-diol (2): Dark-brown oil; IR (neat) ν_{max} 3413 (br), 2970, 2913, 1416, 1187 cm^{-1}; UV/Vis (MeOH) λ_{max} 229, 299 nm. HRESIMS: *m/z* 231.1496 [M − H]$^-$ (calcd for C$_{15}$H$_{19}$O$_2$, 231.1385).

6-(3-hydroxy-6-methyl-1,5-heptadien-2-yl)-3-methylbenzene-1,4-diol (3): Yellow amorphous solid; $(\alpha)_D^{25}$ +0.72 (*c* 0.484, CH$_3$OH); IR (MeOH) ν_{max} 3314 (br), 2943, 2831, 1033 cm^{-1}; UV/Vis (CH$_3$OH) λ_{max} 195, 299 nm. ^{1}H-NMR (400 MHz, CDCl$_3$) and ^{13}C-NMR (100 MHz, CDCl$_3$) see Table 1; HRESIMS: *m/z* 247.1344 [M − H]$^-$ (calcd for C$_{15}$H$_{19}$O$_3$, 247.1334), *m/z* 149.0575 (M − C$_6$H$_{11}$O)$^-$ (calcd for C$_9$H$_9$O$_2$, 149.0602).

4-hydroxy-3,7-dimethyl-7-(3-methylbut-2-en-1-yl)benzofuran-15-one (4): Yellow amorphous solid; $(\alpha)_D^{25}$ +2.2 (*c* 0.115, MeOH); IR (MeOH) ν_{max} 3313 (br), 2944, 2832, 1656, 1451, 1035 cm^{-1}; UV/Vis (MeOH) λ_{max} 196, 294 nm. ^{1}H-NMR (400 MHz, CDCl$_3$) and ^{13}C-NMR (100 MHz, CDCl$_3$) see Table 1; HRESIMS: *m/z* 245.1126 [M − H]$^-$ (calcd for C$_{15}$H$_{17}$O$_3$, 245.1177).

1,8-epoxy-1(6),2,4,7,10-bisaborapentaen-4-ol (5): Yellow amorphous solid; IR (neat) ν_{max} 3266 (br), 2915, 1437, 1168, 805, 434 cm^{-1}; UV/Vis (MeOH) λ_{max} 203, 257, 297 nm. HRESIMS: *m/z* 229.1234 [M − H]$^-$ (calcd for C$_{15}$H$_{17}$O$_2$, 229.1229).

6-(2-methoxy-5-methylhept-4-en-2-yl)-3-methylbenzene-1,4-diol (6): Dark-brown oil; $(\alpha)_D^{25}$ +5.0 (*c* 0.0337, CH$_3$OH); IR (MeOH) ν_{max} 3339 (br), 2926, 1453, 1374, 1183, 1051 cm^{-1}; UV/Vis (CH$_3$OH) λ_{max} 196, 297 nm. ^{1}H-NMR (400 MHz, CDCl$_3$) and ^{13}C-NMR (100 MHz, CDCl$_3$) see Table 2; HRESIMS: *m/z* 263.1610 [M − H]$^-$ (calcd for C$_{16}$H$_{23}$O$_3$, 263.1647).

9-(3,3-dimethyloxiran-2-yl)-1,7-dimethyl-7-chromen-4-ol (7): Green crystals; $(\alpha)_D^{25}$ −10.4 (*c* 0.0322, CH$_3$OH); IR (neat) ν_{max} 3388 (br), 2926, 1412, 1178, 994, 829, 597 cm^{-1}; UV/Vis (CH$_3$OH) λ_{max} 194, 217, 330 nm. ^{1}H-NMR (400 MHz, CDCl$_3$) and ^{13}C-NMR (100 MHz, CDCl$_3$) see Table 2; HRESIMS: *m/z* 245.1126 [M − H]$^-$ (calcd for C$_{15}$H$_{17}$O$_3$, 245.1177).

3.4. Biological Activities

3.4.1. Cytotoxicity

The cytotoxic activity of compounds **1–7** was tested against A-549 human lung carcinoma cells, MDA-MB-231 human breast adenocarcinoma cells, HT-29 human colorectal carcinoma cells, and PSN1 human pancreatic adenocarcinoma cells. The four cell lines were provided by the American Type Culture Collection (ATCC): A549 from ATCC CCL-185, MDA-MB-231 from ATCC HTB-26, HT-29 from ATCC HTB-38 and PSN-1 from ATCC CRM-CRL-3211. The concentration giving half maximum inhibitory concentration (IC$_{50}$) was calculated according to the procedure described in the literature [32]. Cell survival was estimated using the National Cancer Institute (NCI) algorithm [33]. Dose-response parameters were determined at three different concentrations of each one of the compounds.

3.4.2. Zebrafish Nile Red Fat Metabolism Assay

The lipid reducing activity of the compounds was analyzed using the zebrafish Nile red fat metabolism assay as previously described [16,25]. Approval by an ethics committee was not necessary for the presented work since the procedures used are not considered animal experimentation according to EC Directive 86/609/EEC for animal experiments. In brief, zebrafish embryos were raised from 1 DPF (days post fertilization) in egg water (60 µg/mL marine sea salt dissolved in distilled H$_2$O) with 200 µM PTU (1-phenyl-2-thiourea) to inhibit pigmentation. From 3 DPF to 5 DPF, zebrafish larvae were exposed to compounds at a final concentration of 10 µM with the daily renewal of water and compounds in a 48 well plate with a density of 6–8 larvae/well (*n* = 6–8). A solvent control (0.1% DMSO) and positive control (REV, resveratrol, final concentration of 50 µM) were included in the assay. Lipids were stained with Nile red overnight at the final concentration of 10 ng/mL. For imaging, the larvae were anesthetized with tricaine (MS-222, 0.03%) for 5 minutes and fluorescence analyzed

Mar. Drugs **2019**, *17*, 375

with a fluorescence microscope (Olympus BX43, Hamburg, Germany). Fluorescence intensity was quantified in individual zebrafish larvae by ImageJ [34]. Effective concentrations 50% (EC_{50}) values were determined in further assays by dose-response curves by using a 1:2 v/v dilution series from 20 μM to 312.5 nM (final concentrations) in 7 dilution steps.

4. Conclusions

This work represents the first isolation and structural elucidation of novel compounds **3**, **4**, **6**, and **7**. It is also the first report of the isolation of compounds **1**, **2**, and **5** from marine sources. Besides being a known and wide-spread class of compounds, the structures of the new compounds isolated present unique structural features. The isolation of these novel compounds, as well as related analogs previously found in marine-derived organisms, raises the question of who is the real metabolite producer, the host or the associated-microorganisms. Further studies are needed in order to answer that question. All of the isolated compounds except for **1** and **6**, showed significant lipid-reducing activity when tested in the zebrafish Nile red fat metabolism assay, but no general toxicity, reinforcing their biotechnological potential. More studies are needed in order to relate the bioactivity with structural features.

Supplementary Materials: The following are available online at http://www.mdpi.com/1660-3397/17/6/375/s1. Figure S1: Picture of the fresh sponge; Figures S2–S44: HRESIMS and NMR spectra of compounds **1–7**; Figure S45: MS fragmentation pattern of compound **7**.

Author Contributions: M.C. performed the isolation and structural elucidation of the compounds and wrote the paper. L.C. performed the organic extractions. R.U. conducted the zebrafish Nile red fat metabolism assay. M.P. and M.T. designed and guided the experiments. All the authors read, reviewed, and agreed with the structure and content of the manuscript.

Funding: The research leading to these results received funding from the Marie Curie Actions of the European Union's Seventh Framework Programme FP7/2007-2013/ under REA grant agreement No. 607786, BluePharmTrain, and by the European ERA-NET Marine Biotechnology project CYANOBESITY (ERA-MBT/0001/2015), financed by national funds through FCT (Foundation for Science and Technology, Portugal), RANNIS (Icelandic Center of Research, Iceland), and FCT strategic fund UID/Multi/04423/2019. Ralph Urbatzka was supported by FCT grant SFRH/BPD/112287/2015.

Acknowledgments: The authors gratefully acknowledge the help of their PharmaMar colleagues and all the assistance given, including R. Fernández for revising the spectroscopic data and the manuscript and J.M. Dominguez for the cytotoxicity assays. The authors would also like to thank Andalas University (Indonesia) for helping with the sponge collection.

Conflicts of Interest: The authors declare no conflict of interest.

References

1. Haefner, B. Drugs from the deep: Marine natural products as drug candidates. *Drug Discov. Today* **2003**, *8*, 536–544. [CrossRef]
2. Blunt, J.W.; Carroll, A.R.; Copp, B.R.; Davis, R.A.; Keyzers, R.A.; Prinsep, M.R. Marine natural products. *Nat. Prod. Rep.* **2018**, *35*, 8–53. [CrossRef] [PubMed]
3. Blunt, J.W.; Copp, B.R.; Keyzers, R.A.; Munro, M.H.G.; Prinsep, M.R. Marine natural products. *Nat. Prod. Rep.* **2017**, *34*, 235–294. [CrossRef] [PubMed]
4. Mehbub, M.F.; Lei, J.; Franco, C.; Zhang, W. Marine sponge derived natural products between 2001 and 2010: Trends and opportunities for discovery of bioactives. *Mar. Drugs* **2014**, *12*, 4539–4577. [CrossRef] [PubMed]
5. Jansen, B.J.M.; de Groot, A. Occurrence, biological activity and synthesis of drimane sesquiterpenoids. *Nat. Prod. Rep.* **2004**, *21*, 449–477. [CrossRef] [PubMed]
6. Xue, D.-Q.; Liu, H.-L.; Chen, S.-H.; Mollo, E.; Gavagnin, M.; Li, J.; Li, X.-W.; Guo, Y.-W. 5-Alkylpyrrole-2-carboxaldehyde derivatives from the Chinese sponge *Mycale lissochela* and their PTP1B inhibitory activities. *Chin. Chem. Lett.* **2017**, *28*, 1190–1193. [CrossRef]
7. Miller, S.L.; Tinto, W.F.; McLean, S.; Reynolds, W.F.; Yu, M. Bisabolane Sesquiterpenes from Barbadian *Pseudopterogorgia* spp. *J. Nat. Prod.* **1995**, *58*, 1116–1119. [CrossRef]

8. Jin, A.; Wu, W.-M.; Yu, H.-Y.; Zhou, M.; Liu, Y.; Tian, T.; Ruan, H.-L. Bisabolane-Type Sesquiterpenoids from the Whole Plant of *Parasenecio rubescens*. *J. Nat. Prod.* **2015**, *78*, 2057–2066. [CrossRef] [PubMed]

9. Yegdaneh, A.; Putchakarn, S.; Yuenyongsawad, S.; Ghannadi, A.; Plubrukarn, A. 3-Oxoabolene and 1-Oxocurcuphenol, Aromatic Bisabolanes from the Sponge *Myrmekioderma* sp. *Nat. Prod. Commun.* **2013**, *8*, 1355–1357. [CrossRef]

10. Wright, A.E.; Pomponi, S.A.; McConnell, O.J.; Kohmoto, S.; McCarthy, P.J. (+)-Curcuphenol and (+)-Curcudiol, Sesquiterpene Phenols from Shallow and Deep Water Collections of the Marine Sponge *Didiscus flavus*. *J. Nat. Prod.* **1987**, *50*, 976–978. [CrossRef]

11. Peralta-Yahya, P.P.; Ouellet, M.; Chan, R.; Mukhopadhyay, A.; Keasling, J.D.; Lee, T.S. Identification and microbial production of a terpene-based advanced biofuel. *Nat. Commun.* **2011**, *2*, 483. [CrossRef] [PubMed]

12. Hurt, R.T.; Kulisek, C.; Buchanan, L.A.; McClave, S.A. The Obesity Epidemic: Challenges, Health Initiatives, and Implications for Gastroenterologists. *Gastroenterol. Hepatol.* **2010**, *6*, 780–792.

13. Fu, C.; Jiang, Y.; Guo, J.; Su, Z. Natural Products with Anti-obesity Effects and Different Mechanisms of Action. *J. Agric. Food Chem.* **2016**, *64*, 9571–9585. [CrossRef] [PubMed]

14. Hu, X.; Tao, N.; Wang, X.; Xiao, J.; Wang, M. Marine-derived bioactive compounds with anti-obesity effect: A review. *J. Funct. Foods* **2016**, *21*, 372–387. [CrossRef]

15. Castro, M.; Preto, M.; Vasconcelos, V.; Urbatzka, R. Obesity: The Metabolic Disease, Advances on Drug Discovery and Natural Product Research. *Curr. Top. Med. Chem.* **2016**, *16*, 2577–2604. [CrossRef] [PubMed]

16. Noinart, J.; Buttachon, S.; Dethoup, T.; Gales, L.; Pereira, J.A.; Urbatzka, R.; Freitas, S.; Lee, M.; Silva, A.M.S.; Pinto, M.M.M.; et al. A New Ergosterol Analog, a New Bis-Anthraquinone and Anti-Obesity Activity of Anthraquinones from the Marine Sponge-Associated Fungus *Talaromyces stipitatus* KUFA 0207. *Mar. Drugs* **2017**, *15*, 139. [CrossRef] [PubMed]

17. Schmidt, N.G.; Pavkov-Keller, T.; Richter, N.; Wiltschi, B.; Gruber, K.; Kroutil, W. Biocatalytic Friedel–Crafts Acylation and Fries Reaction. *Angew. Chem. Int. Ed.* **2017**, *56*, 7615–7619. [CrossRef] [PubMed]

18. Capon, R.; Ghisalberti, E.; Jefferies, P. New aromatic sesquiterpenes from a *Halichondria* sp. *Aust. J. Chem.* **1982**, *35*, 2583–2587. [CrossRef]

19. Arihara, S.; Umeyama, A.; Bando, S.; Imoto, S.; Ono, M.; Yoshikawa, K. Three New Sesquiterpenes from the Black Heartwood of *Cryptomeria japonica*. *Chem. Pharm. Bull.* **2004**, *52*, 463–465. [CrossRef]

20. Raju, B.; Subbaraju, G.; Rao, C.; Trimurtulu, G. Two New Oxigenated Lobanes from a Soft Coral of *Lobophytum* species of the Andaman and Nicobar Coasts. *J. Nat. Prod.* **1993**, *56*, 961–966. [CrossRef]

21. Duh, C.; El-Gamal, A.; Chiang, C.; Chu, C.; Wang, S.; Dai, C. New Cytotoxic Xenia Diterpenoids from the Formosan Soft Coral *Xenia umbellata*. *J. Nat. Prod.* **2002**, *65*, 1882–1885. [CrossRef] [PubMed]

22. Bishara, A.; Rudi, A.; Goldberg, I.; Benayahu, Y.; Kashman, Y. Novaxenicins A–D and xeniolides I–K, seven new diterpenes from the soft coral *Xenia novaebrittanniae*. *Tetrahedron* **2006**, *62*, 12092–12097. [CrossRef]

23. Davyt, D.; Fernandez, R.; Suescun, L.; Mombru, A.W.; Saldana, J.; Dominguez, L.; Fujii, M.T.; Manta, E. Bisabolanes from the red alga *Laurencia scoparia*. *J. Nat. Prod.* **2006**, *69*, 1113–1116. [CrossRef] [PubMed]

24. Wei, M.Y.; Wang, C.Y.; Liu, Q.A.; Shao, C.L.; She, Z.G.; Lin, Y.C. Five Sesquiterpenoids from a Marine-Derived Fungus *Aspergillus* sp Isolated from a Gorgonian *Dichotella gemmacea*. *Mar. Drugs* **2010**, *8*, 941–949. [CrossRef] [PubMed]

25. Hansson, D.; Menkis, A.; Olson, Å.; Stenlid, J.; Broberg, A.; Karlsson, M. Biosynthesis of fomannoxin in the root rotting pathogen Heterobasidion occidentale. *Phytochemistry* **2012**, *84*, 31–39. [CrossRef] [PubMed]

26. Prompanya, C.; Dethoup, T.; Gales, L.; Lee, M.; Pereira, J.A.C.; Silva, A.M.S.; Pinto, M.M.M.; Kijjoa, A. New Polyketides and New Benzoic Acid Derivatives from the Marine Sponge-Associated Fungus Neosartorya quadricincta KUFA 0081. *Mar Drugs* **2016**, *14*, 134. [CrossRef] [PubMed]

27. Almeida, C.; Kehraus, S.; Prudêncio, M.; König, M.K. Marilones A–C, phthalides from the sponge-derived fungus *Stachylidium* sp. *Beilstein J. Org. Chem.* **2011**, *7*, 1636–1642. [CrossRef] [PubMed]

28. El Maddah, F.; Eguereva, E.; Kehraus, S.; König, G.M. Biosynthetic studies of novel polyketides from the marine sponge-derived fungus *Stachylidium* sp. 293K04. *Org. Biomol. Chem.* **2019**, *17*, 2747–2752. [CrossRef] [PubMed]

29. Urbatzka, R.; Freitas, S.; Palmeira, A.; Almeida, T.; Moreira, J.; Azevedo, C.; Afonso, C.; Correia-da-Silva, M.; Sousa, E.; Pinto, M.; et al. Lipid reducing activity and toxicity profiles of a library of polyphenol derivatives. *Eur. J. Med. Chem.* **2018**, *151*, 272–284. [CrossRef]

30. Costa, M.; Rosa, F.; Ribeiro, T.; Hernandez-Bautista, R.; Bonaldo, M.; Goncalves Silva, N.; Eiriksson, F.; Thorsteinsdottir, M.; Ussar, S.; Urbatzka, R. Identification of Cyanobacterial Strains with Potential for the Treatment of Obesity-Related Co-Morbidities by Bioactivity, Toxicity Evaluation and Metabolite Profiling. *Mar. Drugs* **2019**, *17*, 280. [CrossRef]

31. Jones, K.S.; Alimov, A.P.; Rilo, H.L.; Jandacek, R.J.; Woollett, L.A.; Penberthy, W.T. A high throughput live transparent animal bioassay to identify non-toxic small molecules or genes that regulate vertebrate fat metabolism for obesity drug development. *Nutr. Metab.* **2008**, *5*, 23. [CrossRef] [PubMed]

32. Skehan, P.; Storeng, R.; Scudiero, D.; Monks, A.; McMahon, J.; Vistica, D.; Warren, J.T.; Bokesch, H.; Kenney, S.; Boyd, M.R. New Colorimetric Cytotoxicity Assay for Anticancer-Drug Screening. *JNCI* **1990**, *82*, 1107–1112. [CrossRef] [PubMed]

33. Shoemaker, R.H. The NCI60 human tumour cell line anticancer drug screen. *Nat. Rev. Cancer* **2006**, *6*, 813–823. [CrossRef] [PubMed]

34. ImageJ. Available online: https://imagej.nih.gov/ij/index.html (accessed on 7 September 2018).

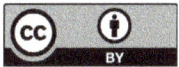

MDPI

St. Alban-Anlage 66

4052 Basel

Switzerland

Tel. +41 61 683 77 34

Fax +41 61 302 89 18

www.mdpi.com

Marine Drugs Editorial Office

E-mail: marinedrugs@mdpi.com

www.mdpi.com/journal/marinedrugs

www.ingramcontent.com/pod-product-compliance
Lightning Source LLC
Chambersburg PA
CBHW051853210326
41597CB00033B/5885